OXFORD MEDICAL PUBLICATIONS

Oxford Handbook of
Neonatology

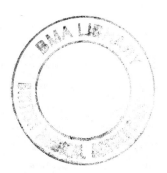

Published and forthcoming Oxford Handbooks

Oxford Handbook of
Neonatology

Second Edition

Dr Grenville Fox
Consultant Neonatologist,
Evelina London Children's Hospital,
Guy's & St Thomas' NHS Foundation Trust,
London, UK

Dr Nicholas Hoque
Consultant Neonatologist,
Queen Charlotte's and St Mary's Hospitals,
Imperial College Healthcare NHS Trust, UK

and

Dr Timothy Watts
Consultant Neonatologist,
Evelina London Children's Hospital,
Guy's & St Thomas' NHS Foundation Trust,
London, UK

OXFORD
UNIVERSITY PRESS

OXFORD
UNIVERSITY PRESS

Great Clarendon Street, Oxford, OX2 6DP,
United Kingdom

Oxford University Press is a department of the University of Oxford.
It furthers the University's objective of excellence in research, scholarship,
and education by publishing worldwide. Oxford is a registered trade mark of
Oxford University Press in the UK and in certain other countries

© Oxford University Press 2017

The moral rights of the authors have been asserted

First Edition published in 2010
Second Edition published in 2017

Impression: 1

Published in the United States of America by Oxford University Press
198 Madison Avenue, New York, NY 10016, United States of America

British Library Cataloguing in Publication Data

Data available

Library of Congress Control Number: 2016945507

ISBN 978-0-19-870395-2

Printed and bound in China by
C&C Offset Printing Co., Ltd.

Preface

The original idea for this handbook arose from files of clinical guidelines from our own neonatal unit. Our ethos in developing these guidelines was that they should avoid dogma and provide practical guidance rather than rigid rules and regulations. These have been rewritten to provide much of the practical advice given in this handbook, with succinct background notes added to each topic. We hope this will provide enough detail to inform medical and nursing staff at all levels and act as an aide-memoire to those with more experience in the specialty. Practical guidance and a suggested approach to different clinical situations have been written using the best available evidence, but we have relied on consensus of opinion where evidence is lacking.

This second edition has a revised chapter order and a new chapter on neonatal endocrinology, with updates to all other sections reflecting recent changes and evidence in the specialty.

Grenville Fox
Nicholas Hoque
Timothy Watts

Acknowledgements

We are grateful to our consultant colleagues, trainees, senior nursing staff, and subspecialty teams at the Evelina London Children's Hospital Neonatal Unit at St. Thomas' Hospital, who have contributed to the guidelines which formed the original idea for this handbook. We are particularly grateful to Michael Champion from the Evelina London Children's Hospital for his contribution to the metabolic section; and to Julia Phillips from King's College Hospital, and Tony Hulse from the Evelina London Children's Hospital for the new endocrinology chapter. We are also grateful to Victoria Barr for rendering of selected illustrations.

Contents

Symbols and abbreviations

<	less than
>	greater than
~	approximately
+/−	with or without
↑	increased
→	leads to
↓	decreased
ΔP	change in pressure
A/C	assist control
AAP	American Academy of Pediatrics
Ab	antibody
ABC(D)	airway, breathing, circulation, (disability)
ACE	angiotensin converting enzyme
AChR	acetylcholine receptor
ACTH	adrenocorticotropic hormone
ADH	antidiuretic hormone
ADHD	attention deficit hyperactivity disorder
ADPKD	autosomal dominant polycystic kidney disease
AED	automatic external defibrillator
AFB	acid-fast bacilli
ALCAPA	anomalous origin of left coronary artery from pulmonary artery
ALP	alkaline phosphatase
ALT	alanine transferase
ALTE	acute life-threatening events
AMH	anti-Müllerian hormone
ANNP	advanced neonatal nurse practitioner
anti-HBe	HB e antibody
AP	antero-posterior
APH	antepartum haemorrhage
APLS	Advanced Paediatric Life Support
APTT	activated partial thromboplastin time
ARDS	acute respiratory distress syndrome
ARPKD	autosomal recessive polycystic kidney disease
ART	antiretroviral treatment
AS	aortic stenosis
ASD	atrial septal defect

AST	aspartate transaminase
AV	atrioventricular
aVF	augmented vector foot (ECG lead)
AVRT	atrioventricular re-entry tachycardia
AVSD	atrioventricular septal defect
AXR	abdominal X-ray
AZT	zidovudine (azidothymidine)
BAPM	British Association of Perinatal Medicine
BCG	bacillus Calmette-Guérin
bd	twice daily
BE	base excess
BMF	breast milk fortifier
BMI	body mass index
BP	blood pressure
BPD	bronchopulmonary dysplasia
BW	birth weight
CCAM	congenital cystic adenomatoid malformation
CDH	congenital diaphragmatic hernia
CF	cystic fibrosis
CFM	cerebral function monitoring
CGA	corrected gestational age
CGH	comparative genomic hybridization
CHAOS	congenital high airway obstruction syndrome
CHARGE	Coloboma, Heart defects, choanal Atresia, Retardation of growth/development, Genital abnormalities, and Ear abnormalities
CHB	complete heart block
CHD	congenital heart disease
CK	creatine kinase
CLD	chronic lung disease
CMV	cytomegalovirus
CNS	central nervous system
CoA	coarctation of the aorta
CONS	coagulase negative staphlyococci
CPAP	continuous positive airway pressure
CPK	creatinine kinase
CPR	cardiopulmonary resuscitation
CRH	corticotropin-releasing hormone
CRP	C-reactive protein
CSF	cerebrospinal fluid
CT	computed tomography

CTG	cardiotocograph
CUSS	cranial ultrasound scan
CVP	central venous pressure
CVS	chorionic villous sampling
CXR	chest X-ray
DAT	direct antiglobulin test
DC	direct current
DDH	developmental dysplasia of the hip
DEAFF	detection of early antigen fluorescent foci
DHEAS	dehydroepiandosterone sulphate
DIC	disseminated intravascular coagulation
DILV	double inlet left ventricle
DMSA	dimercaptosuccinic acid scan
DSD	disorders of sexual differentiation
DTaP	diptheria, tetanus, pertussis (acellular)
DWI	diffusion-weighted imaging
EBM	expressed breast milk
ECG	electrocardiogram
echo	echocardiography
ECMO	extracorporeal membrane oxygenation
ECV	external cephalic version
EDD	expected date of delivery
EDF	end-diastolic flow
EEG	electroencephalogram
EFM	electronic fetal monitoring
EIA	enzyme immunoassay
ELBW	extremely low birth weight
EMG	electromyography
ENT	ear, nose, and throat
ETT	endotracheal tube
EXIT	*ex utero* intrapartum treatment
FBC	full blood count
FDP	fibrin degradation products
FENa	fractional excretion of sodium
FFP	fresh frozen plasma
FGR	fetal growth restriction
FHM	fetal heart rate monitoring
FHR	fetal heart rate
FiO_2	fraction of inspired oxygen
FLAIR	fluid-attenuated inversion recovery

FRC	functional residual capacity
FSH	follicle-stimulating hormone
G6PD	glucose-6-phosphate dehydrogenase
GA	gestational age
GBS	group B streptococcus
G-CSF	granulocyte colony stimulating factor
GFR	glomerular filtration rate
GGT	gamma glutamyl transferase
GH	growth hormone
GI	gastrointestinal
GIT	gastrointestinal tract
GMH	germinal matrix haemorrhage
GOR	gastro-oesophageal reflux
GTN	glyceryl trinitrate
GU	genito-urinary
HAART	highly active anti-retroviral treatment
HAS	human albumin solution
HbA1C	haemoglobin A1C
HBeAg	HB e antigen
HBIG	HB immunoglobulin
HBsAg	HB surface antigen
HBV	hepatitis B virus
hCG	human chorionic gonadotrophin
Hct	haematocrit
HCV	hepatitis C virus
HDN	haemolytic disease of the newborn
HELLP	haemolysis, elevated liver enzymes, and low platelets
HFNC	high-flow nasal cannula
HFOV	high-frequency oscillatory ventilation
HHHF	heated humidified high flow
HIE	hypoxic ischaemic encephalopathy
HIHA	hyperinsulinism hyperammonaemia
HIV	human immunodeficiency virus
HLHS	hypoplastic left heart syndrome
HMA	homovanillic acid
HOOF	Home Oxygen Order Form
HPI	haemorrhagic periventricular/parenchymal infarction
HR	heart rate
HSV	herpes simplex virus
HTLV	human T-cell leukaemia virus

I:E	inspiratory:expiratory ratio
IAA	interrupted aortic arch
IBP	invasive blood pressure
ICP	intracranial pressure
IEM	inborn errors of metabolism
IgG	immunoglobulin class G
IM	intramuscular
iNO	inhaled nitric oxide
INR	international normalized ratio
IPPV	intermittent positive pressure ventilation
IRT	immunoreactive trypsinogen
ITP	immune thrombocytopenia
ITU	intensive care unit
IUGR	intrauterine growth restriction
IV	intravenous
IVC	inferior vena cava
IVDU	intravenous drug user
IVF	*in vitro* fertilization
IVH	intraventricular haemorrhage
IVI	intravenous infusion
IVIG	intravenous immunoglobulin
IVS	intact ventricular septum
LA	left atrium
LBW	low birth weight
LCHAD	long-chain 3 hydroxyacyl CoA dehydrogense
LDH	lactate dehydrogenase
LFT	liver function tests
LH	luteinizing hormone
LMP	last menstrual period
LP	lumbar puncture
LV	left ventricle
LVH	left ventricular hypertrophy
MABP	mean arterial blood pressure
MAP	mean airway pressure
MAPCA	major aorto-pulmonary communicating arteries
MAS	meconium aspiration syndrome
MC&S	microscopy, culture, and sensitivities
MCA	middle cerebral artery
MCAD	medium-chain acyl CoA dehydrogenase deficiency
MCUG	micturating cystourethrogram

MMR	mumps, measles, and rubella (vaccine)
MPH	massive pulmonary haemorrhage
MRI	magnetic resonance imaging
MRSA	meticillin-resistant *Staphylococcus aureus*
MSU	mid-stream specimen of urine
MV	minute volume
NAITP	neonatal alloimmune thrombocytopenia
NAS	neonatal abstinence syndrome
NAVA	neurally adjusted ventricular assist
nBiPAP	nasal bi-level positive airway pressure
NBM	nil by mouth
nCPAP	nasal continuous positive airway pressure
NCS	nerve conduction studies
NEC	necrotizing enterocolitis
NG	nasogastric
NGT	nasogastric tube
NIBP	non-invasive blood pressure
NICE	National Institute for Health and Care Excellence
NICU	neonatal intensive care unit
nIPPV	nasal intermittent positive pressure ventilation
NJT	nasojejunal tube
NNU	neonatal unit
NPASS	Neonatal Pain, Agitation, & Sedation Score
npCPAP	single naso-pharyngeal prong CPAP
NSAID	non-steroidal anti-inflammatory drug
NTD	neural tube defect
OA	oesophageal atresia
OGT	orogastric tube
OI	oxygenation index
PA	pulmonary atresia
PaO_2	partial pressure of oxygen
PAV	proportional assist ventilation
$(Tc)PCO_2$	(transcutaneous) partial pressure of carbon dioxide
PCR	polymerase chain reaction
PCV	packed cell volume
PDA	patent ductus arteriosus
PEEP	positive end expiratory pressure
PEP	post-exposure prophylaxis
PET	pre-eclampsia
PGE_2	prostaglandin E2
PHVD	post-haemorrhagic ventricular dilatation

PICU	paediatric intensive care unit
PIE	pulmonary interstitial emphysema
PIH	pregnancy-induced hypertension
PIP	peak inspiratory pressure
PIVH	peri/intraventricular haemorrhage
PK	pyruvate kinase
PLIC	posterior limb of the internal capsule
PLTC	pressure-limited, time-cycled
PMA	post-menstrual age
PN	parenteral nutrition
po	orally, by mouth
$(Tc)PO_2$	(transcutaneous) partial pressure of oxygen
POCT	point-of-care therapy
PPH	post-partum haemorrhage
PPHN	persistent pulmonary hypertension of the newborn
PPV	positive pressure ventilation
PR	per rectum
PrAP-A	pregnancy associated protein-A
(P)PROM	(preterm) prelabour rupture of membranes
PS	pulmonary stenosis
PSV	pressure-support ventilation
PT	prothrombin time
PTH	parathyroid hormone
PTU	propylthiouracil
PTV	patient-triggered ventilation
PUJ	pelvi-uteretic junction
PUV	posterior urethral valves
PV	periventricular
PVL	periventricular leucomalacia
PVR	peripheral vascular resistance
PVZ	periventricular zone
qds	four times a day
RA	right atrium
RAD	right axis deviation
RBC	red blood cell
RCOG	Royal College of Obstetricians and Gynaecologists
RCPCH	Royal College of Paediatrics and Child Health
RCT	randomized controlled trial
RDS	respiratory distress syndrome
ROM	rupture of membranes
ROP	retinopathy of prematurity

RPD	renal pelvis dilatation
RPR	rapid plasma reagin
RR	respiratory rate
RSV	respiratory syncytial virus
RT	reptilase time
RTI	respiratory tract infection
RV	right ventricle
RVH	right ventricular hypertrophy
RVOT	right ventricular outflow tract
SALT	speech and language therapy
SBR	serum bilirubin
SCBU	special care baby unit
SEM	skin-eye-mouth
SGA	small for gestational age
SGS	subglottic stenosis
SIADH	syndrome of inappropriate antidiuretic hormone
SIDS	sudden infant death syndrome
SIMV	synchronized intermittent mandatory ventilation
SIPPV	synchronized intermittent positive pressure ventilation
SLE	systemic lupus erythematosus
SMA	spinal muscular atrophy
SPA	suprapubic aspiration
SpO$_2$	peripheral oxygen saturation
SpR	specialist registrar
SVC	superior vena cava
SVT	supraventricular tachycardia
SWS	Sturge–Weber syndrome
TAM	transient abnormal myelopoiesis
TAPVC	total anomalous pulmonary venous connections
TB	tuberculosis
tds	three times a day
TFTs	thyroid function tests
TGA	transposition of the great arteries
THAM	tris-hydroxymethyl aminomethane
Ti	inspiratory time
TII	thyroid inhibiting immunoglobulin
TMD	transient myeloproliferative disorder
ToF	tetralogy of Fallot
TOF	tracheo-oesophageal fistula
TORCH	Toxoplasmosis, Rubella, CMV, Herpes simplex

tPA	tissue plasminogen activator
TPN	total parenteral nutrition
TPPA	*Treponema pallidum* particle agglutination
TRH	thryrotropin-releasing hormone
TSH	thyroid stimulating hormone
TSI	TSH receptor-stimulating immunoglobulins
TT	thrombin time
TTN	transient tachypnoea of the newborn
TTTS	twin–twin transfusion syndrome
U&Es	urea and electrolytes
UAC	umbilical artery catheter
URTI	upper respiratory tract infection
US	ultrasound
UTI	urinary tract infection
UVC	umbilical venous catheterization
V/Q	ventilation perfusion
VA	veno-arterial
VACTERL	Vertebral anomalies, Anal atresia, Cardiovascular anomalies, Tracheo-esophageal fistula, Esophageal atresia, Renal and/or radial anomalies, Limb anomalies
VDRL	venereal disease reference laboratory test
VE	ventricular ectopics
VEP	visual evoked potentials
VILI	ventilator-induced lung injury
VKDB	vitamin K deficiency bleeding
VLBW	very low birth weight
VLCAD	very long-chain acyl CoA dehydrogenase deficiency
VMA	vanillylmandelic acid
VP	ventriculoperitoneal
VSD	ventricular septal defect
VT	tidal volume
VTc	ventricular tachycardia
VTV	volume-targeted ventilation
VV	veno-venous
VZIG	varicella zoster immunoglobulin
VZV	varicella zoster virus
WCC	white cell count
XR	X-ray
WPW	Wolff–Parkinson–White syndrome

Antenatal care, obstetrics, and fetal medicine

Routine antenatal screening and diagnosis of fetal anomalies

Routine antenatal screening

- A first antenatal ('booking') appointment is usually arranged at 10–12 weeks gestation. A history, examination (including BP and BMI), and blood/urine tests are carried out to identify women requiring closer surveillance and care during the pregnancy.
- Blood tests for:
  - full blood count (FBC)
  - haemoglobin electrophoresis to exclude haemoglobinopathies
  - maternal blood group and atypical antibodies (red cell allo-antibodies)
  - serology for syphilis, hepatitis B (HBV), HIV (some centres also check for toxoplasma)
- Urine tests (dipstick) for protein, glucose, and blood
- Fetal ultrasound (US) may be done at this stage to determine gestational age
- General health and pregnancy information given, including offering anomaly screening.

Screening for trisomy 21 (Down syndrome) and other trisomies

- Combined test screening uses several independent risk factors, which are combined to calculate a risk. It is important to explain (and provide written information) that screening is not a diagnostic test and that a negative test does not guarantee that there is no fetal anomaly
- Type of screening used and timing may vary between different centres. Screening usually carried out between 11 and 14 weeks gestation
- Risk calculation based on maternal age, blood hormone assays, and ultrasound scan findings
- Commonest combined test uses nuchal thickness measurement from ultrasound scan + blood measurement of pregnancy-associated protein-A (PrAP-A) and free β-human chorionic gonadotrophin (hCG)
- Results usually take 7–10 days
- Trisomy detection rate ~90% with ~5% false positive rate
- Other screening tests may be carried out later (15–22 weeks) if booking too late for nuchal scanning, or according to local centre choice. Accurate ultrasound dating is combined with triple (α-fetoprotein, oestriol, and free β-hCG) or quadruple (same + inhibin A) blood test
- Ultrasound scanning may also be used in some centres to detect hypoplastic nasal bone or tricuspid regurgitation at 11–14 weeks gestation
- Later ultrasound screening for trisomies may be considered in women presenting too late for nuchal scanning or blood tests (i.e. >22 weeks gestation)
- Soft tissue markers assessed on ultrasound scan (usually in fetal medicine department).

Risk of autosomal trisomy increases with maternal age
Risk at birth:
- ~1:1000 if mother is 28 years old
- ~1:100 if mother is 40 years old
- ~1:25 if mother is 45 years old.

Diagnosis of fetal anomalies

Ultrasound diagnosis of fetal anomalies
- 'Anomaly scan' routinely carried out at 18–21 weeks
- % of anomalies detected varies according to gestation, maternal BMI, operator skill/experience, type of anomaly (e.g. ~99% anencephaly diagnosed on 20-week scan)
- Some relatively common findings may be soft markers of generalized anomalies *or* normal variants such as:
  - choroid plexus cysts: ~1% finding in all 20-week scans with very weak association with trisomies, but considered normal variant if findings otherwise normal
  - 'golfballs' (echogenic foci in ventricles of heart), weak association with trisomies, but considered normal variant if findings otherwise normal
  - increased nuchal thickness: increased risk of trisomy or early development of hydrops
  - echogenic bowel: may be normal variant or associated with chromosomal anomalies, cystic fibrosis, and other causes of fetal bowel obstruction
  - single umbilical artery: not significant unless found alongside other anomalies.

Antenatal genetic testing (karyotype, array CGH, or DNA)
- Done by chorionic villous sampling (CVS), amniocentesis, fetal blood sample, or cell free fetal DNA
- Full karyotype results usually take 1–2 weeks, although specific results by polymerase chain reaction available within a few days
- May be offered to women at high risk of fetal genetic disease due to maternal age (usually >36 years), family history, or if 1st trimester screening indicates high risk.

Chorionic villous sampling
- Carried out between 10 and 13 weeks gestation
- Needle aspiration (inserted into maternal abdomen or via cervix under US control) of trophoblast cells
- Miscarriage risk ~1%.

Amniocentesis
- Carried out after 15 weeks gestation
- Needle inserted into maternal abdomen under US control and ~15 ml amniotic fluid removed
- Miscarriage risk up to 1%
- Follow-up studies have suggested that there is a small increased risk of neonatal respiratory problems due to relative temporary oligohydramnios.

Fetal blood sampling
- May be possible after 18 weeks gestation
- Rarely indicated for genetic diagnosis, but may be used in investigation of hydrops (see ➲ Hydrops fetalis, pp. 84–6) to detect anaemia, chromosomal anomalies, or viral infection.

Cell free fetal DNA (cffDNA) testing
- cffDNA, which originates from trophoblasts is fetal DNA which circulates in the maternal blood stream
- Testing for trisomy 21 is possible from around 10 weeks gestation, with high detection and low false positive rates
- Some single gene disorders can also be diagnosed using 1st trimester cffDNA testing
- Current tests are expensive but have a rapid turnaround time and may reduce the need for more invasive testing.

Maternal diabetes

Complications of pregnancy due to maternal diabetes

Risk of fetal/neonatal complications

Increased with worsening maternal glycaemic control:

- Risk of congenital malformations is ~3 times more than in non-diabetic women and related to maternal HbA1C at time of conception (therefore no increased risk in gestational diabetics). Abnormalities include:
  - congenital heart disease
  - sacral agenesis (caudal regression syndrome)
  - microcolon
  - renal tract anomalies
  - neural tube defects
  - microcephaly
- Increased risk of spontaneous miscarriage
- Increased risk of late intrauterine fetal death
- Intrauterine growth retardation (IUGR) 3 times more common than in non-diabetic women due to placental dysfunction with small vessel disease (N.B. risk of IUGR is also increased in gestational diabetes but less so)
- Polyhydramnios (due to fetal polyuria)
- Preterm labour
- Macrosomia due to increased fetal insulin (anabolic and growth factor-like effect) increases risk of instrumental or Caesarean birth, birth trauma, fetal distress, and neonatal encephalopathy
- Hypoglycaemia (due to fetal hyperinsulinaemia—usually resolves within 48 hours; see ➜ Hypoglycaemia: overview, pp. 372–3)
- Surfactant deficiency/transient tachypnoea of newborn (TTN)
- Transient hypertrophic cardiomyopathy (septal)
- Polycythaemia (increases risk of significant jaundice)
- Other biochemical disturbances (hypocalcaemia, hypomagnesaemia).

Management of infants of diabetic mothers

See Infants of diabetic mothers in ➜ Hypoglycaemia: management, p. 375.

Hypertension, pre-eclampsia, eclampsia, and HELLP syndrome

Maternal hypertensive diseases during pregnancy

- **Pre-existing chronic hypertension**
  - may become superimposed with pregnancy-induced hypertension (PIH) or pre-eclampsia (PET)
  - risk of PET is raised
- **Pregnancy-induced hypertension (PIH)** = BP >140/90 in 2nd half of pregnancy with no proteinuria
  - usually little or no risk to the fetus unless severe
  - fetal growth assessment (+/− umbilical artery Doppler studies), amniotic fluid measurement, and monitoring for raised maternal liver enzymes, urate, and lactate dehydrogenase (LDH) may be required, as well as monitoring for proteinuria
- **Pre-eclampsia (PET)** = hypertension + renal involvement (usually proteinuria)
  - increased risk in primips, extremes of maternal age, obesity, maternal illness (diabetes, lupus, hypertension, renal disease) and multiple pregnancy
  - associated with ↑ risk of placental failure → IUGR and the need to deliver preterm
  - varies from mild (~5% pregnancies) to severe (~1% pregnancies); severity worse with earlier onset
  - severe PET associated with ↑ risk of abruption
  - neonates of affected mothers may have polycythaemia, neutropenia, and thrombocytopenia
  - monitor mother and fetus as for PIH
  - in previous pregnancy with severe PET, low-dose aspirin from 16 weeks reduces risk of recurrence by ~20%
  - maternal condition improves after delivery of placenta
- **HELLP syndrome (haemolysis, elevated liver enzymes, low platelets)** = PET (usually severe) + haemolysis, elevated liver enzymes, and low platelets
- **Eclampsia** = seizures associated with hypertension and proteinuria. Risk of fetal hypoxia is high
- Maternal antihypertensive drugs may be associated with side effects in the neonate:
  - **methyldopa**: good safety profile, few side effects in fetus/neonate
  - **hydralazine**: good safety profile, few side effects in fetus/neonate
  - **beta-blockers**: associated with IUGR if used early in pregnancy, hypoglycaemia, bradycardia, and hypotension in high doses
  - **magnesium**: hypotension and hypotonia
  - **angiotensin converting enzyme (ACE) inhibitors**: neonatal renal failure, contraindicated antenatally
- Breastfeeding is safe with most maternal antihypertensives, apart from ACE inhibitors (except safe with captopril).

Systemic lupus erythematosus, thyroid disease, maternal thrombocytopenia, and maternal myasthenia gravis

Systemic lupus erythromatosus (SLE)

Associated with:
- ↑ Risk of recurrent miscarriage (most cases associated with antiphospholipid syndrome)
- IUGR (usually if maternal renal involvement and hypertension)
- 3rd degree heart block due to permanent damage to the cardiac conduction system (His bundle fibrosis) by anti-Ro and anti-La antibodies (see ➲ Arrhythmias: bradyarrhythmias, p. 230)
- Erythematous 'butterfly' facial rash, which resolves spontaneously after a few weeks
- Haematological abnormalities (e.g. thrombocytopenia, neutropenia).

Thyroid disease

- Maternal thyrotoxicosis or maternal hypothyroidism: see ➲ Thyroid disorders, pp. 450–1.

Maternal thrombocytopenia

- If mother has autoimmune thrombocytopenia (auto-ITP), antibodies may cross placenta and cause neonatal thrombocytopenia
- <20% of babies of mothers with ITP have low platelets
- Even if the baby has severe thrombocytopenia, risk of severe haemorrhage is low; therefore, no indication for delivery by Caesarean section
- Baby's platelet count should be checked soon after birth if mother has thrombocytopenia
- Consider treatment with immunoglobulin in well, term babies with platelet count <20–30 × 10^9/l. Threshold for treatment and platelet transfusion should be less if baby is preterm or unwell
- Consider platelet transfusion or systemic steroids if no response to immunoglobulin
- For management of neonatal thrombocytopenia see ➲ Thrombocytopenia, pp. 408–9.

Maternal myasthenia gravis

- Mother has anti-acetylcholine receptor antibodies, which may cross the placenta
- ~10–20% of babies of affected mothers develop transient neonatal myasthenia gravis
- Incidence of neonatal myasthenia ↑ if previous sibling affected
- Neonatal myasthenia gravis may also occur in babies of asymptomatic mothers
- May present antenatally with ↓ fetal movements and polyhydramnios
- Postnatal onset of symptoms within 5 days of birth, usually lasting up to 4 weeks
- → Hypotonia, poor feeding, and respiratory failure
- Edrophonium or neostigmine may be used diagnostically if mother asymptomatic
- Treatment is supportive and neostigmine (anticholinesterase).

Maternal smoking, alcohol, and drug ingestion

Maternal smoking

Associated with IUGR (reducing birth weight by up to 10%) and ↑ risk of sudden infant death syndrome (SIDS).

Alcohol ingestion

Current UK government advice is for women to consume no alcohol during pregnancy.

>3 units/day during pregnancy is associated with ~5% ↓ in birth weight and fetal alcohol syndrome. Features of fetal alcohol syndrome (often difficult to diagnose in immediate postnatal period) include:
- Pre- and postnatal growth failure
- Microcephaly
- Short palpebral fissures
- Maxillary hypoplasia
- Short nose, smooth philtrum, and thin upper lip
- Ventricular septal defect (VSD), atrial septal defect (ASD), or occasionally other congenital heart disease
- Developmental delay/low IQ.

Therapeutic drugs with known teratogenic effects
- **Anticonvulsants:** phenytoin, carbamazepine, valproate
- Cancer chemotherapy drugs
- Warfarin
- Retinoids
- Lithium.

Maternal opiate and other illicit drug use
- Withdrawal reactions (neonatal abstinence syndrome (NAS)) may occur in babies of mothers using opiates and other drugs, including benzodiazepines, antidepressants, and barbiturates
- Management of babies with NAS (see ➲ Care of the baby whose mother is drug dependent, pp. 46–7).

Cocaine and 'crack'
- Associated with late *in utero* death, intracranial haemorrhage, and infarction
- Irritability and poor sleeping as well as seizures may occur. Prolonged withdrawal, similar to opiates, does not occur.

Intrauterine growth restriction and small for gestational age babies

- Small for gestational age (SGA) = weight below a specified centile for gestation. This is usually <10th centile
- SGA fetus may be either:
  - normal SGA (anomaly scan and other investigations normal) ~70% (i.e. constitutionally small)
  - abnormal SGA (fetal abnormalities)
  - fetal growth restriction (FGR)
- Abnormal SGA and FGR fetuses have intrauterine growth restriction (IUGR)
- Fetal abdominal and head circumference used to predict fetal size
- Abdominal and head measurement:
  - *Proportional*: symmetrical IUGR, usually onset in 1st trimester, may be normal SGA, but often associated with fetal abnormalities (abnormal SGA)
  - *Head sparing*: asymmetrical IUGR, usually onset in 2nd/3rd trimesters, usually due to FGR (placental dysfunction).

Causes of IUGR

- Maternal:
  - familial/racial/constitutional
  - low socio-economic status/poor nutrition/smoking, alcohol, and drug use
  - poor health
  - drugs (beta-blockers, phenytoin, steroids)
  - high altitude
- Placental:
  - hypertension/pre-eclampsia/vascular (SLE/antiphospholipid syndrome)
  - multiple births
- Fetal:
  - trisomies (18 > 21, 13)
  - other fetal anomalies (particularly if multiple)
  - infection (cytomegalovirus (CMV), toxoplasmosis, etc.).

If IUGR suspected

Further investigations are likely to include:
- Repeat US measurements (may be as often as 1–2 times per week)
- Doppler blood flow studies of:
  - umbilical artery (or uterine artery) (↑ pulsatility due to ↑ placental resistance, pattern of diastolic blood flow reduced (diastolic notching), → absent → reversed as condition of fetus deteriorates (Fig. 1.1)). Reversed end-diastolic flow (EDF) implies that placental resistance is so high that blood flows away from the placenta and back into the umbilical arteries during diastole
  - umbilical vein (↓ flow)

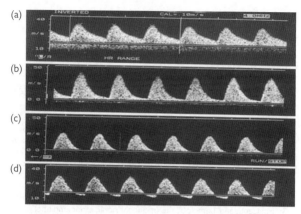

Fig. 1.1 Pulse wave Doppler flow from umbilical artery at 28 weeks gestation showing: a) normal, b) reduced, c) absent, and d) reversed flow as placental function deteriorates with IUGR.

- fetal aorta (↑ pulsatility due to ↑ placental resistance)
- fetal middle cerebral arteries (↓ pulsatility/↓ resistance due to ↑ diastolic brain blood flow—i.e. hypoxia leads to fetal compensatory mechanisms causing redistribution of arterial blood flow to the brain, myocardium, and adrenals)
- Assessment of amniotic fluid volume (amniotic fluid index)
- US of fetal bowel looking for echogenicity
- Cardiotocograph (CTG) assessment (may be daily).

Consideration of early delivery based on assessments and gestation

- Maternal antenatal steroids are usually given if early delivery is likely (absent or reversed EDF, etc.)
- Mode of delivery is more likely to be Caesarean section
- Management of SGA babies (see ⟳ Management of vulnerable babies on postnatal ward and transitional care, pp. 44–5, and ⟳ Enteral feeds: general principles, p. 94).

Multiple births

Incidence of multiple births in the UK:
- Twins: 14.5/1000 live births (UK, 2001)
- Triplets: 1/5000
- Quadruplets: 1/360,000
- Incidence of multiple births is rising and higher in older mothers (partly due to assisted conception).

Twins
- Depending on the number of fertilized oocytes, twins may be mono- or dizygotic (1:2 ratio), although zygosity can only be determined by DNA analysis
- Depending on the timing of splitting of the single embryo, monozygotic twins may have either:
  - 2 placentas and 2 amniotic sacs (dichorionic) ~33% cases
  - 1 placenta and 2 amniotic sacs (monochorionic diamniotic) ~65% cases
  - 1 placenta and 1 amniotic sac (monochorionic monoamniotic) ~1% cases
  - single fused fetus, 1 placenta, and 1 amniotic sac (conjoined twins)
- Outcome is related to chorionicity, rather than zygosity
- Chorionicity can be determined antenatally by 1st trimester US (appearance of chorion at base of inter-twin membrane or 'lambda' sign) or postnatally by examination of the placenta
- ↑ Risk of most complications of pregnancy in multiple pregnancy → perinatal mortality rate 5 times that of singleton pregnancies (~5% in monochorionic, 2% in dichorionic twin pregnancies).

Twin-to-twin transfusion syndrome (TTTS)
TTTS occurs in up to 25% of monochorionic twins via placental vascular connection.

Complications
- Recipient twin:
  - polyhydramnios
  - +/– hydrops
  - +/– polycythaemia
- Donor twin:
  - IUGR
  - oligohydramnios
  - +/– anaemia.
- **Management**: repeated amnio-reduction of recipient twin or laser coagulation of placental vascular connections.
- Death of one twin leads to ↑ risk for surviving twin, particularly of preterm birth. The risk of death or adverse neurodevelopmental outcome:
  - ~5–10% in dichorionic twins
  - ~30% in monochorionic twins
- Cord entanglement: a complication of monoamniotic twin pregnancy with 10–12% risk of intrauterine fetal death after 24 weeks gestation. Elective preterm delivery is recommended in some centres.

Oligohydramnios and polyhydramnios

Oligohydramnios/anhydramnios

- Oligohydramnios: amniotic fluid volume <500 ml
- Fetus is at risk of:
  - pulmonary hypoplasia if onset of oligohydramnios <26 weeks gestation
  - fetal distress during labour.

Causes of oligohydramnios/anhydramnios

- Bilateral fetal renal disease (= oligohydramnios/anhydramnios sequence—severe pulmonary hypoplasia, contractures, and Potter's facies):
  - renal agenesis
  - cystic dysplastic kidneys
  - polycystic kidney disease
  - obstructive uropathy (e.g. posterior urethral valves)
- Placental insufficiency
- Fetal abnormalities (e.g. trisomies)
- **Preterm pre-labour rupture of membranes (PPROM):** risk of pulmonary hypoplasia 20–30% if onset <26 weeks, but very low >26 weeks gestation
- Twin-to-twin transfusion syndrome (TTTS): donor twin.

Management of oligohydramnios

If there are no fetal anomalies, amnio-infusion may ↓ risk of pulmonary hypoplasia.

Polyhydramnios

- Polyhydramnios: amniotic fluid volume >2 l
- ↑ Risk of:
  - preterm birth
  - PPROM
  - malpresentation
  - APH
  - cord prolapse.

Causes of polyhydramnios

- Idiopathic
- Maternal diabetes
- TTTS: recipient twin
- Upper gastrointestinal (GI) atresia (oesophageal atresia +/− tracheo-oesophageal, duodenal atresia). It is suggested that a nasogastric (NG) tube is passed and abdominal X-ray performed in the immediate post-natal period in all cases of severe polyhydramnios
- Congenital diaphragmatic hernia
- Neuromuscular disease (congenital myotonic dystrophy, spinal muscular atrophy, congenital myopathies)
- Chromosomal abnormalities.

Management of polyhydramnios

- **Amnio-reduction:** relieves discomfort for mother and →↓ risk of PPROM and preterm labour
- **Indometacin:** →↓ fetal urine production, →↓ amniotic fluid volume.

Preterm labour and other obstetric complications

Preterm labour

Onset of labour <37 weeks gestation. Causes/associations include:

- Idiopathic (~80% cases)
- Polyhydramnios
- PPROM
- Chorioamnionitis
- APH
- Cervical incompetence
- Low socio-economic status.

Management of preterm labour

- Tests to predict preterm delivery: unlikely to deliver if either -ve fetal fibronectin test or transvaginal cervical length >15 mm
- Tocolytics: atosiban and nifedipine have been shown to increase the number of women with preterm labour not delivered within 48 hours, but benefits to neonatal mortality and morbidity less certain
- Place of birth: outcomes for extreme prematurity improved in babies delivered in higher-volume tertiary centres
- Antenatal corticosteroids
  - given to mothers at risk of preterm birth reduces risk of neonatal death, respiratory distress syndrome (RDS), peri/intraventricular haemorrhage (PIVH), and necrotizing enterocolitis
  - single course (usually IM betamethasone 12 mg, 2 doses 12 hours apart, or dexamethasone 6 mg, 4 doses 6 hours apart) recommended for women between 24^{+0} and 34^{+6} weeks of gestation at risk of preterm birth (and should be considered between 23^{+0}–23^{+6} weeks gestation)
  - also recommended for women with planned elective Caesarean section <38^{+6} weeks gestation, although elective Caesarean section should be delayed until after 39 weeks gestation if possible
  - most effective if birth >24 hours and <7 days after administration of 2nd dose, but mortality ↓ if given <24 hours before birth, therefore still recommended if birth expected within this time
  - repeated courses not usually recommended (e.g. for multiple pregnancy or onset of preterm labour >1 week after the initial course)
- Magnesium sulfate: given to women at risk of early preterm birth reduces the risk of cerebral palsy in surviving babies.

Antepartum haemorrhage (APH)

Major vaginal bleeding >24 weeks gestation.

Causes

- Placental abruption
- Placenta praevia
- Vasa praevia (fetal vessels within membranes close to cervical os), can result in severe anaemia at birth.

Associations
- Preterm labour
- ↑ Perinatal mortality
- Risk of adverse neurodevelopmental outcome.

Preterm pre-labour rupture of membranes (PPROM)

Causes/associations
- Polyhydramnios
- Multiple pregnancy
- Chorioamnionitis
- Amniocentesis/cordocentesis
- Cervical incompetence.

Risks
- Preterm labour (~80% cases)
- Chorioamnionitis
- Pulmonary hypoplasia (if onset <26 weeks; see ➔ Pulmonary hypoplasia, p. 138).

Management
- **Maternal antibiotics:** erythromycin →↑ gestation and better neonatal outcomes if no evidence of chorioamnionitis or broad-spectrum antibiotics (not co-amoxiclav as associated with ↑ risk of necrotizing enterocolitis) if chorioamnionitis suspected (see ➔ Early onset bacterial infection, pp. 328–9, for management of baby following PPROM)
- Antenatal steroids
- **Amnioinfusion:** if high risk of pulmonary hypoplasia.

Umbilical cord prolapse

Obstetric emergency, usually managed by emergency Caesarean section, due to high risk of cord compression or vascular spasm → risk of fetal hypoxia ischaemia. Risk ↑ with:
- Multiple birth
- Polyhydramnios
- PPROM
- Malpresentation (breech, transverse lie).

Problems during labour and birth

Malpresentation

- Breech presentation:
  - incidence ~3% at term
  - external cephalic version →↓ incidence of vaginal breech or elective Caesarean section. Usually performed at 34–36 weeks gestation
  - ↓ risk of perinatal mortality/morbidity with elective Caesarean section
- Transverse lie:
  - risk of cord prolapse and obstructed labour
  - elective Caesarean section recommended
- Brow presentation:
  - risk of obstructed labour
  - elective Caesarean section recommended.

Fetal distress

Recognized by:
- Passage of meconium during labour—a non-specific sign of fetal distress
- Electronic fetal monitoring (EFM) used to determine whether fetal heart rate (FHR) pattern normal, suspicious, or pathological (Tables 1.1 and 1.2).

Table 1.1 Features of fetal heart rate (FHR) pattern used for electronic fetal monitoring (EFM) classification

	Baseline (beats/min)	Variability (beats/min)	Decelerations	Accelerations
Reassuring	110–160	≥5	None	Present
Non-reassuring	100–109 161–180	<5 for 40–90min	Variable decelerations for >50% contractions ≥90min. Single prolonged deceleration up to 3min	Absence of accelerations in otherwise normal cardiotocograph of uncertain significance
Abnormal	<100 or >180 or sinusoidal ≥10min	<5 for >90min	Either atypical variable decelerations >50% contractions or late decelerations both ≥30min. Single prolonged deceleration >3min	

Table 1.2 Electronic fetal monitoring (EFM) classification

Category	Definition
Normal	All 4 features of fetal heart rate (FHR) pattern reassuring
Suspicious	1 feature of FHR pattern non-reassuring, all others reassuring
Pathological	≥2 features of FHR pattern non-reassuring or 1 or more abnormal

- Fetal pH from fetal blood sampling:
  - taken from fetal scalp if concern regarding fetal distress, unless immediate delivery indicated
  - urgent emergency Caesarean section indicated if pH <7.2. Sample should usually be repeated within 30 minutes if 7.21–7.24 or within 1 hour if FHR pattern on EFM remains pathological despite fetal scalp pH ≥7.25.

Failure to progress

Causes

- Malpresentation
- Cephalopelvic disproportion
- Incoordinate/poor uterine contractions.

Management

- Augmentation with oxytocin +/− artificial rupture of membranes
- Caesarean section.

Shoulder dystocia

An inability to deliver the shoulders after delivery of the baby's head.

- Occurs in ~1% term births (↑ incidence if fetus macrosomic/infant of diabetic mother)
- Obstetric emergency due to risk of acute cord compression and fetal hypoxia ischaemia
- Also high risk of Erb's palsy and other brachial plexus injuries
- Obstetrician may need to fracture baby's clavicle(s).

Further information

Doyle LW, Crowther CA, Middleton P, Marret S, Rouse D. Magnesium sulphate for women at risk of preterm birth for neuroprotection of the fetus. *Cochrane Database Syst Rev* 2009. ℘ www.onlinelibrary.wiley.com/doi/10.1002/14651858.CD004661.pub3/abstract

The Fetal Medicine Foundation: ℘ www.fetalmedicine.org/var/uploads/Doppler-in-Obstetrics.pdf

National Institute for Health and Care Excellence (2015) NICE guidelines (NG25). Preterm labour and birth. ℘ www.nice.org.uk/guidance/ng25

National Institute for Health and Care Excellence (2015) NICE quality standard (QS105). Intrapartum care. ℘ www.nice.org.uk/guidance/qs105

Roberts D, Dalziel SR. Antenatal corticosteroids for accelerating fetal lung maturation for women at risk of preterm birth. *Cochrane Database Syst Rev* 2006. ℘ www.onlinelibrary.wiley.com/doi/10.1002/14651858.CD004454.pub2/abstract

Chapter 2

Management at birth and routine postnatal care

Resuscitation of the newborn

Approximately 5–10% of all neonates require some resuscitation after birth. Midwifery and obstetric staff who attend all births should be trained in basic life support of newborn babies and neonatal unit staff should be trained in advanced life support.

Births that neonatal unit staff should attend

At least one member of the neonatal unit team, competent in resuscitation of the newborn, should attend high-risk births. Opinion regarding what defines 'high-risk' varies and so recommendations differ from unit to unit. A suggested list is:

- Emergency Caesarean section
- Elective Caesarean section—only if under general anaesthetic or if there are complications
- Instrumental delivery (forceps and ventouse)
- Breech vaginal delivery
- Meconium-stained amniotic fluid
- Fetal distress
- Antepartum haemorrhage (APH)
- Multiple pregnancy (one member of staff for each baby)
- Preterm birth (below 37 completed weeks gestation)
- Known congenital abnormality
- Significant maternal disease, which may have an immediate adverse effect on the baby (e.g. congenital myotonia, myasthenia gravis).

Resuscitation guidelines

Fig. 2.1 is taken from the Resuscitation Council (UK), Resuscitation Guidelines, 2015, for newborn life support.

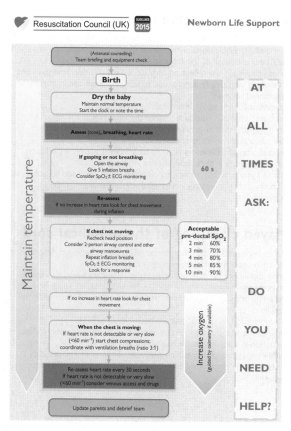

Fig. 2.1 Newborn life support.
Reproduced with the kind permission of the Resuscitation Council (UK).

Umbilical cord blood gases

Umbilical cord blood gas analysis may be recommended after all births where there is suspicion of intrapartum hypoxia ischaemia and is a useful guide to the condition of the fetus at the time of birth.
- Cord venous pH is a reflection of placental gas transfer, whereas cord arterial pH indicates fetal response to labour—therefore important to take paired samples
- Cord venous pH usually > arterial pH (by >0.02)
- Cord arterial PCO_2 usually > venous (by >0.5 kPa)
- Cord compression or prolapse likely to lead to larger differences (venous-arterial pH difference >0.15)
- Venous-arterial differences likely to be smaller if placental perfusion compromised (e.g. abruption, uterine rupture)
- Risk of hypoxic ischaemic encephalopathy (HIE) and poor neurological outcome only significantly increased if cord arterial pH <7.05 (<7.0 in preterm).

Delayed clamping of the umbilical cord

Evidence from randomized controlled trials suggests benefit in delaying cord clamping in uncomplicated term pregnancies.
- Cord should not be clamped earlier than necessary based on clinical assessment
- Delayed cord clamping >30 seconds decreases risk of anaemia/iron deficiency at 4 months
- No increased risk of post-partum haemorrhage (PPH)
- Benefits may be greater in preterm babies—additional possible effect of reduction in intraventricular haemorrhage (IVH)
- Early cord clamping may still be necessary if there is PPH, placenta praevia, cord tight around baby's neck or if immediate resuscitation required.

Meconium-stained amniotic fluid

See ➔Meconium aspiration syndrome, pp. 120–1.

- Meconium-stained amniotic fluid may occur secondary to fetal distress in more mature pregnancies without evidence of fetal distress (unusual in preterm; approximately 35% of pregnancies >42 weeks)
- Routine suction of the oropharynx/nasopharynx is *not* recommended. Meconium and amniotic fluid should be removed from the baby's face and mouth immediately after the baby's head has been delivered
- If the baby is in good condition (i.e. establishes regular respirations quickly, crying, normal heart rate, well perfused, active, and no signs of respiratory distress), no further intervention is necessary
- If further resuscitation is required, positive pressure ventilation should be avoided until it is confirmed that the airway is clear by visualizing the vocal cords directly with a laryngoscope
- If the airway is not clear of meconium (or secretions/blood), use suction from the oropharynx and above the cords, under direct vision with a laryngoscope. Then proceed to intubation with the appropriate sized endotracheal tube (ETT)—usually 3.5 mm for a term baby. Clearing the airway of meconium can then be performed either by:
  - attaching suction tubing via a connector directly onto the ETT so that the ETT is used as the suction device
  - applying suction via a large bore (8 French) suction catheter placed down the ETT. Withdrawing the ETT with suction catheter in situ may improve clearance of thick meconium. This may need to be done 2 or 3 times
- Insert NG tube and empty the stomach of meconium-stained fluid
- Monitor for signs of respiratory distress for at least the next 4–6 hours. This may be carried out on the postnatal ward or neonatal unit, depending on the baby's condition. A longer period of observation may be necessary if concerns persist.

Delivery room management of congenital anomalies

In many cases, these are antenatally diagnosed, allowing postnatal management to be planned, usually in a tertiary centre, where the relevant sub-specialty team is on site. Most babies with antenatally diagnosed congenital anomalies should be resuscitated as required and admitted to the neonatal unit once initial stability is achieved.

See individual sections on congenital anomalies for specific guidance for management of each condition.

Routine postnatal newborn care

Risk assessment at birth

All babies should have a risk assessment for complications requiring observation or neonatal input. A care plan should be documented either by the midwife, or the neonatal team.

Infection
Viral
- Babies born to mothers with known viral infections should have a postnatal plan
- If there are no booking bloods, urgent virology for Hepatitis B and HIV should be sent. Ensure this is followed up and acted upon
- See ➔ Chapter 12, Infection, for individual congenital infections.

Bacterial
- Babies are at risk of bacterial infection in the immediate newborn period. Refer to ➔ Early onset bacterial infection, pp. 328–9 for risk factors, investigation, and management
- If the baby is to stay with mother, ensure clear plans for observation and treatment are documented.

Gestation
- Many babies born less than 37 weeks gestation can be looked after on the postnatal ward. Most local guidelines will have gestation and birth weight guidance for admission to the neonatal unit (e.g. <34 weeks gestation or <1800 g)
- Ensure particular attention is paid to avoiding hypothermia (e.g. skin-to-skin, hat) and observation for hypothermia, hypoglycaemia, etc.

Hypoglycaemia
Babies at risk of hypoglycaemia (e.g. preterm (<37 weeks); babies with intrauterine growth retardation (IUGR), and infants of diabetic mothers) can be managed on the postnatal ward. See ➔ Hypoglycaemia: management, pp. 374–5.

IUGR
Ensure you are aware of baby's birth weight and centile. IUGR babies are at risk of hypothermia, hypoglycaemia, and poor feeding.

Jaundice
Look at mother's blood group, presence of atypical antibodies, and history of significant jaundice in previous babies.

Postnatal observation
- Within the first hour of birth all babies should have an initial examination by the midwife including weight and head circumference, which should be plotted on the appropriate centile chart.
- Initial observations of temperature, pulse, respirations, and colour should also be documented.
- A full newborn examination should be carried out within 72 hours of birth. See ➔ Examination of the newborn, pp. 28–30.

- The neonate should be observed in the first 24 hours for
  - skin colour: jaundice/cyanosis/pallor/rashes
  - assessment of respiratory distress
  - tone
  - movement and activity
  - feeding
  - passage of meconium/urine
  - umbilicus/clamp.

Feeding

Breastfeeding

Women should be offered skin-to-skin contact with their babies as soon as possible after birth to help optimize milk production and bonding. They should have continued skilled breastfeeding support to ensure comfortable positioning of mother and baby and ensure good attachment is achieved. Unrestricted breastfeeding frequency and duration should be encouraged.

Support

- Additional support should be available for women after Caesarean section or anaesthetic. Mothers should be made aware of how to access the breastfeeding support in hospital and in the community. Information regarding supplementation of feeds can be given if there is anxiety about milk supply. Mothers can express their breast milk which can then be given by cup or bottle.
- Difficulties can arise because of poor attachment, nipple pain, engorgement or mastitis, inverted nipples, or tongue tie.

Assessment

- Indicators of good attachment include:
  - mouth wide open
  - less areola visible underneath the chin than above
  - chin touching the breast, lower lip rolled down and the nose free
  - no pain
- A successfully breastfeeding baby will demonstrate
  - audible and visible swallowing
  - sustained rhythmic suck
  - relaxed arms and hands
  - moist mouth
  - regular soaked nappies.

Tongue tie

- Tongue tie occurs in up to 10% of newborns, depending on definition
- There is growing consensus that tongue tie can lead to breastfeeding difficulties in some circumstances. There is evidence to suggest that division of tongue tie can improve feeding
- The decision to divide the tongue tie should be based on expert feeding assessment only and not for aesthetic reasons. Local referral pathways will vary
- The risks associated with tongue tie repair are bleeding, infection, and reoccurrence.

Transitional care

See ➔ Management of vulnerable babies on postnatal ward and transitional care, pp. 44–5.

Transfer to the community

- All babies should be assessed as well at discharge by an appropriately-qualified professional:
  - detailed newborn examination will normally be done prior to discharge
  - if this has not occurred, ensure arrangements for examination within 72 hours of birth
- All babies should have been assessed as feeding adequately by the chosen method of feeding
- In mothers who wish to breastfeed, breastfeeding technique should be taught and actively assessed as adequate by a midwife trained in breastfeeding support
- All babies should be weighed by 5 days of age (whether in hospital or in the community) to ensure there has not been excessive weight loss and/or dehydration
- All mothers should be given information on the following prior to transfer:
  - temperature control (including pyrexia and low temperature)
  - feeding and signs of poor feeding or feeding failure, such as lethargy, lack of changing stool by day 4/5
  - jaundice
  - respiratory difficulties
  - SIDS and co-sleeping guidance
  - newborn blood spot screening tests (Guthrie) to be performed at 5–7 days.

Examination of the newborn

Aims
- To detect abnormalities and clinical problems that have an effect on morbidity and institute a plan of management
- To impart advice and reassurance to parents.

When and by whom?
- Trained personnel, usually neonatal/paediatric medical staff, midwives, GPs, advanced neonatal nurse practitioners
- Within first 72 hours (in hospital, usually within first 24 hours)
- If there are no problems, this examination need not be repeated before discharge.

What is needed?
- A well-lit room that can be darkened to study red reflexes
- Stethoscope
- Ophthalmoscope
- Tape measure
- Maternal and neonatal records.

Pre-examination
- Introduce yourself and obtain consent from mother (or both parents if present) to examine the baby. Explain the purpose of the examination.
- Check maternal notes for:
  - family history
  - maternal medical or social problems
  - booking blood results and any other blood tests during pregnancy (e.g. thyroid function, viral infections)
  - fetal scan results
  - antenatal details, including maternal and fetal wellbeing, presentation (e.g. breech)
  - risk factors for infection
  - details of labour
- Check baby's notes for:
  - resuscitation details
  - birth weight
  - condition of baby since birth (feeding, passed urine/meconium, etc.)
  - any management plans already made
- Ask parents about family history of congenital deafness and congenital dislocation of the hip.

Examination
The description here is very systematic—in reality, be opportunistic (e.g. ophthalmoscopic examination as soon as the baby's eyes open; listen to the heart while baby is not crying). Some observations should be made while talking to mother and while undressing the baby.

The baby should be completely undressed for the examination and appropriate attention given to maintenance of its temperature. The following list is not exhaustive:
- General appearance: is baby dysmorphic? (check parents)
- Size of baby: plot weight and head circumference on centile chart
- Colour of baby: pink, cyanosed, jaundiced, pale
- Spontaneous activity of baby
- Birth marks and rashes
- Cardiac apex and impulse
- Heart sounds and murmurs
- Femoral pulses
- Patency of the upper airway
- Inspection *and* palpation of the palate
- Respiratory distress
- Auscultation of the lungs
- Observation of the abdomen
- General and organ-specific palpation of the abdomen
- Examination of hernial orifices
- Palpation of the testes, inspection of penis/observation of the vulva
- Inspection of the anus (patency and position)
- Examination of the limbs: count digits, palmar creases
- Elicit head control by pull-to-sit
- Examine truncal tone in ventral suspension
- Inspect midline of back from anterior fontanelle: skin defects, naevi (particularly lower end for lumps, birthmarks, pits, hairs, and fistulae)
- Elicit Moro reflex
- Palpate anterior fontanelle
- Examine for hip stability (Barlow and Ortolani tests)
- Elicit red reflex in both eyes.

Discharge
- Provide detailed documentation and record if baby is fit for discharge
- If a problem has been identified, ensure that there is a management plan instituted and a letter to the GP has been completed
- Discuss any need for outpatient follow-up with the senior staff
- Inform parents clearly of any follow-up arrangements and why they are needed
- **Early discharge:** for babies who are discharged to the community within 6–24 hours, parents should be warned to look out for:
  - jaundice (particularly within 24 hours of birth)
  - respiratory difficulty
  - feeding difficulty
  - delay in passage of urine or meconium beyond 24 hours.

Further information

National Institute for Health and Clinical Excellence (2006) NICE guidelines (CG37). Postnatal care up to 8 weeks after birth. ℘ www.nice.org.uk/guidance/cg37

National Institute for Health and Care Excellence (2014) NICE guidelines (CG190). Intrapartum care for healthy women and babies. ℘ www.nice.org.uk/guidance/cg190

NHS Newborn & Infant Physical Examination Programme. ℘ www.gov.uk/topic/population-screening-programmes/newborn-infant-physical-examination

Resuscitation Council. *Newborn Life Support: Resuscitation at birth*, 4th ed. Resuscitation Council, London, 2016.

Resuscitation Council. *Resuscitation and support of transition of babies at birth* (Guidelines and NLS algorithm) 2015. ℘ www.resus.org.uk/resuscitation-guidelines/

Vain NE, Szyld EG, Prudent LM, et al. Oropharyngeal and nasopharyngeal suctioning of meconium-stained neonates before delivery of their shoulders: multicentre, randomised controlled trial. *Lancet* 2004; **364**: 597–602.

Wiswell TE, Gannon CM, Jacob J, et al. Delivery room management of the apparently vigorous meconium-stained neonate: results of the multicenter international collaborative trial. *Pediatrics* 2000; **105**: 1–7.

Chapter 3

Problems on the postnatal ward

Approach to the dysmorphic baby

History
- Ask for relevant family history
- Check antenatal history, particularly screening tests and antenatal ultrasound scans
- Observe parental features.

Examination
- Examine the baby thoroughly and record all the dysmorphic features clearly and systematically in the notes
- Record the weight, head circumference, and length on the appropriate centile chart
- Consider passing an NG tube into stomach and check patency of both nostrils to exclude oesophageal and choanal atresia
- Seek senior review +/− genetics opinion.

Possible further investigations (depending on other findings)
- Genetics: tests ordered will depend on local guidelines, which might include:
  - array comparative genomic hybridization (CGH)
  - chromosomal analysis
  - rapid PCR test (polymerase chain reaction) for specific disorders (particularly trisomy 13, 18, and 21) if available
  - DNA analysis (seek prior genetics opinion if necessary, so that specific test can be arranged)
- X-rays: chest, abdomen, and spine
- Cranial, renal, and abdominal US
- Echocardiogram
- Eye examination by paediatric ophthalmologist
- Ensure hearing screen is performed.

Communication with parents
- This is often difficult, particularly if a diagnosis is not clear, as parental and staff anxiety will be high
- Be sure to involve senior medical staff
- Try to ensure any difficult news is imparted to both parents or at least with another supportive person present
- Be open and honest with parents; if you are not sure, say so.

Down syndrome

Background

- Caused by the presence of all or part of an extra chromosome 21
- 1 in 800–1000 live births
- Increased risk with increasing maternal age: risk under 30 years <1 in 1000; risk at 35 years 1 in 400; risk at 42 years 1 in 60. However, 75% of babies with Down syndrome are born to mothers <35 years old
- Underlying genetics may be:
  - trisomy 21 (95%) (usually maternal non-dysjunction)
  - mosaicism (1–2%)
  - translocation (2–3%) where parent may carry balanced translocation; parental chromosome analysis is indicated.

Postnatal assessment

Diagnosis made antenatally

- Check fetal echocardiogram findings for evidence of congenital heart disease
- Full clinical examination, particularly of cardiovascular system
- Check result of antenatal karyotype
- Ensure the baby is seen by senior medical staff.

Diagnosis suspected postnatally

- See early and perform full examination, particularly of cardiovascular system
- Seek immediate senior medical review
- Be sensitive to parents' anxiety and, if necessary, say you are asking a more senior doctor to see the baby
- Take blood for genetics and request urgent PCR (if available) for trisomy 21.

Once confirmed or if diagnosis likely on clinical grounds

- Check FBC and blood film to exclude polycythaemia, transient abnormal myelopoiesis (TAM, also called Transient Leukaemia of Down Syndrome, or TL-DS), and thrombocytopenia. If TAM is present (occurs in up to 10% of babies with Down syndrome), the baby has a high risk (20–30%) of later myeloid leukaemia—refer to haematologist
- Refer to paediatric cardiologist: congenital heart disease occurs in 45%; commonest diagnosis is atrioventricular septal defect (AVSD)
- Consider presence of associated problems, e.g. duodenal atresia, Hirschsprung's disease
- Ensure appropriate feeding assessment and support
- Ensure parents receive appropriate counselling from consultant (see next section, **➔** Information that may be given to the parents, pp. 34–5).

Information that may be given to the parents

- Confirmation of the diagnosis, with discussion of the genetics (consider referral for geneticist follow-up)
- Developmental delay and learning difficulties
- High incidence of congenital heart disease

- Potential for feeding problems, hypotonia, visual impairment (e.g. squint and cataracts), hearing impairment, duodenal atresia, hypothyroidism (1%), leukaemia (<1%), short stature, and recurrent upper respiratory tract infections and otitis media
- Requirement for follow-up in the community with paediatrician and therapists
- Written information about Down syndrome and support groups.

Follow-up
- Neonatologist (within a few weeks of discharge):
  - to ensure adequate feeding and growth
  - explore how parents and family are coping with diagnosis
  - further discuss implications and answer questions
  - ensure appropriate referrals (particularly to community services) have been made
- Ensure hearing screening performed
- Speech and language therapist (if there are significant feeding problems)
- Local special needs support if available
- Referral to community paediatrician
- Inform GP and health visitor by phone, and supply typewritten discharge summary
- Ophthalmologist (3–6 months).

Delayed passage of meconium

- Most healthy babies pass meconium within 24 hours of birth. Delay beyond 24 hours is unusual and underlying pathology should be considered
- Possible aetiologies are:
  - Hirschsprung's disease
  - meconium ileus
  - meconium plug
  - intestinal dysmotility, particularly in growth restricted baby
  - imperforate anus
  - prematurity.

Management

- Review full history with mother and midwives; ensure that no meconium was passed prior to delivery
- Examine maternal notes for any evidence of polyhydramnios or other abnormalities on antenatal scans (e.g. dilated loops of bowel)
- Take feeding history and elicit history suggestive of obstruction (e.g. bilious vomiting, abdominal distension)
- Fully examine baby, particularly for clinical state of the baby (perfusion, etc.), abdominal distension, tenderness, and check anus is patent
- If <24 hours old, baby is well with no vomiting, and normal examination then observe closely
- If >24 hours old; or <24 hours but with concerning features in the history or on examination: consider bowel obstruction, Hirschsprung's disease, enterocolitis, and sepsis:
  - admit to the neonatal unit
  - seek senior medical review
  - request AXR and discuss with consultant +/– paediatric surgeon
- If a baby has been given a suppository to aid passage of meconium then this baby should still be discussed with a paediatric surgeon in view of the possibility of Hirschsprung's disease
- If a meconium plug is passed, IRT (spot of blood on Newborn bloodspot screening card) and cystic fibrosis genetic studies should be checked. Hirschsprung's disease should also be considered.

Common skin problems in the newborn: naevi

Capillary naevi/port wine stains

- Incidence 0.3%
- Usually larger and darker than salmon patches (see **➲** p. 39); present at birth; grow with infant and do not fade or darken with age
- Seek senior medical review
- If face and orbital area involved, consider Sturge–Weber syndrome (SWS)
- If naevus is in the region of the ophthalmic region of trigeminal nerve 25% have SWS. Consider:
  - neuroimaging +/− neurology referral for cerebral arteriovenous malformation
  - ophthalmological review for glaucoma
- Consider dermatology referral, as pulsed dye laser therapy may be indicated for significant lesions.

Capillary haemangiomas: 'strawberry' naevi

- Common (incidence up to 10%); male:female ratio 2:1. More common in preterm
- Uncommonly visible at birth, but usually appear by 4 weeks
- Course variable, but usually increase in size over 3–9 months, then involute, and resolve completely
- Rarely, a large haemangioma may involve a large proportion of a limb, or cause haemorrhage, ulceration, or thrombocytopenia
- If complicated (large or multiple):
  - seek senior review if uncertainty about diagnosis or if further assessment needed (e.g. if vision may be obstructed)
  - dermatology referral may be warranted and treatment with beta-blockers considered
  - if multiple, further investigation may be necessary to rule out visceral involvement (e.g. abdominal ultrasound).

Congenital melanocytic naevi

- Brown/black lesions present at birth; incidence 1%
- Small, medium-sized, large, or giant
- Giant melanocytic naevus ('bathing trunk' naevus):
  - rare
  - seek senior medical review
  - refer to dermatologist
  - there is a small risk of later malignant change to melanoma (perhaps 5% over a lifetime).

Sebaceous naevi (naevus of Jadassohn)

- Yellow-brown sebaceous fleshy slightly raised lesions present at birth and most common on scalp; incidence 0.3%
- Persist and become more nodular in adolescence. Have very small risk of malignant change later in life (predominantly basal cell carcinoma)
- Refer to dermatologist.

Common skin problems in the newborn: other

Erythema toxicum

Also known as erythema neonatorum or urticaria neonatorum:

- Common and benign (>50% newborn in first 2 weeks). More common if term or post-term
- Variable erythematous patches with small eosinophilic 'pustules' (less pustular than *Staphylococcus* spots)
- Reassure.

Transient neonatal pustular melanosis

- Present at birth, more common in black infants (in whom the incidence is up to 5%)
- Benign, superficial, non-erythematous, vesiculopustular rash, which may rapidly dry, leaving hyperpigmented macules that fade in weeks
- Reassure.

Milia

- Common (>50% newborn) and benign
- Obstructed sebaceous glands
- 1–2 mm yellow-white spots, most common on nose and face that resolve after 2 months
- Reassure.

Miliaria

- Obstructed sweat ducts
- Pinpoint vesicles on forehead, scalp, and skin folds that resolve by 1–2 weeks
- Reassure.

Staphylococcal skin infection

Presentation

- **Mildest form:** a few pustules on erythematous base
- **Severe form:** cellulitis and scalded skin appearance.

Management

- If diagnosis is in doubt, puncture a lesion and send contents for MC&S (microscopy, culture, and sensitivities)
- If systemically well in mild cases, start oral flucloxacillin
- If systemically unwell or extensive skin changes (i.e. with cellulitis or skin loss):
  - admit to neonatal unit (NNU)
  - send FBC, CRP, blood culture
  - start IV antibiotics (e.g. flucloxacillin and gentamicin).

Salmon patches/stork marks
- Very common, incidence up to 50%
- Circumscribed lesions usually at back of neck, nuchal fold, eye-lids, forehead, and above upper lip
- Fade with time, therefore reassure.

Mongolian blue spot
- Common and benign, found in 90% Asian and Afro-Caribbean babies and 5% Caucasian
- Blue/grey irregular patches, most commonly on the lower back, but can extend over whole back and on extensor surfaces of limbs
- Should not be mistaken for bruising
- Usually fade, but may persist.

Skin tags
- Check for other dysmorphic features. If near the ear, check external auditory meatus patency and arrange hearing screening
- Refer to plastic surgeon.

Polydactyly and accessory digits
- Common, with a higher incidence in black babies; often positive family history (usually autosomal dominant)
- Check no other dysmorphic features
- Historically, these have been tied off with a suture and left to fall off. However, this is associated with neuromas at the site, so refer to plastic surgeon.

Talipes equinovarus

Background
- Incidence of 1 in 1000 births, male preponderance
- May be isolated or associated with syndromes (e.g. trisomy 13, 18), intrauterine restriction of movement (e.g. oligohydramnios) or neuromuscular disorders.

Assessment
- Check mother's antenatal notes and ultrasound scan results and ask about fetal movements
- Look for any other abnormalities with particular attention to neuromuscular, spinal, and hip examination
- Positional talipes:
  - passively corrects beyond the neutral position
  - baby also is able to actively correct foot posture
  - parents can be reassured that posture will fully correct without any further input
  - no physiotherapy or specialist follow-up required
- Structural talipes *does not* correct beyond the neutral position.

Management of structural talipes
- Examine the hips carefully and arrange a hip ultrasound scan to exclude congenital dislocation of the hips
- Refer to physiotherapy and paediatric orthopaedic surgeons
- Management is by foot stretches, splinting, strapping, or casting as required
- Manipulation and application of well-moulded plaster casts may correct mild to moderate deformities and can improve severe deformities, making subsequent surgery easier
- Casting is most effective when commenced in the first few days
- Arrange for orthopaedic surgeons to assess the baby either prior to or soon after discharge
- Early surgery may induce fibrosis, scarring, and stiffness, and thus is likely to be delayed until at least 3 months.

Neonatal hip problems: developmental dysplasia and congenital dislocation of the hip

Background
- Spectrum from shallow acetabulum to frank dislocation
- 1% of babies will have developmental dysplasia of the hip (DDH), 1 in 1000 will have persistent dislocation
- Female preponderance.

Risk factors
- Family history, especially first degree relative
- Breech presentation at or after 36 weeks gestation, or at delivery if this is <36 weeks
- Oligohydramnios
- Sternomastoid tumour and torticollis
- Talipes deformities, including equinovarus, calcaneovalgus, metatarsus adductus
- Congenital myopathies and neurological disease.

Management

Screening
This is recommended for family history and breech presentation (see ➋ Risk factors, p. 41). (See ➋ Further information, p. 50.) Some units will also recommend for other risk factors
- Hip ultrasound scan at 4–6 weeks
- Refer to orthopaedics if ultrasound abnormal.

Abnormal clinical hip examination
Findings may include positive Ortolani or Barlow tests, clicky hips, asymmetrical creases, or limited abduction:
- Seek senior medical review
- If hip examination confirmed to be abnormal:
  - discuss with paediatric orthopaedics team
  - arrange early hip ultrasound scan (should be completed by 2 weeks of age)
  - arrange early orthopaedic referral.

Orthopaedic treatment
- Pavlik harness
- Hip spica
- Surgical reduction.

Lower spinal abnormalities: sacral dimples, pits, and spinal dysraphism

Natal dimples or pits

- Very common within or just above the natal cleft
- If skin overlying the defect is intact and there are no other abnormalities on examination then reassure
- If there is uncertainty as to whether the skin is intact and there is no sinus or discharge:
  - check that neurological examination is normal
  - seek senior medical review
  - arrange ultrasound scan of the lower spinal cord (+/− kidneys and bladder) as an outpatient
  - arrange outpatient follow-up.

Spinal dysraphism

See ➙ Malformations of the central nervous system, pp. 318–21.

- Any lesion at any spinal level with a fat pad, significant hairy patch, atretic skin, sinus, or swelling—or if there are associated lower limb neurological signs or bladder dysfunction—warrants early investigation
- Seek senior medical review
- Arrange early AP and lateral X-rays of the lumbosacral spine and ultrasound scan of the lower spinal cord, kidneys, and bladder. If this is abnormal then it will be necessary to investigate further with an MRI scan. Discuss further follow-up with paediatric neurology or neurosurgical team
- There is a small risk of recurrence and the advice is to take high dose folic acid pre-conception and during early pregnancy in subsequent pregnancies.

Brachial plexus palsies

- Risk factors include: being large for gestational age, infant of diabetic mother
- Usually precipitated by shoulder dystocia at birth.

Types of brachial plexus palsy

- Erb's palsy
  - C5–C6 nerve roots
  - 'waiter's tip' position: decreased or absent shoulder abduction with elbow extension, forearm internal rotation, and wrist flexion
- Klumpke's palsy (rare)
  - C8–T1 nerve roots
  - 'claw hand': intrinsic muscles of the hand involved, along with wrist and finger flexors, sympathetic nerves leading to Horner's syndrome, and also hyperabduction of shoulder
- Erb-Duchenne-Klumpke palsy
  - C4–T1 nerve roots
  - entire arm paralysed
  - raised hemidiaphragm may occur if extensive enough lesion to involve C4.

Assessment

- Look for signs of fracture of humerus or clavicle; if in doubt do X-ray of limb and shoulder
- Assess and record full neurological examination of affected limb
- Assess for signs of respiratory distress (implying diaphragm involvement) or unequal pupils (Horner's syndrome) which may indicate a worse prognosis
- CXR if lesion extensive or if C4 likely to be involved
- Parents should be spoken to by senior doctor regarding prognosis and recovery.

Management

Refer to physiotherapy for advice on positioning and handling, sensory stimulation, and passive stretches of the hand, wrist, and elbow. Will need outpatient physiotherapy and medical follow-up.

Prognosis

- 80–90% chance of full recovery in all but most extensive lesions
- Onward referral for specialist assessment should be considered if no biceps recovery evident at 6 weeks or if weakness persists >3 months.

Management of vulnerable babies on postnatal ward and transitional care

- Babies who require more than 'routine' postnatal care are increasingly cared for on postnatal wards, due to restricted capacity on NNUs and the desire to keep mothers and babies together
- Some units will have a Transitional Care (TC) Unit for such babies. This may involve higher midwifery ratios, or staffing with neonatal nursing staff. What constitutes TC and the model of care used will vary between hospitals
- Babies considered 'vulnerable' or qualifying for TC may include:
  - 'late' preterm (e.g. 34–37 weeks)
  - low birth weight (LBW) (i.e. BW <2.5 kg)
  - small for gestational age (SGA, <10th centile for gestational age)
  - babies with reported feeding difficulties
  - infants of diabetic mothers
  - babies requiring phototherapy
  - babies with medical problems (e.g. cleft palate, Down syndrome)
  - babies of drug using mothers (see ➔ Care of the baby whose mother is drug dependent, pp. 46–7)
  - mothers with social concerns (e.g. depression, psychiatric disturbance, contact with social services, learning difficulties)
  - multiple births
  - babies transferred from NNU.

Assessment

- Review maternal and pregnancy history:
  - evidence of placental insufficiency if LBW or SGA
  - maternal illness during pregnancy if suspecting congenital infection
  - infection risk factors, particularly if preterm
- Take a good feeding history from midwives and mother
- **On examination:** signs of congenital infection or dysmorphism if symmetrically SGA
- Complications include hypoglycaemia, hypothermia, hypocalcaemia, polycythaemia, poor feeding, and jaundice
- Consider viral serology and/or karyotype if suspected from examination, especially if significantly SGA.

Management

- Regular observations (temperature, heart rate, respiration rate, activity level, feeding)
- Avoid hypothermia by ensuring the baby is adequately wrapped and has a hat on, or using overhead heater if necessary. Criteria for admission to NNU vary, but most babies below 1800 g will not be able to maintain their temperature adequately on the postnatal wards
- Encourage early and frequent (every 3–4 hours initially) breastfeeding, or, if formula feeding, ensure adequate volumes are being taken (60–90 ml/kg/day initially, increasing over the first few days)

- Monitor for and treat hypoglycaemia according to guidelines. This will pertain only to those considered at risk such as infants of diabetic mothers, preterm, LBW, SGA (see ⮕ Hypoglycaemia: overview, pp. 372–3, Hypoglycaemia: management, pp. 374–5)
- Consider the presence of polycythaemia if baby SGA; and check PCV (packed cell volume) with FBC if suspected, or if hypoglycaemia or jaundice becomes a problem
- Careful assessment of fitness for discharge is required
- For babies who are preterm or LBW:
  - ensure that feeding is adequate regardless of whether the baby is breast or bottle fed
  - babies should be weighed prior to discharge
  - if a baby is below birth weight at discharge, the percentage weight loss should be calculated. Babies with weight loss of 5–10% may need to stay longer to assess feeding and ensure that weight does not fall further. If weight loss >10% birth weight: assess state of hydration and review fluid intake. Consider looking for hypernatraemic dehydration
  - if a baby is ≥10 days old and still below birth weight, there should be at least 2 weights to show that weight gain is ≥10 g/kg/day. Ideally, babies should have started to gain weight prior to discharge.
  - earlier discharge can be considered if there is enhanced community support available
- Ensure appropriate support in community after discharge. Consider neonatal outreach and/or outpatient follow-up.

Care of the baby whose mother is drug dependent

- This may include mothers on opiates, cocaine and derivatives, benzodiazepines, and excessive alcohol
- Monitoring is necessary to detect and treat withdrawal symptoms, and to assess the mother's ability to adequately care for her baby.

General postnatal care

- **Neonatal review after birth:** attention to what drugs the mother has been taking, by what route, and how recently
- Check mother's HIV, hepatitis B (HBV), and hepatitis C (HCV) status, and act accordingly
- Some units will recommend HBV vaccination regardless of maternal status
- If the mother is taking opiates, naloxone should not be used as there is some evidence that it may provoke a serious withdrawal reaction
- Inform the appropriate allocated or duty social worker of the birth as soon as possible
- The baby should be kept with mother on the postnatal ward unless it has seizures, or withdrawal symptoms cannot be controlled, or a social services assessment recommends separation
- Mothers may breastfeed unless there is another contraindication (e.g. multiple drug use), although the adequacy of the milk supply may be affected by narcotics in particular
- All babies should be kept in hospital for at least a week or until symptoms have been controlled and maternal care is adequately assessed or appropriate alternative care is organized for the baby
- Regular observations (temperature, heart rate, respiration) and drug withdrawal symptoms should be scored regularly from birth. Most units will have a 'drug withdrawal chart', which will score the baby according to withdrawal symptoms (although scoring systems and guidelines vary). An example of a 'Neonatal abstinence chart' is shown in Fig. 3.1
- Minimal handling
- Send urine (or urine dipstick) for toxicology
- Decision for discharge should involve multidisciplinary input, with maternity, neonatal, and social services involvement. A case conference may need to be organized before discharge
- Inform GP/health visitor of discharge
- There is evidence that babies who withdraw may have long-term developmental concerns. Arrange outpatient follow-up for neurodevelopmental assessment.

Relevant drugs

Opiates

- May be illicit or prescribed. May include morphine, heroin, pethidine, and methadone. Also be aware of mothers who have had prolonged analgesia (e.g. in sickle cell disease)
- Withdrawal symptoms in the baby may occur from day 1 up to day 7, and in mothers dependent on methadone, seizures may occur even later (methadone has a long half-life)
- Symptoms of withdrawal include:
  - *central nervous system*: irritability, high-pitched cry, sleep disturbance, seizures
  - *autonomic nervous system*: yawning, sneezing, sweating, hiccups
  - *gastrointestinal*: poor feeding, disordered suck, vomiting, diarrhoea
  - *respiratory*: tachypnoea.

Treatment

- Indications:
  - withdrawal score persistently high
  - seizures
  - inability to feed, sleep, or gain weight
- Oral morphine is the drug of choice for babies withdrawing from narcotics. Dose should be adequate to control symptoms. Length of withdrawal process is very variable and may take many weeks. Weaning should be gradual and according to baby's needs
- Consider discharge on medication (e.g. morphine if baby is stable and the community support is appropriate).

Cocaine

- Features of withdrawal typically occur during first 5 days of life
- Signs are usually mild (in contrast to opiate withdrawal)
- Effects of fetal cocaine exposure may include:
  - *vasoconstriction*: fetal hypoxia and stillbirth, placental abruption, preterm labour, intrauterine growth retardation (IUGR), microcephaly, intracerebral ischaemic lesions, limb reduction defects
  - *increased neurotransmission*: hyperactivity, irritability, abnormal sleep patterns, increased tone
- Postnatal cranial ultrasound scan should be done prior to discharge.

Cannabis

- Inconsistent clinical signs in infant
- May cause IUGR, preterm delivery, and some neurobehavioural problems.

NEONATAL ABSTINENCE CHART

Baby's name
Hospital number
Date of birth
(place patient's sticker here)

Mother's name

Ward

Consultant

Date										
Time										
High-pitched cry										
Tremors										
Hypertonicity										
Convulsions										
Hyperthermia > 38°C Tachypnoea >60/min										
Vomiting Diarrhoea										
Yawning Hiccoughs										
Salivation Stuffy nose Sneezing										
Sweating Dehydration										
Total score										

The presence of any one feature within any group of the listed observations would result in a total score of 1 for that group of items. The total score possible is therefore 10. Treatment is likely to be required for any score ≥6, or for convulsions and possibly vomiting, diarrhoea or inability to sleep.

Fig. 3.1 Neonatal abstinence chart..

Further information

American Academy of Pediatrics Committee on Drugs. Neonatal drug withdrawal. *Pediatrics* 1998; **101**: 1079–1088.

Down's Syndrome Association. ✆ www.downs-syndrome.org.uk/.

Hudak ML, Tan RC, The Committee on Drugs and the Committee on Fetus and Newborn. Neonatal Drug Withdrawal. *Pediatrics* 2012; **129**: e540.

National Institute for Health and Clinical Excellence (2006) NICE guidelines (CG37). Postnatal care up to 8 weeks after birth. ✆ www.nice.org.uk/guidance/cg37

NHS Population screening programmes guidance, Newborn & Infant Physical Examination: ultrasound scan for hip dysplasia. ✆ www.gov.uk/government/publications/newborn-and-infant-physical-examination-ultrasound-scan-for-hip-dysplasia

Admission, discharge, and outcome

Admission to the neonatal unit

Criteria for admission

Different neonatal units (NNUs) will have different criteria for admission. The following will apply to most:

- Preterm <34 weeks gestation
- Birth weight <1800 g
- Signs of respiratory distress (see ➲ Initial management of babies presenting with respiratory distress, pp. 108–9)
- Neonatal encephalopathy (see ➲ Neonatal encephalopathy, p. 280)
- Seizures (see ➲ Neonatal seizures, pp. 290–3)
- Suspected perinatal asphyxia (especially if cord pH <7.0 or base deficit <–15)
- Sepsis (see ➲ Early onset bacterial infection, pp. 328–9)
- Hypoglycaemia (see ➲ Hypoglycaemia: overview, pp. 372–3; ➲ Hypoglycaemia: management, pp. 374–5)
- Haemolytic disease of newborn (see ➲ Haemolytic disease of the newborn, pp. 402–3)
- Significant congenital abnormality
- Unstable baby of drug using mother (see ➲ Care of the baby whose mother is drug dependent, pp. 46–7)
- Others (e.g. hydrops).

Admission documentation

- Essential history includes:
  - maternal medical, family, and obstetric history
  - last menstrual period (LMP) and expected date of delivery (EDD); whether EDD is certain, and whether based on LMP or scans
  - booking bloods, including blood group and antibody screen, and infection screen
  - history of this pregnancy, including screening for Down syndrome and antenatal ultrasound scans
  - indications for delivery, including maternal illness and risk factors for neonatal sepsis
  - birth history, need for resuscitation, resuscitation events in detail (e.g. time to spontaneous respiration and first heart rate, intubation +/– surfactant administration, staff present), Apgar score
  - postnatal course leading up to admission
- Clinical examination
- Diagnoses (or differentials)
- Problem list—enter all diagnoses/problems
- Management plan
- Complete growth chart (weight and occipito-frontal circumference)
- Complete results sheets, including blood test results and microbiology
- Document information given to parents.

If baby has been transferred from another unit, document:

- Neonatal course leading up to transfer
- Significant events during transfer
- Investigations that need to be chased at the referring unit.

Clinical

- **Thorough clinical examination to rule out any congenital malformation:** remember that if there is one, or more than one congenital anomaly, always look hard for others. In particular, exclude anorectal malformations and cleft palate
- **Relevant observations:** heart rate, respiratory rate, O_2 saturation, BP, temperature
- Arrange relevant investigations:
  - *blood tests:* may include blood sugar, FBC and blood film, C-reactive protein (CRP), blood cultures, blood gas—urea and electrolytes (U&Es) at birth not necessary as they only reflect mother's results
  - *X-rays:* chest X-ray if signs of respiratory distress; can wait 4 hours for clearance of lung fluid unless required to make urgent diagnosis (e.g. pneumothorax), or check position of endotracheal tube (ETT) or umbilical lines
- Establish intravenous +/− arterial access as necessary
- Ensure that vitamin K has been prescribed and given (intramuscular is recommended)
- Prescribe any other necessary medications (e.g. antibiotics, caffeine)
- Prescribe IV fluids if necessary or advise nursing staff about feeds required
- Discuss baby's clinical condition with the parents at the earliest opportunity and document the conversation
- If baby is not ready to feed, encourage mother to express breast milk
- If indicated (e.g. preterm), perform initial cranial ultrasound.

Babies with surgical conditions

Along with the clinical requirements, these babies may have other requirements (e.g. gastroschisis, duodenal atresia):

- Inform surgeon, anaesthetist, and theatre staff
- May need group and save (or cross-match) along with admission bloods. Blood banks in some hospitals will require maternal blood as well as baby's blood
- May require wide bore nasogastric tube (NGT) +/− free drainage
- Cover protruding abdominal contents with cling film or other proprietary product to prevent heat and fluid loss
- Consider abdominal X-ray
- May need to be nil by mouth (depending on diagnosis).

Routine monitoring

- All babies, regardless of gestation or birth weight, should be monitored on admission to the unit
- All observations should be clearly recorded on the appropriate observation chart.

Commonly monitored vital signs
- **Heart rate:** normal 120–160/min
- **Respiratory rate +/– apnoea:**
  - normal respiratory rate 40–60/min
  - apnoea alarms are usually set to alarm after 20 seconds
- Blood pressure:
  - non-invasive blood pressure should be recorded on admission for all babies. It is important to use the correct sized cuff for this
  - invasive blood pressure monitoring from an indwelling peripheral or umbilical arterial line is the preferred method of monitoring for any unstable baby
  - mean blood pressure should be > corrected gestational age in weeks
- Oxygen saturation:
  - target saturations depend on gestational age and the baby's underlying condition
  - evidence shows that in extremely preterm babies low saturation limits are associated with increased mortality, whilst high saturations/hyperoxia lead to retinopathy of prematurity (ROP)
  - babies <32 weeks should have saturations of 88–95%. N.B. saturations do not distinguish high oxygen tension
  - babies with congenital heart disease should have individualized alarm limits
- Temperature:
  - method used for central temperature varies (e.g. axilla or rectal)
  - may be intermittent or continuous, usually by a skin probe. Continuous monitoring with a rectal probe is often used in therapeutic hypothermia. Servo-control setting of the baby's temperature in the incubator is particularly useful in preterm babies
  - comparison of central and peripheral temperature measurement is useful in sick neonates as an indicator of peripheral perfusion
  - the thermoneutral range is 36.5–37.5°C.

Other continuous monitoring sometimes employed
- **Transcutaneous O_2 and CO_2 tension:** useful in babies on respiratory support for continuous monitoring (particularly babies on high frequency oscillatory ventilation (HFOV)) and to reduce blood loss from frequent blood gases
- **End tidal CO_2:** may not be accurate in newborns due to ETT leak (uncuffed) and large anatomical dead space
- **Central venous pressure:** may be monitored via an umbilical venous catheter in the inferior vena cava.

Assessment of gestational age of the newborn

- In infants without congenital anomalies, outcome is most closely determined by gestation, and the incidence of complications increases with falling gestation (e.g. necrotizing enterocolitis (NEC), intraventricular haemorrhage, ROP)
- Knowing the gestation of extremely preterm babies accurately:
  - assists with prognosis, which is important for perinatal decisions and parental guidance
  - allows comparison of unit figures with national and international data, also important for audit
  - is useful for some surveillance programmes by gestational triggers (e.g. ROP screening below 32 weeks)
  - may be useful to assess the gestation of seemingly mature, but low weight infants who may feed poorly as a consequence of unanticipated prematurity
- Gestational age assessment can be by mother's menstrual dates, or obstetric ultrasound dating (see ➲ Obstetric dating, in this chapter, p. 56). The NICE Antenatal Care guideline recommends using ultrasound dating between 10^{+0} and 13^{+6} weeks in preference to maternal dates to calculate estimated date of delivery
- Clinical assessment of the newborn baby is less accurate. The only indication for this is if the mother is completely uncertain of her dates and there has not been an early obstetric scan.

Definitions

- Gestation is expressed as completed weeks following the LMP
- The 'average' duration of pregnancy is 40 weeks
- Preterm is <37 weeks. There is no standard definition of extreme vs. mild or moderate prematurity
- Term 37–42 weeks
- Post-term >42 weeks
- After *in vitro* fertilization (IVF), etc., the exact date of conception is known, and about 2 weeks should be added to extrapolate to the theoretical previous LMP
- A baby born after 26 weeks gestation is 26 weeks post-menstrual age (PMA); 10 weeks later he is 36 weeks PMA (also referred to as corrected gestational age (CGA)).

Obstetric dating

- Fetal ultrasound estimation of gestation is considered accurate if the scan is carried out at 10–19 weeks.

Neonatal assessment

- Consistent patterns of development of neurological and 'external' or 'physical' characteristics have been observed in preterm infants and have been used in scoring schemes to assess gestation (Dubowitz, Ballard, etc.)
- Limitations of scoring schemes:
  - time-consuming, disturbs the sickest of patients, and are subjective
  - consistently have an accuracy of ±2 weeks
  - few of them have been validated on infants <32 weeks gestation, the most important group to classify
  - need to be performed within 12–48 hours of birth to be reasonably valid
- Nerve conduction velocity, the appearance of the anterior vascular capsule of the lens, and the appearance of cranial ultrasound characteristics have also been used to assess gestation. All of these methods are time consuming and the accuracy is ±2 weeks.

Sedation and analgesia

- Evidence suggests that the fetus develops pain perception by the third trimester
- Babies are often subjected to painful and unpleasant stimuli in the postnatal period, particularly on the neonatal unit. It is increasingly recognized as important to monitor, alleviate, or attenuate the discomfort associated with these experiences whenever possible
- Painful/uncomfortable stimuli on NNU include:
  - intubation
  - blood sampling—capillary sampling is thought to be more painful than venepuncture
  - line insertion
  - ETT suction
  - clinical conditions (e.g. NEC, extravasation injuries, abscesses).

Assessment of neonatal pain

- Structured scoring systems can be useful in assessing infant pain and their requirement for, and response to, sedation and analgesia
- Several have been formulated and validated e.g. NPASS (Neonatal Pain, Agitation & Sedation Score)
- These assessments tend to use a combination of physiological and behavioural factors, such as:
  - crying/irritability
  - arousal state
  - facial expression
  - changes in vital signs (heart rate, BP, SaO_2).

Pharmacological approaches

See Table 4.1.

Pre-medication for intubation

(See also ➲ Endotracheal intubation, pp. 494–5.)

- Should always be used unless there are specific contraindications or intubation is being performed as part of cardiopulmonary resuscitation
- There is no consensus amongst NNUs as to which drug(s) to use, although account should be taken of analgesia, sedation, paralysis, and potential need for vagal blockade (especially to avoid bradycardia)
- Commonly used medications are a narcotic for analgesia/sedation (e.g. fentanyl, morphine); a hypnotic (e.g. midazolam); a short-acting paralytic agent (e.g. suxamethonium), and atropine (see Table 4.1).

Non-pharmacological approaches

(See also ➲ Developmental care, p. 62.)
  These should be used before and with medication.

- Quiet, calm environment (reduce noise and bright light)
- Reducing handling
- Positioning (swaddling, nesting)
- Comforting handling (containment holding, skin-to-skin 'kangaroo' care)

Table 4.1 Sedation and analgesia used on NNU. Always refer to local or national formulary guidance for dosages

Drug	Use	Advantages	Disadvantages
Morphine	Common Sedative and analgesic Particularly ventilated babies Bolus +/− infusion	Well tolerated Oral or IV	Respiratory depression Hypotension Withdrawal
Fentanyl	Most often for sedation/analgesia prior to intubation	Well tolerated Short-acting	May cause 'rigid chest syndrome' if not used with muscle relaxant
Midazolam	Sedative		No analgesic properties Respiratory depression
Clonidine	Sedative Morphine sparing properties	Oral or IV	Little evidence for use in newborn
Paracetamol	Pain relief in term babies Oral or IV	Oral or IV No respiratory depression	
Chloral hydrate	Sedative Oral or suppository	Oral preparation Little/no respiratory depression No habituation	No analgesic properties Gastric irritation
Paralysing agents, e.g. pancuronium, vecuronium	When sedation ineffective, especially when baby fighting ventilation Pancuronium—boluses Vecuronium—infusion	Useful in active term babies with difficult ventilation, e.g. meconium aspiration, persistent pulmonary hypertension of newborn (PPHN)	May increase ventilatory requirements Oedema Increased secretions May have prolonged recovery time
Suxamethonium	Preintubation	Short-acting	May cause bradycardia

- Oral comfort:
  - non-nutritive sucking (finger or dummy/pacifier)
  - feeding, particularly breastfeeding.

Oral sucrose
- Increasingly used for analgesia during painful procedures in term and near-term babies e.g. phlebotomy, cannulation, lumbar puncture, IM injection, wound/dressing care, ROP screen

- Evidence shows reduction in pain scores when used; breast milk used in the same way is as effective, as is breastfeeding during procedures if practically possible
- Ineffective if given by nasogastric or orogastric tube
- Best used with pain scoring system and non-pharmacological calming techniques.

Administration
- Give orally: 0.2 ml aliquots onto tongue or by dummy/pacifier dips 2 minutes prior to procedure
- Up to 2 ml can be given per procedure in term babies
- Short-acting, may need repeated doses for single procedure.

Developmental care

There is increasing understanding that the newborn, particularly preterm, baby gains benefits from close attention to their behavioural responses.
Developmental care:
- Aims to improve physiological stability, reduce neonatal stress, and provide appropriate sensory experiences for babies, thereby improving developmental outcomes
- Tends to be nurse-led; all staff have responsibility to be aware
- Provides opportunities for parental involvement, improved parent satisfaction, and confidence.

Aspects of developmental care
- Recognizing neonatal stress
  - important for staff to recognize neonatal behavioural cues to reduce distress and discomfort
  - may include bradycardia, gagging, startling, hypo- or hypertonia, facial grimacing
- Positioning
  - nesting
  - regular repositioning
  - promotes normal posture, development, self-regulation, reduces musculoskeletal deformity (e.g. plagiocephaly)
- Attention to light and sound
  - reduced lighting
  - pay attention to quiet time, take care when closing incubator doors, using waste bins, etc.
- Handling
  - reduce handling and procedures, cluster interventions
  - be gentle
- Oral stimulation
  - neonates are subject to unpleasant oral stimulation (intubation, NGT insertion); can result in aversive behaviours (e.g. inability to orally feed)
  - promote non-nutritive sucking, positive facial touch, etc.

Kangaroo care
- Also referred to as 'skin-to-skin'
- Should be encouraged as soon as baby is considered sufficiently stable—this can include babies that still require intensive care
- Has been shown to:
  - increase breastfeeding outcomes
  - stabilize physiological parameters
  - improve parent involvement, bonding, satisfaction.

Perioperative management

Pre-operative preparation

- Ensure appropriate investigations:
  - blood count and biochemistry will normally be required within 24 hours of operation
  - coagulation profile should be checked before any major surgery or if clotting abnormalities are expected (ensure that baby has received vitamin K if surgery necessary in first few days of life)
  - CXR taken and available to anaesthetists and surgeons if baby ventilated
- Group and save or cross-match blood:
  - guided by surgeons and proposed operation
  - follow local transfusion guidelines
  - baby may need packed cells, platelets, or fresh frozen plasma, depending on clinical circumstances
- Liaise with anaesthetists, particularly if baby is unstable or complex
- Detailed clinical review on the day to check that baby is fit and stable for the operation
- Fasting guidelines vary: commonly 4 hours in breastfed and 6 hours in formula-fed babies
- Ensure that there is secure IV access (usually two cannulae; consider the need for central venous access) and start 10% glucose + additives at the time of the 1st omitted feed (usually 4–8 hours pre-operatively)
- Consider inserting an arterial line prior to major operation
- Ensure that the operating surgeon has obtained written informed consent.

Post-operative management

- Post-operative blood tests as necessary depending on operation (e.g. blood count, biochemistry, blood gas)
- Careful management of fluid:
  - strict input and output charts should be maintained
  - maintenance fluids will usually be reduced after general anaesthetic to approximately two-thirds of previous requirement for at least 24 hours post-operatively as there is often increased antidiuretic hormone (ADH) secretion
  - further fluid restriction may be necessary and should be carefully evaluated at least once daily
  - use regular (at least daily) weights to assess
- Read the anaesthetic record, particularly for fluids and medications (including antibiotics) that have been given intraoperatively
- Read the surgeon's operative notes carefully and follow instructions as indicated.

Initial management of the extremely preterm infant

- This refers to babies of <26 weeks gestation, i.e. near the limits of viability
- Senior medical input should always be available for these babies
- A detailed review of clinical circumstances leading to the premature birth should be made, and plans made in the light of this
- An experienced member of the team should speak to the parents before birth wherever possible to explain the possible outcomes and potential problems, and agree a plan of management
- Difficulties may occur when gestation is not accurately known, but most NNUs will not offer intensive care to babies <23 weeks
- Increasing evidence indicates that these babies have lower mortality if born and cared for in level 3 NICUs.

Resuscitation at birth

- Decisions regarding initiation and continuation of resuscitation should be made by experienced staff in consultation with parents
- An extremely preterm baby who is in poor condition at birth with a low heart rate and no respiratory effort, +/– severe bruising must already have suffered considerable hypoxic-ischaemic insult, which is likely to have affected the fragile brain
- If the baby is apnoeic at birth, it is usually reasonable to attempt lung inflation, with further management guided by heart rate response
- If there is no response to attempted lung inflation, cardiac resuscitation (i.e. cardiac massage and/or adrenaline) is unlikely to be helpful at these gestations
- Guidance from the British Association of Perinatal Medicine and the Nuffield Council of Bioethics suggests the following approach:
  - *<23^{+0} weeks*: no active resuscitation
  - *23^{+0}–23^{+6} weeks*: resuscitate with lung inflation if parents agree, although a decision not to resuscitate is appropriate
  - *24^{+0}–24^{+6} weeks*: resuscitate with lung inflation initially, unless there is evidence of significant fetal compromise
  - *≥25^{+0} weeks*: active resuscitation recommended
- If a decision has been made not to start or continue active resuscitation, full humane care must continue until the baby dies
- The parents should be kept informed at all times.

Fluid balance

- The skin of the <26-week newborn is unkeratinized and extremely thin, leading to massive evaporative water and heat loss
- To reduce loss of water and heat, the baby should put in a plastic bag (or proprietary wrap) from birth without prior drying at least until on NNU
- Nurse babies in high humidity (about 90%) in a closed environment (usually a servo-controlled incubator). Humidity can be reduced after about one week.

Initial respiratory support

- Although the majority of babies at this gestation will require initial ventilatory support, non-invasive support (e.g. continuous positive airway pressure (CPAP)) is increasingly used
- Early exogenous surfactant at resuscitation is recommended in babies who require intubation to improve the outcome of respiratory distress syndrome (RDS)
- Babies may have initial minimal ventilation ('honeymoon period'), but may still progress to severe chronic lung disease
- Oxygen tension should be tightly controlled, avoiding both hyperoxia and hypoxia. Start resuscitation in air (i.e. FiO_2 0.21). Aim for saturations 88–95%
- Attention should be focused on reducing ventilator-induced lung injury and the incidence and severity of chronic lung disease:
  - early use of CPAP is increasingly used in even these most preterm babies
  - start with lower peak inspiratory pressures than in older babies (e.g. 20 cmH_2O)
  - monitor and control tidal volumes in addition to ventilatory pressures.

Other aspects of initial care on NNU

- Most babies will require insertion of an arterial line for BP and blood gas monitoring and a central venous line, for inotropic support if required, or early parenteral nutrition (e.g. umbilical)
- Babies should be handled as little as possible (minimal handling)
- Initial cranial ultrasound should be performed within 4 hours.

Discharge from the neonatal unit

All babies being discharged (to home, postnatal ward, or another hospital or ward) will need the following:

- A thorough clinical examination with discharge weight and head circumference (plotted on their centile chart)
- Ongoing feeding plan
- Where available, a hand-held Child Health Record with relevant sections completed
- Discharge summary completed, with a copy provided to parents. A copy should also be sent to GP, health visitor, community midwife, referring obstetricians, and/or paediatricians
- Discharge medications prescribed
- Parents informed regarding follow-up arrangements
- General advice given to parents regarding avoidance of cot death, and how and when to seek medical advice if there are any concerns, with contact numbers where necessary.

Additionally, in some babies, the following should be done/arranged as relevant:

- Cranial ultrasound
- Immunizations
- Hearing screening
- Screening for ROP
- Hip ultrasound (e.g. if family history of developmental dysplasia of the hip (DDH) or breech delivery)
- Referral to appropriate services, such as physiotherapy and speech and language therapy
- Referral to other specialties, such as cardiology, orthopaedics, plastic surgery
- Teaching of basic resuscitation to parents.

Special circumstances

- If the baby is discharged home on oxygen then the relevant equipment and safety measures should be in place with input from outreach or community nurses
- Consider any extra community support that may be required for vulnerable families, including referral to social services if required. If there are significant social concerns, a named social worker should be identified prior to discharge
- Parents of babies with extra needs will need appropriate support and training prior to and after discharge, for example:
  - basic resuscitation
  - nasogastric or gastrostomy tube feeding
  - tracheostomy (including skills in care and tracheostomy tube replacement)
- If babies are being discharged for palliative care, detailed advance care directives should be carefully planned, parents will need appropriate care and counselling prior to discharge, and community nurses and GP must be informed.

Follow-up

- If the admission is brief, many babies will not require specific neonatal or paediatric follow-up
- Very low birth weight and babies born significantly preterm should have regular follow-up designed to pick up developing problems:
  - growth and feeding
  - neurodevelopment
  - other medical problems
- Babies <1500 g or <32 weeks gestation should be followed up until at least 2 years corrected age with detailed developmental assessment
- Additional plans regarding vaccination may be required in some babies—for example, respiratory syncytial virus (RSV) or influenza vaccination in winter for babies with respiratory or cardiac problems (see Immunizations relevant to the neonatal unit, pp. 366–8).

Outcome after preterm birth

- Preterm birth is associated with increased mortality and morbidity compared with birth at term
- Adverse outcomes increase with increasing prematurity
- Outcome data must be interpreted with caution for many reasons, including:
  - mortality at gestations >24 weeks has reduced over the last 10–15 years and there is a lag between this trend and publication of up-to-date data
  - studies of outcome have shown significant variation even between developed countries
  - at extremely low gestations, particularly <25 weeks, the practice of offering resuscitation and intensive care may vary
- Survival data will also be affected by the population studied (e.g. whether the data includes all births including stillbirths; or all live born babies; or only babies admitted to neonatal intensive care units (NICU) and therefore not including babies who die on labour wards)
- Outcomes are better for babies cared for in units that provide tertiary neonatal care; babies who are not transferred *ex utero* for intensive care; girls; singletons; babies exposed to antenatal steroids; and those of higher birth weight for gestation.

Neurodevelopmental disability

- Figures in Table 4.2 include mild, moderate, and severe disability
- In addition to motor and cognitive deficits, preterm babies have increased incidence of visual and hearing deficits, communication disorders (e.g. autism), and behavioural problems (e.g. attention deficit hyperactivity disorder (ADHD)).

Other long-term outcomes

- Chronic lung disease:
  - approximately 3 out of 4 babies <26 weeks are still requiring oxygen at 36 weeks corrected age
  - many require domiciliary oxygen, but most are out of oxygen by 1 year
  - higher rates than the general population for readmission for viral respiratory tract infection (especially RSV), admission to paediatric intensive care unit (PICU), and mortality
  - abnormalities on lung function testing persist for years
- Feeding and growth:
  - feeding difficulties due to aversion may require speech and language therapy input
  - growth often remains poor following discharge.

Table 4.2 Preterm birth survival rates and neurodevelopmental problems

Gestation	Survival %	Neurodevelopmental problems	
		Cognitive delay %	Cerebral palsy %
22	<1		
23	15–30	75	25
24	35–50	40–50	15–20
25	55–70		
26	70–80		
27	90	30–40	10–15
28	95		
29	95		
30	97	25–35	5–10
31	98		
32	98		

Figures are for live births and are composites from the studies listed in Further information, p. 70.

Further information

The BOOST II United Kingdom, Australia and New Zealand Collaborative Groups. Oxygen satura-tions and outcomes in preterm infants. *N Engl J Med* 2013; **368**: 2094–2104.

Costeloe KL, Hennessy EM, Haider S, Stacey F, Marlow N, Draper ES. Short term outcomes after extreme preterm birth in England: comparison of two birth cohorts in 1995 and 2006 (the EPICure studies). *BMJ* 2012; **345**: e7976 doi.

Larroque, B, Ancel PY, Manet S, et al. Neurodevelopmental disabilities and special care of 5 year old children born before 33 weeks of gestation (the EPIPAGE Study) and longitudinal cohort study. *Lancet* 2008; **371**: 813–820.

Lemons JA, Bauer CR, Oh W, et al. Very low birth weight outcomes of the National Institute of Child Health and Human Development Neonatal Research Network, January 1995 through December 1996. *Pediatrics* 2001; **107**: E1.

Marlow N, Wolke D, Bracewell MA, et al. Neurologic and developmental disability at six years of age after extremely preterm birth. *N Engl J Med* 2005; **352**: 9–19.

Moore T, Hennessy EM, Myles J, et al. Neurological and developmental outcome in extremely pre-term children born in England in 1995 and 2006: the EPICure studies. *BMJ* 2012; **345**: e7961 doi.

National Institute for Health and Care Excellence (2008, updated 2016). NICE guidelines (CG62) Antenatal care for uncomplicated pregnancies. ℘ www.guidance.nice.org.uk/CG62

Nuffield Council on Bioethics. Critical decisions in fetal and neonatal medicine: ethical issues (2006). ℘ www.nuffieldbioethics.org/neonatal-medicine

SUPPORT Study Group of the Eunice Kennedy Shriver NICHD Neonatal Research Network. Target ranges of oxygen saturations in extremely preterm infants. *N Engl J Med* 2010; **362**: 1959–1969.

Wilkinson AR, Ahluwalia J, Cole A, et al. BAPM. The Management of Babies Born Extremely Preterm at less than 26 weeks of gestation: a Framework for Clinical Practice at the Time of Birth (2008). ℘ www.bapm.org/publications/documents/guidelines/Approved_manuscript_preterm_final.pdf

Fluids and electrolytes

Fluid balance: background

Fluid management in the newborn baby is dependent on an understanding of the requirement to compensate for fluid loss (output) and the requirement to provide energy and nutrition.

Output

Renal losses

- Renal function undergoes rapid changes in the first postnatal days with glomerular filtration rate (GFR) increasing over the first 24–48 hours
- After relatively low urine output in the first day, it is normal for babies to have a diuresis. This is precipitated by sodium loss (natriuresis) after release of atrial natriuretic peptide following cardiopulmonary adaptation. This leads to the normal postnatal weight loss associated with a contraction in extracellular fluid of about 10%
- In babies who are unwell, with or without respiratory distress syndrome (RDS), natriuresis/diuresis may be delayed and its onset usually coincides with clinical improvement
- Preterm babies may have ongoing tubular immaturity with a poor ability to excrete excessive electrolyte load, conserve electrolytes, or concentrate urine.

Transepidermal insensible water losses—May be high in the extremely preterm baby in the first week and it is very important to nurse these babies in high humidity to reduce this.

Babies with respiratory distress—Irrespective of the need for respiratory support, there may be relatively high insensible loss from the respiratory tract.

Input

Enteral feeds

- These are the input of choice in well babies with mature gut
- Full-term babies have physiological mechanisms to cope with the small milk volume that they will receive from normal breastfeeding in the first 24 hours of life
- Stricter, more generous feed volumes may be required in babies at risk of hypoglycaemia or poor feeding (e.g. low birth weight)
- Babies who are unwell and/or have respiratory distress may need to have feeds withheld in the initial phase of illness.

Intravenous fluids

- Start with 10% glucose
- Monitor blood glucose—some babies (e.g. those with intrauterine growth retardation, or infants of diabetics) will require an increase in maintenance fluid or more concentrated glucose. 12.5% glucose can run peripherally, higher concentrations should be via a central line—a percutaneously inserted central catheter or umbilical venous catheter (UVC)
- Additives are generally not required in IV fluids for the first 24–48 hours of life

- After day 2, sodium and potassium will normally be required (see ➜ Sodium balance, pp. 76–7, and Table 5.1). It may not be necessary to add calcium to IV fluids in a well baby if enteral feeds are likely to be established within the first 4–5 days. Be guided by plasma electrolytes
- Parenteral nutrition should be considered in all babies who are unlikely to be fed in the first week. Preterm babies should be started early (within the first 2 days; see ➜ Parenteral nutrition, pp. 90–2).

Table 5.1 Basic electrolyte requirements. IV additives (mmol/kg/day) for well babies

	Sodium	Potassium	Calcium
Term	2–3	2	0.5
30–36 weeks	4	2	0.5–1.5
<30 weeks	4–8	2–4	1.5

Fluid balance: general guidelines for fluid intake

Normal term uncomplicated babies

- **Day 1:** 60 ml/kg/day
- **Day 2:** 90 ml/kg/day
- **Day 3:** 120 ml/kg/day
- **Day 4:** consider increasing to 150 ml/kg/day, although 120 ml/kg/day will often be adequate.

Considerations for babies on the neonatal unit

The fluid regimen for normal term babies may alter depending on:

- **Gestation:** very premature babies, especially those <28 weeks, have high insensible losses and may require more fluid than this. Incubator humidification is very important in these babies
- **Clinical state:**
  - may need to increase fluids more slowly (or reduce them) if baby is sick or oedematous
  - may need to increase fluids faster if baby hypoglycaemic or dehydrated, although avoid increasing more than 1 day in advance of the guidelines for term babies
  - assessment of a baby's general state of hydration is crucial—use clinical examination, weight, urine output, plasma sodium and urea, base deficit
- **Perinatal hypoxia ischaemia:** baby may have acute renal dysfunction or raised antidiuretic hormone (ADH) levels requiring fluid restriction. May become hypocalcaemic early and require supplementation
- **Plasma sodium:** in the first few days of life, can be used as a guide to hydration. Hyponatraemia indicates water excess; hypernatraemia indicates dehydration (see ➔ Sodium balance, pp. 76–7).
- **Weight:**
  - daily weights are advised in all babies needing intensive care
  - beware of increasing fluids and consider fluid restriction in any baby that has gained weight from birth during the first week of life, as there is evidence that preterm babies' respiratory outcome is likely to be worse if sodium is added before natriuresis and weight loss has started
  - weight loss from birth will usually indicate that the baby has started to have an obligatory sodium requirement
- **Urine output:** should be monitored carefully in all babies needing intensive care. Aim for >1 ml/kg/h.

Monitoring fluid balance

Electrolytes

- Daily: if on clear IV fluids; in babies <30 weeks for first 3 days (at least) and in babies with perinatal hypoxia ischaemia in the first 3 days
- 2–3 times daily: in extremely preterm (<26 weeks) in first 3 days
- May be less frequent thereafter if stable
- **Weight**: measure daily in babies cared for in the intensive care unit (ITU) in the first week of life unless very unstable. Can be less frequent thereafter if baby is stable
- **Urine output**: measure in all babies in ITU during the first week of life. If baby stable this can be measured by weighing nappies. If there are any concerns urine should be caught in a bag or catheterize.

Sodium balance

Background

See also ➜ Fluid balance: background, pp. 72–3; ➜ Fluid balance: general guidelines for fluid intake, pp. 74–5.

- Newborn babies do not have an obligatory sodium requirement in the first 24–48 hours of life
- The predominant route of sodium loss in babies is renal. This starts with a natriuresis on day 2–3 of life. Preterm babies may have large ongoing urinary sodium loss due to tubular immaturity
- A positive sodium balance (over and above replacement of losses) is required for normal growth.

Abnormalities in sodium balance

As extracellular fluid is predominantly sodium and water, fluid and sodium balance should always be assessed using plasma sodium and baby's weight together.

Hyponatraemia

- **Hyponatraemia**: plasma sodium <135 mmol/l
- **Severe hyponatraemia**: plasma sodium <120 mmol/l
- Preterm infants may have a marked natriuresis from day 2–3 lasting 2–3 weeks.

General principles of management

> Hyponatraemia + weight gain = excess water → fluid restrict
>
> Hyponatraemia + weight loss = sodium (and water) depletion → give more sodium (and water)

- It may be easy to underestimate sodium deficit, particularly if the baby's weight is not taken into account:
  - serum sodium only falls late in total body sodium depletion
  - it should be remembered that normonatraemic weight loss indicates both water and sodium deficit
- Measuring urine sodium may be useful in hyponatraemia, although in preterm babies it may be high even if total body sodium is low due to the kidneys' reduced ability to conserve sodium
- Sodium deficit = (138 – plasma Na$^+$) × 0.6 × weight (kg)
  Replace 1/3 over 8 hours, next 1/3 over 16 hours, and final 1/3 over next 24 hours. **NB** include ongoing requirements in your calculations.

Hypernatraemia

- **Hypernatraemia**: plasma sodium >145 mmol/l
- **Severe hypernatraemia**: plasma sodium >160 mmol/l.

General principles of management

> Hypernatraemia + weight loss = water depletion → give more water (with adequate sodium)

- Hypernatraemic dehydration is common in the newborn period
  - transepidermal water loss in extremely preterm babies in first 1–2 days of life
  - breastfeeding failure in term or near-term babies
- Rehydration in preterm hypernatraemia will usually be achieved by adding extra fluid as 5 or 10% glucose on top of maintenance. It is important to provide maintenance sodium intake to replace losses once natriuresis/diuresis and weight loss have commenced, even if baby has high serum sodium
- In hypernatraemic dehydration hypotonic fluids and fluids with low sodium concentrations should be avoided in order to avoid cerebral oedema
- Rehydration in hypernatraemic term babies is best achieved with feeds.

Hypernatraemia in term or near-term babies
- Common in breastfed babies, often leads to readmission from the community at 5–7 days of life
- Incidence: serum sodium >160mmol/l in 7 in 100,000 live births
- Invariably associated with weight loss, usually >10% of birth weight; jaundice is often present
- Risk factors: first time breastfeeding mothers, Caesarean (particularly elective) or instrumental birth, preterm or small for gestational age, early discharge from postnatal ward
- Due to inadequate breast milk intake due to low milk volumes or problems with technique
- Serious sequelae are rare; seizures, sinus thrombosis and death have been described
- Management: usually only requires supplemental feeds and breastfeeding support on postnatal ward; may require admission to neonatal unit (NNU) if severe or baby unwell. Avoid IV rehydration if possible.

  Hypernatraemia + weight gain = excess sodium intake → reduce sodium intake (+/− reduce fluids)

- It is important to remember 'hidden' sodium intake in preterm babies (e.g. 0.9% saline flushes, heparinized saline being given through arterial lines (0.5 ml/h, 0.45% heparinized NaCl = 1 mmol Na^+/day)).

Hyperkalaemia

- Usually defined as a serum potassium level of ≥7.0 mmol/l
- Potentially life-threatening condition, which if untreated can lead to arrhythmias and death.

Pathophysiology

- Most commonly seen in extremely preterm infants
- Serum potassium levels usually peak at around 24 hours after birth, and return to normal values by 72 hours of age
- Particularly in the extreme preterm, underlying factors are likely to be:
  - increased potassium release from catabolized cells and a shift of intracellular potassium ions into the extracellular space
  - low renal excretion due to impaired renal function, immaturity of the renal tubular mechanisms for potassium secretion, and reduced glomerular filtration rate
- Antenatal steroids reduce the incidence of non-oliguric hyperkalaemia in extremely low birth weight infants
- Babies tend to tolerate higher serum potassium levels than children or adults.

Risk factors

- Extreme prematurity: occurs in up to 60% of infants born at <28 weeks gestation
- Low systemic blood flow
- Acute renal failure (e.g. after perinatal asphyxia)
- Haemolysis
- Sepsis
- Double volume exchange transfusion (when 'old blood' has been used)
- Chronic renal failure (e.g. congenital renal abnormalities).

Complications

Progressive cardiac dysrhythmia with increasing plasma potassium:
- Tall, peaked T wave
- Ventricular arrhythmias, widening of the QRS complex, then sine-wave QRS complexes
- Cardiac arrest.

The reported mortality of neonates with hyperkalaemia is 15–80%, even with treatment, although this is likely to be due to its association with other problems (e.g. extreme prematurity, renal failure, etc.).

Diagnosis

- Infants who are at risk of hyperkalaemia should have early and regular serum potassium levels
- Haemolysis (e.g. in a 'squeezed' heel prick sample) can give a falsely elevated result. Specimen should be from a free-flowing sample (arterial or venous)
- If plasma K^+ >6 mmol/l, send a further sample urgently

- Assess ECG trace on the monitor for abnormally peaked T wave, and widened or abnormal QRS complexes
- If plasma K^+ ≥7.0 mmol/l and/or ECG shows abnormality, treat immediately; do not wait for the repeat sample result.

Treatment

- Stop any infusions containing potassium immediately
- Correct metabolic acidosis with sodium bicarbonate
- Intravenous salbutamol. Give 4 µg/kg diluted to 10 µg/ml solution slowly over at least 5 minutes or as infusion. Can be repeated 2-hourly
- Intravenous insulin with glucose. Insulin at 0.3–0.6 units/kg/h (**NB** This is a higher dose than used for treating hyperglycaemia). Change maintenance fluids to 20% glucose connected to a central line. Monitor blood glucose levels closely. Fluid restriction in renal failure may make it difficult to provide adequate glucose intake for use of insulin for hyperkalaemia
- If ECG changes are present, give calcium gluconate to stabilize the myocardium. Give 0.5 ml/kg of 10% calcium gluconate (0.1125 mmol/kg) as slow IV injection; or as infusion diluted to 1 in 5 and administered at 0.22 mmol/kg/h (i.e. over approximately 30 min)
- Calcium Resonium® given rectally as 0.125–0.25 g/kg; dose can be repeated 6-hourly if needed. This is a slow-acting ion exchange resin. More likely to be used in bigger babies with renal failure than in preterm hyperkalaemia. Potential complication of rectal impaction and perforation.

Acid-base balance

Background

- Maintenance of a stable pH is crucial to normal cellular function and the body has complex processes with which to do this
- Acid-base balance is maintained by buffering systems and renal and respiratory regulation
- Newborn, particularly preterm, babies commonly have acid-base imbalance:
  - greater acid (H^+) production due to high growth rates, high protein turnover, and bone mineralization
  - inefficient regulatory systems.

Buffering systems

- These are natural mechanisms that absorb or release H^+ and work immediately to maintain pH where there are acute changes in acid-base status
- The three main systems are bicarbonate (HCO_3^-), phosphate (PO_4^-), and protein; they reversibly bind H^+ due to their negative charge
- The bicarbonate system is extracellular and modulates pH by the following reactions: $H^+ + HCO_3^- \leftrightarrow H_2CO_3 \leftrightarrow H_2O + CO_2$
- The phosphate and protein systems are intracellular. H^+ is exchanged across the cell membrane for intracellular Na^+ and K^+. This mechanism can result in hyperkalaemia in acute metabolic acidosis.

Renal regulation

- The kidneys are responsible for excretion of H^+ and reabsorption of HCO_3^- resulting in urine acidification
- This produces a relatively delayed compensatory response to changes in pH
- Reduced tubular function in newborn, particularly preterm, babies impairs their ability to compensate for acidosis.

Respiratory regulation

- Changes in pH are modulated by altering respiratory drive, leading to changes in the clearance of CO_2 from the lungs. CO_2 and H^+ are related via HCO_3^-/H_2CO_3 reaction (shown under buffering systems)
- In acidosis, H^+ stimulates respiratory chemoreceptors and increased ventilation clears more CO_2
- This produces a relatively quick regulatory response (minutes to hours) to changes in pH.

Assessment of acid-base balance

Blood gas analysis

- An indispensable test on NNU, as part of initial assessment and for ongoing monitoring in babies requiring intensive care, particularly if ventilated

- A blood gas result needs to be interpreted knowing which blood sample has been taken:
  - venous blood only gives an accurate result for pH
  - capillary blood will usually be accurate for pH and PCO_2 (although PCO_2 may be falsely increased if peripheral perfusion is poor, particularly in term or near-term babies—avoid making decisions on intubation and ventilation on capillary PCO_2 in such babies)
  - arterial blood will give accurate results for pH, PO_2 and PCO_2 (PO_2 needs to be interpreted in the context of a baby's O_2 saturation at the time the sample is taken)
- Blood gas machines measure pH, PO_2 and PCO_2 and calculate HCO_3^- and base excess (BE) from these measured values
- Acceptable values for these vary with clinical circumstances, but Table 5.2 gives general guidance:
  - correlate PO_2 with saturations; higher is usually acceptable in term babies; beware hyperoxia in preterm babies
  - low CO_2 causes cerebral vasoconstriction (with risk of periventricular leucomalacia (PVL) in preterm babies); usually accept higher values in chronic lung disease if pH acceptable
- Many modern blood gas machines also provide other useful information, including lactate (see ➔ Interpreting metabolic acidosis, pp. 81–2), anion gap, Hb, electrolytes (sodium, potassium, chloride, corrected calcium)
- Interpret blood gases in conjunction with clinical state; attempt to conclude both the underlying diagnosis and the degree of compensation for it.

Interpreting metabolic acidosis

You can interpret the degree of metabolic acidosis and its underlying basis using the following:

- **Base excess (BE)**: derived by the blood gas machine from pH and PCO_2, this is the calculated amount of base required to correct the pH to 7.40 at a PCO_2 of 40 mmHg (5.3 kPa). Negative BE (also called 'base deficit') indicates metabolic acidosis; positive BE indicates metabolic alkalosis

Table 5.2 Guidance for normal values of acid-base parameters in newborns

Parameter	Normal range	Normal range
pH	7.30–7.40 pH as low as 7.25 acceptable in preterm babies	
PO_2	6.0–8.0 kPa	45–60 mmHg
PCO_2	4.5–6.5 kPa	35–50 mmHg
HCO_3^-	20–24 mmol/l	
Base excess (BE)	−3 to +3 BE as low as −10 may be acceptable in preterm babies	

- **Anion gap:** measured difference between anions (negative charge) and cations (positive charge); normal range <16 mmol/l
  - anion gap = $(Na^+ + K^+) - (HCO_3^- + Cl^-)$
  - helps with diagnosing the underlying cause of acidosis. Raised anion gap indicates accumulation of additional acid (e.g. lactate and other tissue acids, metabolic acidaemias)
- **Lactate:** normal range ≤2.0 mmol/l; produced by anaerobic metabolism; raised with tissue hypoxia; causes acidosis. Measurement is required when assessing significant metabolic acidosis.

Clinical situations of acid-base imbalance

Physiological and biochemical changes can be primary or compensatory. Compensation in the newborn is rarely complete.

Respiratory acidosis

- Reduced alveolar ventilation causes ↑CO_2 which dissolves in plasma driving formation of H^+
- Causes:
  - upper airway obstruction
  - lung problems: RDS, meconium aspiration, congenital abnormalities (not normally TTN)
  - hypoventilation: encephalopathy, neuromuscular conditions
  - inadequate ventilatory management
- Management: treat the cause; review level of respiratory support.

Metabolic acidosis

- Common on NNU from pathological processes and reduced clearance of acid load (see ➜ Metabolic acidosis: overview, p. 378)
- Causes:
  - lactic acidosis: shock, sepsis, hypotension, necrotizing enterocolitis, perinatal hypoxia ischaemia, blood loss (raised anion gap)
  - excessive chloride intake (hyperchloraemic acidosis): particularly in the first few days in extremely preterm; due to chloride load in total parenteral nutrition (TPN), saline used in arterial lines, flushes, and fluid boluses
  - bicarbonate loss: usually renal due to tubular immaturity; may occasionally be gastrointestinal (normal anion gap)
  - inborn errors of metabolism, renal failure (raised anion gap)
- Management
  - treat the cause
  - correction with sodium bicarbonate should be reserved for significant acidosis due to hyperchloraemia or low bicarbonate, or with significant sequelae of acidosis (e.g. persistent pulmonary hypertension of the newborn, or during resuscitation)
  - half correction of BE: ml of 4.2% bicarbonate required = BE (mmol/l) × 0.4 × weight
  - low dose bicarbonate infusion through an arterial line may be useful in extremely preterm babies with hyperchloraemic acidosis in the first days of life: 1.5 ml 8.4% sodium bicarbonate made up to 20 ml with water for injections (with heparin) gives equivalent sodium concentration to 0.45% saline.

Respiratory alkalosis
- Hyperventilation resulting in ↓ CO_2
  - usually iatrogenic (excessive mechanical ventilation), but may be spontaneous particularly in cerebral irritability (e.g. hypoxic-ischaemic encephalopathy)
  - normal compensatory response to metabolic acidosis.

Metabolic alkalosis
- Uncommon—usually seen as compensation for respiratory acidosis.
- Also occurs from diuretic use.

Hydrops fetalis

Background

- Defined by presence of excess fluid in ≥ two body compartments (ascites, pleural and pericardial effusions, and subcutaneous oedema)
- Often associated *in utero* with polyhydramnios and placental thickening (>6 cm)
- Abnormal flow of fluid from the capillary plasma to extravascular tissues or its subsequent removal may be due to any of the following mechanisms:
  - ↑ capillary hydrostatic pressure
  - ↓ plasma colloid osmotic pressure
  - ↑ capillary permeability
  - ↓ lymph flow.

Classification

Non-immune hydrops fetalis

- ~75% of cases fall into this category
- Incidence ~1 per 3000 deliveries
- Prognosis guarded: fetal death in ~50% of all cases diagnosed *in utero*; ~50% survival in live born hydropic infants.

Immune hydrops fetalis

- Due to alloimmune haemolytic disease (e.g. Rh iso-immunization) (see ➔ Haemolytic disease of the newborn, pp. 402–3)
- Uncommon since introduction of anti-D prophylaxis
- Principles of treatment for non-immune hydrops apply
- Also note the following:
  - hyperbilirubinaemia likely—low threshold for exchange transfusion
  - if *in utero* transfusion has been performed use irradiated blood for transfusion/exchange transfusion due to (small) risk of graft versus host disease.

Differential diagnosis

- Haematologic:
  - fetal alloimmune haemolytic anaemia (see ➔ Immune hydrops fetalis in classification of Hydrops fetalis, p. 84)
  - α-thalassaemia
  - fetomaternal or twin-to-twin transfusion
- Congenital infections:
  - parvovirus B19
  - cytomegalovirus
  - toxoplasma
  - syphilis
- Cardiovascular:
  - arrhythmias (e.g. supraventricular tachycardia (SVT), complete heart block)
  - cardiomyopathy
  - lesions that result in increased right atrial pressure and volume (e.g. Ebstein's)

- left-sided obstructive lesions
- haemangiomas (hepatic, Klippel–Trenaunay–Weber syndrome)
- more uncommon problems include absent ductus venosus, premature closure of arterial duct, intracardiac tumours (tuberous sclerosis), chorioangioma (placenta, chorionic, or umbilical vessels)
- Lymphatic abnormalities:
  - lymphangiectasia
  - cystic hygroma
  - chylothorax
  - in association with Turner's or Noonan's syndromes
- Pulmonary abnormalities:
  - cystic adenomatoid malformation
  - hypoplasia
- Other:
  - renal, such as obstructive uropathy, congenital nephrotic syndrome
  - chromosomal abnormalities (trisomy 15, 18, 21)
  - neoplasms
  - storage diseases
- Idiopathic.

Investigation

Antenatal
- Maternal blood group and antibodies, Kleihauer (investigating alloimmunization), FBC, and Hb electrophoresis
- Fetal medicine ultrasound/fetal echocardiography results
- Maternal serology for congenital infection
- Amniotic fluid analysis with cultures/PCR
- Fetal cordocentesis—FBC, blood group, direct antiglobulin test (DAT), Hb electrophoresis
- Fetal karyotype.

Postnatal
- CXR/AXR
- ECG
- Ultrasound: head, abdomen, and chest
- Echocardiography
- Blood tests
  - FBC, blood film, blood group, and DAT
  - Kleihauer test (maternal blood)
  - karyotype
  - biochemistry and LFTs
  - haemoglobin electrophoresis
  - bacterial and viral cultures, PCR, and/or serology for congenital infections (maternal and infant)
- Diagnostic thoracocentesis and/or paracentesis
- Placental anatomy and histology.

Treatment

- Antenatal treatment:
  - fetal thoracocentesis/paracentesis
  - intrauterine transfusion
  - pharmacological treatment through mother (e.g. arrhythmia)
- Postnatal: predominantly focused on cardiorespiratory stabilization
  - PPHN common, therefore aggressive ventilatory management often necessary including high frequency oscillatory ventilation (HFOV) and inhaled nitric oxide (iNO)
  - thoracocentesis, paracentesis, and fluid and albumin replacement as needed
  - inotropic support as indicated
  - fluid restriction and diuretics
  - specific therapy based on underlying aetiology (e.g. transfusion/exchange transfusion for anaemia).

Chapter 6

Nutrition

Nutritional requirements in neonates

- Well, full-term babies require little in the way of fluid and calorie intake during the first few days of life. Subsequently, average fluid/calorie/protein intake over the next few months varies, but is approximately:
  - fluid: 150 ml/kg/24 h
  - calories: 85–105 kcal/kg/24 h
  - protein: 1.5 g/kg/24 h
- Daily nutritional requirements per kg for stable, growing preterm babies are approximately as given in Table 6.1.

Table 6.1 Daily nutritional requirements per kg for stable, growing preterm babies (after initial postnatal diuresis)

Protein	3.0–3.8 g
Energy	110–120 kcal
Carbohydrates	3.8–11.8 g
Fat	5–20% calories
Sodium	4–5 mmol (after initial postnatal diuresis)
Potassium	2–3 mmol
Calcium	2–3 mmol
Phosphate	1.9–4.5 mmol

+ Other minerals (iron, zinc, copper, etc.), trace elements (selenium, manganese, etc.), and vitamins.

Parenteral nutrition

This may be partial, if the baby is taking some enteral feeds, or total parenteral nutrition (TPN) if not on any enteral feeds.

Indications for parenteral nutrition

- Support of growth from birth in preterm babies <30 weeks gestation
- Poor gut motility (common in extreme prematurity)
- Ileus due to sepsis
- Necrotizing enterocolitis (NEC)/suspected NEC
- Peri-operative (congenital malformations, NEC, etc.)
- Chylothorax
- Short gut (post-surgical resection/NEC).

Composition of parenteral nutrition

Water
- Total fluid = enteral fluid + fluid as PN + fluid as drugs
- Requirement for total fluid is estimated using clinical assessment of state of hydration, weight (and weight change), urine output and other fluid losses (including insensible losses), serum sodium and urea levels.

Protein
- Needed to provide nitrogen requirement for growth (aiming for equivalent rate to match *in utero* growth rate) along with non-protein calories (>25 kcal/g protein = energy necessary for growth)
- Term babies require up to 2.5 g/kg/day amino acids (mainly essential amino acids)
- Preterm babies may require up to 3.5 g/kg/day amino acids. This is usually increased daily over the first few days, starting at 1–1.5 g/kg/day in order to increase fluids and non-protein calories, so that metabolic and fluid balance disturbances are avoided.

Carbohydrates
- Needed to maintain blood glucose (>2.6 mmol/l) and to provide energy for growth
- Given as 5–20% glucose. PN should be administered via a central venous line if glucose concentration >12.5%
- Minimum of 4–6 mg/kg/min glucose is required. Some preterm babies may require as much as 12–14 mg/kg/min
- Extremely preterm babies are more likely to have glucose intolerance and require insulin especially in the first 1–2 weeks.

Lipids
- Soya bean oil emulsions (e.g. Intralipid®) in PN are used to provide:
  - essential fatty acids
  - a concentrated source of calories
  - a vehicle for delivering fat-soluble vitamins
- 20% Intralipid® is tolerated better than 10%
- SMOF lipid (Soya, MCT, Olive oil, Fish oil) may have some advantages over standard soya oil preparations (e.g. Intralipid®) in reducing cholestatic jaundice/PN induced liver disease

- Regular monitoring of plasma lipid levels is essential to avoid hyperlipidaemia
- **Minerals:** sodium, potassium, calcium, phosphate, magnesium
- **Trace elements:** zinc, copper, manganese, selenium, etc.
- **Water-soluble vitamins**
- **Fat-soluble vitamins.**

Prescription of parenteral nutrition
- Usually prescribed daily or, once stable, every 48 hours
- Prescriptions may be individualized or standard preparations may be used
- Usually given via a central venous line, although peripheral venous line may be used if glucose concentration <12.5%
- Advantages of PN are likely to be minimal if used for <5 days, even in extremely preterm
- Minimal enteral feeds ('trophic' feeds) during PN administration have benefits:
    - stimulate gut hormone production ↑ gut motility/adaptation
    - promote normal gut flora
    - ↑ bile concentration, which may →↓ cholestasis (i.e. helps reduce risk of PN cholestasis; see ➲ Complications of parenteral nutrition in neonates, this chapter, pp. 91–92)
- Blood electrolytes and fluid requirements should be monitored daily whilst on PN, as well as regular blood glucose monitoring
- Blood lipid levels should be monitored 2–3 times/week. Triglyceride levels >2 mmol/l should probably be avoided, although this is controversial
- Trace elements should be monitored every few weeks in babies on long-term PN (>4 weeks).

Complications of parenteral nutrition in neonates
- Sepsis:
    - mainly IV line related
    - bacterial (particularly coagulase negative staphylocci)
    - fungal (*Candida* spp., *Malassezia furfur*)
- IV line extravasation
- Venous thrombosis (line-related)
- Fluid/electrolyte imbalance
- Hypoglycaemia
- Hyperglycaemia
- **Metabolic acidosis:** may be related to high chloride load in extremely preterm babies, which may be reduced by replacing some of sodium chloride in PN with sodium acetate
- Hyperlipidaemia
- **Nutritional deficiencies:**
    - metabolic bone disease due to insufficient phosphate in PN (reduce risk by maximizing PN phosphate input)
    - vitamin deficiencies
    - trace element deficiencies (monitor vitamin levels and trace elements every few weeks if on PN >4 weeks)

- Cholestatic jaundice/PN induced liver disease risk increased by:
  - prematurity
  - duration of PN
  - sepsis
  - reduced bile production
- Cholestatic jaundice/PN induced liver disease risk decreased by:
  - trophic feeds
  - SMOF lipid
  - ursodeoxycholic acid (→↑ bile flow).

General issues/general principles

Enteral feeds: general principles

Breastfeeding should be encouraged in healthy term babies, and use of mother's own breast milk should usually be preferable to donor milk or formula in sick or preterm babies.

- Recommended milk intake for formula-fed healthy term babies is approximately:
  - *day 1*: 60 ml/kg/day
  - *day 2*: 90 ml/kg/day
  - *day 3*: 120 ml/kg/day
  - *day 4*: 150 ml/kg/day
  - this remains approximately the same for the next few months, but varies considerably.

Preterm, sick term, and intrauterine growth retardation (IUGR) babies should have their fluid intake prescribed individually, following clinical assessment.

- Consider starting trophic feeds even in sick, preterm babies with umbilical lines if:
  - there is no abdominal distension
  - bowel sounds are present
  - there are minimal clear aspirates
- Increase feeds slowly (20–30 ml/kg/day) and as tolerated if there are risk factors for NEC
- Once full enteral feeds are tolerated in preterm babies, consider increasing fluid volume to 180–220 ml/kg/day
- Preterm formula, breast milk fortifier, or other supplements may be used to maximize nutritional intake once full volume feeds are tolerated, if concerns regarding weight gain persist:
  - *breast milk fortifier*: contains additional protein, calories, sodium, calcium, and phosphate
  - *Duocal®*: contains fat and carbohydrate
  - *Maxijul®*: contains carbohydrate only
  - *Maxipro®*: contains protein only
  - *Calogen®*: contains fat only.

Breast milk and breastfeeding

Physiology

- Rapid ↑ maternal prolactin (from anterior pituitary) occurs immediately post-partum → stimulation of milk production via prolactin receptors in breast
- Baby suckling stimulates prolactin receptors in breast and oxytocin release (from posterior pituitary)
- Oxytocin facilitates milk 'let-down' reflex by → contraction of breast myoepithelial cells
- Colostrum is produced over the first 2–4 days. Subsequent milk production is controlled mainly by the amount of suckling or expression.

Composition of breast milk

See ● Composition of infant formulae and breast milk, p. 102.

Benefits of breastfeeding

- ↓ Risk of infection (particularly gastroenteritis, but also respiratory infection)
  - breast milk contains secretory IgA, lymphocytes, macrophages, complement, etc.
  - risk of NEC ↓ 6 to 10-fold in preterm babies
- Better tolerated in preterm babies
  - reach full enteral feeds quicker
- Possible enhancement of neurodevelopment (particularly in preterm babies)
- Possible ↓ risk of SIDS
- Possible ↓ incidence/severity of colic
- ↓ Risk of later onset disease:
  - atopic eczema
  - diabetes
  - hypertension
  - obesity
  - lymphoma
- Maternal health benefits:
  - ↑ postnatal weight loss
  - enhanced mother-infant bonding
  - ↓ incidence pre-menopausal breast cancer.

Contraindications to breastfeeding

Maternal drugs

- Most maternal medications appear in breast milk, but as few have adverse effect on the baby, breastfeeding is rarely contraindicated
- Table 6.2 shows maternal drugs that may contraindicate breastfeeding and others that should be used with caution or monitored. Local guidelines and advice from pharmacists or drug information services should also be taken into consideration.

Table 6.2 Maternal drugs that may contraindicate breastfeeding and those that should be used with caution or monitored

Breastfeeding contraindicated	Breastfeed with caution or monitor
Amiodarone	Carbamazepine
Atropine	Carbimazole
Chemotherapy drugs	Clonidine
Chloramphenicol	Co-trimoxazole
Dapsone	Ethambutol
Doxepin	Isoniazid
Ergotamine	Gentamicin
Gold	Metronidazole (alters taste of milk)
Indometacin	Oral contraceptives
Iodides	Phenytoin
Lithium	Primidone
Nitrofurantoin (in babies with G6PD deficiency)	Theophyllines
Oestrogens (if high dose)	Thiouracil
Phenindione	
Sulfonamides (in babies with G6PD deficiency)	
Tetracyclines	
Vitamins A and D	

Maternal drug abuse

See ⊃ Care of the baby whose mother is drug dependent, pp. 46–7.
- **Opiates**: breastfeeding should usually be encouraged unless the mother is known to be HIV positive, or if HIV status is unknown and she is known or suspected to be an intravenous drug user. Low-dose maternal opiates may lead to a lower incidence of postnatal withdrawal symptoms. Very high-dose maternal opiates may be a relative contraindication to breastfeeding, depending on the severity of symptoms in the baby
- **Cocaine**: breastfeeding should be discouraged in mothers who continue to use cocaine postnatally, due to potential risk of seizures.

Maternal infection

- **HIV**: breastfeeding is contraindicated in the UK if mother is HIV positive
- **TB**: baby should be managed according to local guidelines. This usually requires treating the baby, and only separating mother and baby if the risk of transmission from the mother is particularly high. Breastfeeding is therefore not usually contraindicated

- **Chickenpox:** breastfeeding should be encouraged in babies exposed to maternal chickenpox. If the mother has chickenpox lesions close to the nipple, milk should be expressed until the lesions have crusted. The baby should be protected from chickenpox with varicella zoster immunoglobulin (VZIG), and so can receive expressed breast milk (see ➲ Perinatal chickenpox, pp. 362–3).

Possible complications of breastfeeding/breast milk administration

Mother
- Breast engorgement
- Breast abscess
- Poor milk production.

Baby
- Poor weight gain/initial excessive weight loss, dehydration
- Breast milk jaundice (see ➲ Neonatal jaundice, pp. 386–7)
- Baby inadvertently given wrong breast milk (see ➲ Infants inadvertently receiving incorrect breast milk, p. 463).

Unfortunately the latter is not an infrequent error on neonatal units, usually when milk is stored for tube-feeding preterm babies. The risk of error may be reduced by robust checking procedures, including double checking of labels and ID bands, the use of warning stickers if babies have similar names, or using technology such as bar-coding, etc.

If a baby is inadvertently given the wrong breast milk, a thorough investigation should be undertaken following local guidelines, parents informed (both donor and recipient) and, with consent, checking both mothers (and recipient baby) for possible transmitted viral infections (hepatitis B and C, HIV).

Donor human milk

Because of the advantages of breast milk in preterm babies, many neonatal units have set up facilities to provide donor breast milk to those whose mothers are unable to provide breast milk for their preterm baby. Breast milk is donated by mothers who have breast milk surplus to their own baby's requirements.

- Donor breast milk is usually only used for those most at risk of complications of prematurity/VLBW (NEC, sepsis, etc.), that is <26 weeks gestation, <1000 g birth weight, profound IUGR with antenatal Doppler study abnormalities. Consideration of donor breast milk use may also be given in more mature babies with congenital abnormalities of the gut (gastroschisis, intestinal atresia) or those with congenital heart disease
- All donors are screened carefully with a questionnaire and serological testing for syphilis, hepatitis B (HBV) and hepatitis C (HCV), HIV 1 and 2, and human T-cell leukaemia virus (HTLV) 1 and 2
- Informed consent is used for both donor and recipient mother
- Donated milk is screened for pathogenic organisms and then pasteurized (heated to 62.5°C for 30 minutes). This temperature is viricidal for HIV, and kills bacteria and *Mycobacterium tuberculosis*
- Post-pasteurization milk is screened once again for the presence of any bacteria.

Composition of infant formulae and breast milks

See Table 6.3.

Table 6.3 Composition of infant formulae and breast milk

Per 100 ml	Preterm breast milk (in first 2–3 weeks)	Preterm breast milk + BMF (2.2 g sachet/100 ml)	Typical preterm formula	Typical follow-on preterm formula	Term breast milk (>2 weeks)	Typical term formula
Protein source	Casein, lactalbumin	Casein, lactalbumin	Casein, lactalbumin	Casein, lactalbumin	Casein, lactalbumin	Casein, lactalbumin
Carbohydrate source	Lactose	Lactose, maltodextrin	Lactose, glucose	Lactose, glucose	Lactose	Lactose
Fat source	LCT	LCT (BMF is fat free)	LCT, MCT, fish oil	LCT, MCT, fish oil, egg lipid	LCT	LCT, fish oil
Osmolality (mOsmol/kgH$_2$O)	275–295	450	375	340	275	340
Energy (kcal)	65	80	80	75	70	66
Protein (g)	1.5	2.6	2.6	2.0	1.3	1.3
Fat (g)	3.5	3.5	3.9	4.0	4.1	3.5
Carbohydrate (g)	6.9	9.6	8.4	7.4	7.2	7.3
Sodium (mg)	28.5	63.5	70	28	15	17
Potassium (mg)	49.6	72.6	82	77	58	65
Calcium (mg)	25.4	91.4	94	87	34	47
Phosphate (mg)	14.2	52.2	62	47	15	26

BMF: breast milk fortifier; LCT: long chain triglycerides; MCT: medium chain triglycerides.

Composition of specialized infant formula milks

See Table 6.4.

Table 6.4 Composition of specialized infant formula milks

Per 100 ml	Pepti-junior®	Pregestimil®	Neocate®	Monogen®
Indications	Malabsorption; post-NEC; short gut; milk intolerance	Short gut; milk intolerance	Short gut; protein intolerance; malabsorption; intractable diarrhoea; cow's milk protein allergy	Chylothorax; steatorrhoea; abetalipo-proteinaemia; intestinal lymphangiectasia; hyperlipo-proteinaemia 1
Protein source	Hydrolysed whey	Casein hydrolysate	Synthetic amino acids	Whey
Carbohydrate source	Glucose syrup	Glucose polymer, modified corn starch, dextrose, maltodextrin	Glucose syrup	Glucose syrup, lactose
Fat source	Corn oil, MCT, fish oil	Sunflower oil, coconut MCT, soya oil, corn oil	Coconut oil, sunflower oil, canola oil	MCT (90%), LCT (10%) (coconut oil, walnut oil)
Osmolality (mOsmol/kg H_2O)	210	330	360	280
Energy (kcal)	66	68	70	74
Protein (g)	1.8	1.9	1.9	2.0
Fat (g)	3.5	3.8	3.4	2.1
Carbohydrate (g)	6.8	6.9	7.9	12
Sodium (mg)	18	29	18	35
Potassium (mg)	65	74	62	63
Calcium (mg)	50	78	69	45
Phosphate (mg)	28	51	50	35

LCT: long chain triglycerides; MCT: medium chain triglycerides; NEC: necrotizing enterocolitis.

Further information

Agostini C, Buonocore G, Carnielli VP, et al. Enteral nutrient supply for preterm infants: Commentary from the European Society for Paediatric Gastroenterology, Hepatology, and Nutrition Committee on Nutrition. *JPGN* 2010; **50**: 85–91.

Respiratory problems

Causes of respiratory distress

- Respiratory distress syndrome (RDS)—surfactant deficiency
- Pneumothorax
- Pneumonia
- Meconium aspiration syndrome (MAS)
- Transient tachypnoea of the newborn (TTN)
- Persistent pulmonary hypertension of the newborn (PPHN)
- Chronic lung disease
- Pulmonary haemorrhage
- Upper airway obstruction:
  - Pierre–Robin sequence
  - subglottic stenosis
  - choanal atresia
  - laryngomalacia
- Congenital chest/lung anomalies:
  - congenital diaphragmatic hernia (CDH)
  - tracheo-oesophageal fistula (TOF)
  - congenital cystic adenomatoid malformation (CCAM)
  - congenital lobar emphysema
  - small chest syndromes
  - pulmonary hypoplasia
  - congenital abnormalities of surfactant
- Non-respiratory causes:
  - metabolic acidosis
  - perinatal asphyxia
  - congenital heart disease
  - severe anaemia.

Initial management of babies presenting with respiratory distress

- **ABC resuscitation** (see ➲ Resuscitation of the newborn, p. 20) and initiate measures to ensure temperature stability (see ➲ Initial management of the extremely preterm infant, pp. 64–5)
- **Review history**: gestation, time of rupture of membranes (ROM), type of delivery, meconium-stained amniotic fluid, maternal diabetes, etc.
- **Examine the baby:**
  - well/unwell, pink/pale/cyanosed, perfusion
  - check chest wall movement
  - auscultate chest
- **Start transcutaneous oxygen saturation monitoring**: maintain saturations at 90–95% if <34 weeks gestation (due to balance of risk between retinopathy of prematurity and mortality and neurodevelopmental morbidity)
- **Check BP**
- **Check temperature**
- **Establish IV access**
- **Blood tests:**
  - blood glucose
  - FBC/C-reactive protein
  - blood culture
  - blood gas—preferably arterial, a capillary sample is only acceptable if peripheral perfusion adequate, arterial access should be obtained if fraction of inspired oxygen (FiO_2) >0.3
- **Start IV fluids** (usually 60 ml/kg/day, initially 10% dextrose)
- **Start IV antibiotics**: a broad-spectrum combination, such as benzylpenicillin and gentamicin (unless *Listeria* suspected, then use amoxicillin and gentamicin). Check local guidelines
- **Chest X-ray (CXR):** if mild respiratory distress not needing ventilatory support, this can be delayed until 4 h. Otherwise, request CXR on admission.

Respiratory support

Guided by clinical state, oxygen requirement, and blood gases.

Ambient/headbox/nasal cannula O_2

If baby:
- Looks comfortable
- FiO_2 <0.3
- Blood gas normal (pH >7.25; PCO_2 <6.5).

If baby has moderate recession or worse, is having apnoea, FiO_2 >0.3 and/or acidotic (pH <7.25), they will need increased respiratory support.

Nasal continuous positive airway pressure (nCPAP)

Consider for any of the following:

- >30 weeks, >1000 g
- Baby looks well
- FiO_2 <0.4
- pH >7.20, PCO_2 <7.0–7.5.

Positive pressure ventilation

Consider for any of the following:

- No improvement on CPAP
- <30 weeks, <1000 g
- Baby unwell, marked recession
- FiO_2 >0.4 in preterm or >0.5–0.6 in term infants
- pH <7.20, PCO_2 >7.5
- **NB** Nasal CPAP may be considered as an alternative to positive pressure ventilation via an endotracheal tube (ETT) at any gestation, weight, or postnatal age, provided the baby is stable enough to tolerate this. Guidelines and practice regarding this may vary considerably between different neonatal units
- Transcutaneous (Tc) PO_2 and PCO_2 monitoring is recommended for any baby requiring ventilatory support or unstable on nCPAP
- Consider surfactant (see ➲ Surfactant, pp. 112–13).

Respiratory distress syndrome

Risk of RDS, also referred to as hyaline membrane disease, decreases with advancing gestational age and is therefore rare in term babies. Other risk factors for RDS include:
- Male gender
- Maternal diabetes
- Maternal hypertension
- IUGR in babies born <29 weeks
- Delivery by Caesarean section
- Perinatal hypoxia/ischaemia/acidosis
- Sepsis
- Hypothermia
- Second twin
- Family history of babies with RDS
- Poor maternal nutrition
- MAS
- Congenital pneumonia
- Severe haemolytic disease of the newborn (HDN).

Risk of RDS is reduced in:
- Female gender
- IUGR in babies born >28 weeks
- Some ethnic groups (risk in white approximately 1.5× black)
- Maternal drugs and smoking (opiates, cocaine, alcohol, and smoking, although risks of any of these heavily outweighed by any possible benefit).

Risk/severity of RDS is reduced with maternal corticosteroids: betamethasone or dexamethasone
- Evidence from randomized controlled trials (RCTs) carried out in the 1970s and 1980s suggests reduction of incidence of RDS and mortality due to RDS by approximately 40%
- Maximum benefit achieved if two doses are given 12 hours apart, between 24 hours and 7 days of the baby's birth (full course)
- Lesser benefit if maternal corticosteroids are received outside these times (partial course)
- Current Royal College of Obstetricians and Gynaecologists (RCOG) recommendations state that every effort should be made to initiate antenatal corticosteroid therapy in women between 24 and 34 weeks gestation (and also consider the same for 35 and 36 weeks) with any of the following:
  - threatened preterm labour
  - antepartum haemorrhage
  - preterm ROM
  - any condition requiring elective preterm delivery.

Recent estimates of incidence of RDS are from populations where maternal corticosteroids and prophylactic surfactant are commonly used. Approximate incidence is:
- 50% <30 weeks
- 37% at 31–32 weeks
- 12% at 33–34 weeks
- 2% at 35–36 weeks.

Pathophysiology of RDS

Surfactant deficiency leads to:

- Alveolar collapse, particularly at end-expiration due to increased surface tension
- Low lung compliance (i.e. volume change small per unit increase in pressure)
- Low lung volumes—functional residual capacity as low as one-tenth of normal. See CXR in Fig. 7.1, showing RDS with typical low lung volumes and generalized 'ground glass' opacification
- Increased work of breathing—exacerbated by low muscle bulk and compliant rib cage in preterm babies
- Delayed postnatal fall in pulmonary vascular resistance leading to ↑ right to left shunting
- Hypoxia →↓ cardiac output → hypotension. This may cause metabolic acidosis, renal failure, and fluid retention
- Reduced tidal ventilation → hypercarbia
- Endogenous surfactant production usually becomes sufficient by 48–72 h of age in preterm babies with RDS. This is not inhibited by treatment with exogenous surfactant
- Clinical improvement usually coincides with endogenous surfactant production, along with marked diuresis.

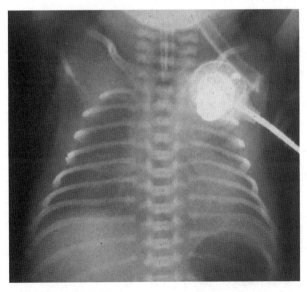

Fig. 7.1 CXR showing RDS with typical low lung volumes and generalized 'ground glass' opacification.

Surfactant

Since the 1980s randomized controlled trials have shown that the use of surfactant to treat neonatal RDS decreases morbidity and mortality. It increases lung compliance and volumes, as well as increasing effective pulmonary blood flow.

Composition of surfactant

- Lipid (mostly phospholipids ~90%)
- Protein (surfactant proteins A, B, C, and D ~10%).

Preparations available

- Two currently available preparations in the UK (both 'natural' i.e. animal derived) are:
  - Curosurf® (poractant alfa)—a porcine lung extract
  - Survanta® (beractant)—a bovine lung extract with added phospholipids
- Previously available synthetic preparations (Exosurf and ALEC) are no longer available as they have been found to be less effective
- 'New generation' synthetic surfactants (e.g. aerosolized KL4) have been used in clinical trials recently with some promising early results.

Schedules for surfactant treatment for neonatal respiratory distress syndrome

- **Prophylactic:** elective intubation at birth with the administration of surfactant in the first few minutes of life before clinical or radiological confirmation of RDS
- **Early selective:** as prophylactic, but only if the baby is already ventilated (i.e. not intubated for the purpose of giving surfactant only)
- **Rescue:** surfactant administered to ventilated infants with clinical +/– radiological signs of RDS:
  - early selective treatment is suggested in preterm babies <30 weeks gestation (given as early as possible after birth) and rescue treatment in those ≥30 weeks
  - it may be justified in spontaneously ventilating babies with significant RDS to intubate and ventilate specifically to give surfactant
  - local policies should be checked carefully as they may vary considerably regarding surfactant administration.

Administration of surfactant

- Discuss the need for surfactant with senior medical staff before use
- Check dose of surfactant according to baby's weight (or estimated weight) and local guidelines
- If a baby requires surfactant (or if the birth of a baby <30 weeks gestation is known to be imminent), remove correct size vial of surfactant from the fridge
- Warm the vial to ambient temperature by holding in the hand for a few minutes and gently turn upside down, without shaking, in order to obtain a uniform suspension

- Equipment required for administration of surfactant:
  - surfactant administration tube supplied with vial (or nasogastric tube (size 6 Fr))
  - sterile 19 G needle and appropriate size syringe
  - scissors or stitch cutter
  - alcohol swabs
  - tape measure
  - sterile gloves
- Prepare the vial by inverting gently a few times, without shaking, to obtain a uniform suspension. Remove outer cap and sterilize inner cap by wiping with an alcohol swab
- Cut the nasogastric tube to the correct length (if not using surfactant administration tube), that is 1 cm shorter than the length of the ETT (including ETT connector, etc.)
- Attach the syringe to the nasogastric tube. To avoid contamination, remember to handle the tube with a sterile glove. Push the surfactant to the end of the nasogastric tube with the syringe, ready for administration
- Monitor oxygenation during and after surfactant administration using saturation monitor (+/– $TcPO_2$/$TcPCO_2$)
- Adjust ventilator peak inspiratory pressure (PIP) and FiO_2 to ensure adequate chest inflation and oxygenation
- Disconnect from ventilator, insert NGT into ETT and inject surfactant down ETT
- Once all surfactant has been administered, remove syringe, and NG tube from ETT
- Reconnect ventilator, adjust PIP and FiO_2 to ensure adequate chest inflation and oxygenation
- Avoid suction for approximately 4 h if possible
- Lung mechanics may change very rapidly (within minutes) and necessitate rapid adjustments of ventilator settings; therefore, observe baby carefully for approximately 30 min after administration
- Repeat blood gas after 30 min
- Consider second and subsequent surfactant doses according to ventilatory requirements. This should always be discussed with senior medical staff. In general, a second dose should be considered 6–12 h after the first in babies <30 weeks gestation, with FiO_2 >0.3 despite adequate ventilator pressures. If a baby has high or increasing ventilator requirements <12 h after the first dose, consider giving the second dose earlier, but exclude other important causes of worsening respiratory function prior to this (e.g. blocked or dislodged ETT or pneumothorax, etc.).

Other indications for surfactant treatment

Surfactant is denatured by fatty acids in meconium and also by certain proteins. Therefore, in the following conditions, if high ventilatory requirements persist, surfactant may be helpful:
- MAS
- Congenital pneumonia
- Pulmonary haemorrhage
- ARDS
- Congenital diaphragmatic hernia.

Transient tachypnoea of the newborn

- Occurs due to delay in clearance of fetal lung fluid
- Increased incidence after elective Caesarean section
- Presents with tachypnoea +/− minimal other signs of respiratory distress
- CXR shows 'wet'-looking lung fields with fluid in fissures
- May require supplementary oxygen, rarely requires positive pressure ventilation (PPV)
- Usually resolves within 24 hours.

Pneumonia

Usually part of more widespread infection. Diagnosis often uncertain due to:
- Isolation of bacteria, viruses, or fungi not synonymous with pneumonia
- CXR changes non-specific.

Early-onset or intrauterine pneumonia

- Onset of symptoms within 48 h of birth
- Incidence 1.5–2 per 1000 live births
- Approximately 70% of cases due to Group B *Streptococcus* (GBS)
- Other causes:
  - *Haemophilus influenzae*
  - *Escherichia coli*
  - *Streptococcus pneumoniae*
  - *Klebsiella pneumoniae*
  - *Listeria monocytogenes*
- Other rarer causes include:
  - *Chlamydia trachomatis*
  - viruses (e.g. cytomegalovirus (CMV), herpes simplex virus (HSV))
  - fungi (e.g. *Candida albicans*)
- Infection is usually a result of infected amniotic fluid or vaginal secretions. Therefore, often associated with pre-labour rupture of membranes (PROM) and evidence of chorioamnionitis
- In preterm infants: presents as RDS, but may produce focal opacities on CXR
- In term infants: presents with signs of respiratory distress; PPHN common
- Treatment with respiratory support and antibiotics (usually penicillin and gentamicin, unless *Listeria* suspected, then use amoxicillin).

Late-onset or nosocomial pneumonia

- Onset of symptoms >48 h after birth
- Common in ventilated babies (ventilator-associated pneumonia), presenting with deterioration in respiratory status, increased ETT secretions and non-specific signs of infection
- Causes similar to early-onset pneumonia (but Gram-negative bacilli are more common) + *Staphylococcus aureus* and *S. epidermidis*, respiratory syncytial virus (RSV), fungi, mycoplasma, etc.
- Treatment with broad-spectrum antibiotics, modified to cover organisms isolated from ETT secretions
- Lung abscess is a rare complication.

Pneumothorax and other pulmonary air leaks

A pulmonary air leak occurs as a result of alveolar over-distension and subsequent rupture. Over-distension is exacerbated in preterm infants due to the reduced number of the pores of Kohn. Air tracks along perivascular spaces into the pleural space to cause pneumothorax, or to the mediastinum to cause pneumomediastinum, and may even enter the pericardial space. In preterm infants, the relatively large amount of connective tissue and water in the lung interstitium predisposes to air remaining here to cause pulmonary interstitial emphysema (PIE).

Tension pneumothorax occurs when intrapleural pressure is greater than atmospheric pressure.

Pneumothorax

- Pneumothorax may occur spontaneously in up to 1% of babies around the time of birth
- More likely to occur in babies with other lung pathology (RDS, MAS, pneumonia, etc.)
- Associated with long ventilator inspiratory times (>0.5 s) and I:E ratios >1:1
- Clinical signs: respiratory distress, increasing oxygen and ventilation requirements, reduced air entry on the affected side, increased PCO_2, hypotension, bradycardia, metabolic acidosis
- Diagnosis: trans-illumination—may be unreliable in term babies or if on high frequency oscillatory ventilation (HFOV), but is useful in most cases of tension pneumothorax for emergency management (Fig. 7.2). CXR is more useful in cases of non-tension pneumothorax and after emergency management
- Treatment:
  - small, asymptomatic pneumothorax: close observation even if ventilated. Try 100% oxygen for 1–2 h in term babies to 'wash out' nitrogen
  - needle drainage: may be used if urgent decompression is required (i.e. in case of tension pneumothorax with poor oxygenation and hypotension)
  - chest drain insertion: required for all tension pneumothoraces, and ventilated or preterm infants with deterioration due to a non-tension pneumothorax (see ➲ Intercostal (chest) drain insertion, pp. 498–9).

Pneumomediastinum

- Usually associated with other forms of air leak
- Air is near the heart with elevation of thymus and lucency between the heart and sternum
- Specific treatment is rarely required, but high inspired oxygen may facilitate more rapid resolution, if used in term infants. Attempts at drainage should be reserved for babies with severe cardiovascular compromise as complications of drain insertion are common.

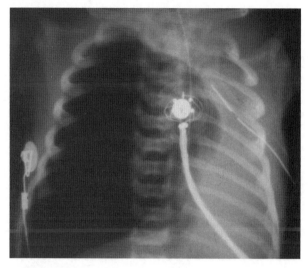

Fig. 7.2 CXR showing right-sided tension pneumothorax. Note the chest drain on the left side from a previous left-sided pneumothorax.

Pneumopericardium

- Air tracks from the mediastinum or pleural space and surrounds the heart, often with associated shock (tamponade)
- Electrocardiogram (ECG) becomes low voltage
- Needle aspiration via a subxiphoid route with US guidance may be considered if symptoms of tamponade persist despite 100% oxygen and reducing ventilator pressures.

Pulmonary interstitial emphysema

- Air leak from alveoli, but contained within interstitial space (Fig. 7.3)
- Incidence is inversely related to gestational age
- CXR appearance typical with tiny 'bubbles' of air throughout affected area
- Usually generalized distribution, but may be lobar
- Associated with a high mortality risk and chronic lung disease in survivors
- Management:
  - attempt to reduce PIP, positive end expiratory pressure (PEEP), and inspiratory time if on conventional ventilation or use a 'low volume' strategy on HFOV. Otherwise ventilate as clinical condition and blood gases determine
  - consider increasing sedation or starting muscle relaxant if baby is 'fighting the ventilator'.

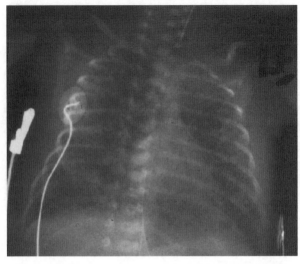

Fig. 7.3 CXR showing bilateral, widespread pulmonary interstitial emphysema (PIE).

Meconium aspiration syndrome

- Approximately 5% of babies develop MAS if there is meconium-stained amniotic fluid (1–5/1000 live births)
- *In utero* hypoxia may induce passage of meconium and associated gasping, increasing the risk of aspiration
- Meconium may be aspirated before, during, or just after birth
- MAS occurs following aspiration of meconium due to several mechanisms:
    - ball-valve obstruction of airways leading to over-inflation of some areas of lung, and predisposing to air leaks and atelectasis of other areas
    - chemical pneumonitis contributing to respiratory distress and leading to inactivation of endogenous surfactant
    - hypoxaemia due to right to left shunting as a result of pulmonary hypertension
    - secondary infection.

Prevention

For management of meconium-stained amniotic fluid see ➋ Meconium-stained amniotic fluid, p. 23.

Clinical signs

- Usually term or post-term baby
- Skin, nails, and umbilical cord may be meconium-stained
- Signs of respiratory distress +/– PPHN
- May have signs of neonatal encephalopathy
- CXR: generalized over-inflation with patchy collapse/consolidation. Pneumothorax and/or pneumomediastinum common (Fig. 7.4).

Management of MAS

Follow the basic guidelines on respiratory distress (see ➋ Initial management of babies presenting with respiratory distress, pp. 108–9), with some specific points:

- Consider nasal continuous positive airway pressure (nCPAP) in babies with mild respiratory distress secondary to MAS, but nCPAP may exacerbate air trapping and increase risk of pneumothorax
- Consider early intubation and PPV in babies with signs of early severe respiratory distress or rapidly worsening respiratory status (e.g. if ambient FiO_2 reaches 0.4 or low flow oxygen requirement is >0.5 l/min and rising, evidence of CO_2 retention, or markedly increased work of breathing)
- Aim for O_2 saturation >98% to decrease pulmonary vascular resistance
- Consider early placement of arterial line (e.g. if ventilated, or if FiO_2 >0.3 and rising, or if early CO_2 retention)—CO_2 retention indicates significant distress in hyperventilating baby
- High PEEP is likely to increase the risk of pneumothorax, but may improve oxygenation
- Use long expiratory times (>0.5–0.6 s) to reduce the risk of exacerbation of gas trapping

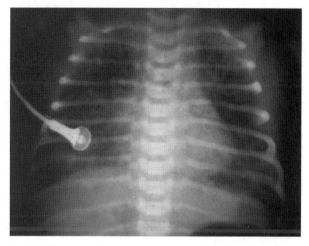

Fig. 7.4 CXR showing meconium aspiration syndrome with typical areas of collapse/consolidation and over-inflation.

- Consider early use of adequate sedation in all ventilated babies with MAS and muscle relaxants in those with an increasing or high ventilatory requirement
- Consider HFOV in severe MAS
- Surfactant has been shown to reduce the risk of air leak, decrease the time on PPV, and reduce the need for extracorporeal membrane oxygenation (ECMO). 3–4 repeat doses up to 6-hourly should be considered in severe MAS
- **Antibiotic therapy:** although meconium itself is usually sterile, secondary pneumonia may occur. Broad-spectrum antibiotics (e.g. penicillin and gentamicin) should be started
- ECMO if intractable hypoxaemia. The UK Collaborative ECMO trial suggested that in babies with severe MAS (oxygenation index (OI) >40), survival was increased by approximately 50%.

Complications of MAS
- Pneumothorax (drain)
- Pneumomediastinum (usually requires no treatment)
- PPHN (may need nitric oxide—see ➜ Persistent pulmonary hypertension of the newborn, pp. 122–3)
- Chronic lung disease—this is rare and associated with severe MAS. Recurrent cough and wheeze and lung function abnormalities have been demonstrated in a minority of school age children who were ventilated for MAS in the neonatal period.

Persistent pulmonary hypertension of the newborn

Persistent pulmonary hypertension of the newborn is a failure of the normal postnatal fall in pulmonary vascular resistance leading to ongoing right to left shunting across the fetal channels (patent foramen ovale and patent ductus arteriosus (PDA)) and resultant hypoxia. In many babies with PPHN, the major shunting occurs at an intrapulmonary level.

PPHN may be:
- **Primary**: idiopathic
- **Secondary**: complicating other lung pathology:
  - surfactant deficiency
  - MAS
  - congenital diaphragmatic hernia
  - other causes of pulmonary hypoplasia
  - perinatal hypoxia ischaemia
  - congenital pneumonia/sepsis (particularly GBS).

Consider diagnosis if:
- Hypoxaemia is out of proportion to the severity of parenchymal lung disease on the CXR
- Hypoxaemia and wide swings in arterial PO_2
- Preductal (e.g. right radial artery) PO_2 higher than post-ductal (umbilical artery or lower limb arterial line) PO_2 by at least 3 kPa
- High OI is also an objective measure of the degree of respiratory failure and is used to determine the need for referral to an ECMO centre in term infants. OI >25 indicates severe respiratory failure. OI >40 suggests that ECMO should be considered (see ➲ Extracorporeal membrane oxygenation, pp. 162–3).

Oxygenation index

Mean airway pressure × FiO_2 (as %)/post-ductal PO_2 (in kPa) × 7.6

Echocardiography

This allows accurate assessment of PPHN and should be requested and performed as soon as possible if PPHN is suspected in order to exclude cyanotic congenital heart disease. It may also be useful to estimate the pulmonary artery pressure, and define the presence and magnitude of shunts at atrial or ductal level. If echocardiography is not immediately available, treatment should not be delayed.

Management

The aim is to maintain normal arterial oxygen levels and normal tissue oxygenation. The two most potent natural pulmonary vasodilators are oxygen and lung inflation.
- **Oxygen**: aim to maintain relatively high PO_2 (suggest 10–13 kPa (in infants >34 weeks corrected gestational age), 7–9 kPa (in preterm infants <34 weeks corrected gestational age) by using appropriate FiO_2)
- **Ventilation**: use appropriate pressures to achieve and maintain good lung inflation
- Aim to maintain PCO_2 in normal to low normal range (i.e. 4.5–5 kPa)

- Consider exogenous surfactant in order to optimize lung inflation and compliance. Consider additional doses, particularly in PPHN complicating severe RDS or MAS
- Sedate and consider paralysis to optimize efficiency of ventilation
- Minimize handling
- Ensure suction of secretions from ETT as required and consider using an 'in-line' suction catheter so that hypoxic episodes during suction are avoided
- Treat underlying cause
- Consider inducing relative metabolic alkalosis with a sodium bicarbonate infusion (or THAM (tris-hydroxymethyl aminomethane) if serum sodium level is high). Aim for a pH >7.4, as this may help reduce pulmonary vascular resistance
- Identify and correct other metabolic abnormalities, such as hypoglycaemia, hypocalcaemia, hypothermia, anaemia, and polycythaemia
- Optimize cardiac output and blood pressure with use of volume and inotropes. Try to avoid inotropes that vasoconstrict (e.g. dopamine, particularly at high dose) as they may worsen PPHN. There is some evidence that noradrenaline (norepinephrine) may be more appropriate than adrenaline (epinephrine) in PPHN, as noradrenaline is less likely to have a pulmonary vasoconstrictive effect
- **High frequency oscillatory ventilation**: may be particularly useful in babies with secondary PPHN and should be considered if oxygenation is still problematic despite optimal conventional ventilation and surfactant (see ➔ High frequency oscillatory ventilation, pp. 160–1)
- Inhaled nitric oxide (iNO):
  - should be considered in any baby with severe hypoxic respiratory failure, despite maximal respiratory support
  - check platelet count and clotting screen if not done in previous 12 h. Correct as necessary
  - suggest start iNO at 5 ppm and increase in steps of 5 ppm approximately every 15 min (up to a maximum 20 ppm) until PO_2 is consistently within the target range (i.e. 10–13 kPa for infants >34 weeks corrected gestational age)
  - if responding, continue inhaled nitric oxide at required concentration to maintain the PO_2 within the target range, until FiO_2 can be weaned to <0.5. Then wean iNO in steps of 1–2 ppm hourly as tolerated. Consider slower weaning (i.e. by 1 ppm every 4 h) from 5 ppm, particularly if iNO has been used for a prolonged period of time
  - whilst on iNO, monitor methaemoglobin levels. Most modern blood gas machines will analyse this. Avoid methaemoglobin levels >4%
  - if response to high concentrations of iNO is poor, consider:
    —ECMO referral (see ➔ Extracorporeal membrane oxygenation, pp. 162–3)
    —adenosine (50 µg/kg/min continuous IVI)
    —magnesium sulfate ($MgSO_4$) (200 mg/kg IV slow bolus). Ensure that BP is optimized prior to giving magnesium sulfate.

Prognosis
Dependent on underlying cause of PPHN.

Pulmonary haemorrhage

- Small bleeds from the upper airway are common secondary to local trauma from suction or intubation
- True or massive pulmonary haemorrhage usually occurs due to increased pulmonary blood flow or pulmonary venous congestion (= haemorrhagic pulmonary oedema), in extremely preterm infants or more mature babies with severe lung disease.

Incidence

~12% very low birth weight (VLBW) babies.

Clinical signs

- Massive pulmonary haemorrhage (MPH) usually associated with an acute deterioration with sudden cardiorespiratory collapse, with poor perfusion, tachycardia, hypotension, worsening respiratory status, and copious amounts of blood from the ETT, mouth, and nose
- Often requires extensive resuscitation and is associated with high mortality
- Clinical signs of PDA are often present
- CXR usually shows bilateral uniform opacification (often 'white out').

Management

- ABC of resuscitation as required. Airway/ETT suction with a wide-bore suction catheter may be necessary to avoid obstruction
- Intubate and commence positive pressure ventilation if baby is not already ventilated
- Use relatively high PEEP (i.e. 6–8 cmH$_2$O)
- Adjust PIP so that the chest wall has adequate movement, and tidal volumes (if monitored) are adequate. Further adjustment may be required according to subsequent CXR and (arterial) blood gases
- Consider HFOV if oxygenation is problematic
- Consider inserting arterial line if not already in place. Adjust ventilation according to arterial blood gases, clinical signs, and respiratory monitoring
- Check FBC, clotting profile, and serum biochemistry. Correct any abnormalities and transfuse packed red blood cells according to local guidelines, or if haemoglobin has fallen acutely secondary to MPH
- Send blood for culture and start broad-spectrum IV antibiotics according to antibiotic protocol if sepsis suspected
- Once the acute haemorrhage has stopped, consider treating with exogenous surfactant if FiO$_2$ has increased significantly (i.e. >0.1) following MPH or if new changes suggesting surfactant deficiency are seen on CXR

- Initial fluid resuscitation (blood or fresh frozen plasma) is likely to be required initially following MPH, but then:
  - restrict fluids if there are signs of fluid overload, congestive cardiac failure, or PDA. This needs to be individualized, but suggest reducing total fluid input by ~ one-third
  - consider IV furosemide 1–2 mg/kg bd if there are signs of fluid overload or congestive cardiac failure
- If there are signs of PDA (or if echocardiography is available and confirms PDA), consider starting either ibuprofen or indometacin, if there are no contraindications to treatment.

Apnoea

- Pauses in breathing lasting up to 20 s are a common phenomenon in neonates and most occur without other physiological changes, ending spontaneously without intervention
- **Definition of apnoea:** pause in breathing >20 s, or <20 s associated with bradycardia and/or cyanosis
- Incidence decreases with increasing gestational age, with marked decrease between 30 and 33 weeks gestation (approximately 50% at 30–31 weeks, 7% 34–35 weeks)
- Apnoea may be:
  - *central*: respiratory effort and nasal airflow absent
  - *obstructive*: only nasal airflow absent
  - *mixed*: initially central followed by airway obstruction
- Apnoea may be caused or exacerbated by:
  - *drugs*: sedation, prostaglandins, following immunization, etc.
  - *systemic illness*: sepsis, IVH, necrotizing enterocolitis (NEC), inborn errors of metabolism, anaemia, hypothermia, gastro-oesophageal reflux (GOR), etc.
  - *upper airway obstruction*: choanal atresia, Pierre–Robin sequence, trisomy 21, etc.

Management

- Investigate and treat any possible underlying cause. This should include a full infection screen and starting broad-spectrum antibiotics in babies with worsening episodes of apnoea, bradycardia, and desaturation, unless another cause is overwhelmingly likely
- Cardiorespiratory monitoring (with pulse oximetry, +/– ECG and more invasive monitoring in unstable or extremely preterm) is essential in any baby at risk of significant apnoea
- Document frequency and severity of apnoea, bradycardia, and desaturations using 'apnoea chart'
- If the baby remains apnoeic with a fall in heart rate and/or saturations, intervention is required, initially by gentle stimulation
- Facial oxygen may be required if gentle stimulation fails to re-establish regular respiration. Occasionally, oral suction may be necessary if secretions or milk are present in the upper airway.
- More severe episodes may require PPV via a mask or intubation. Intubation and PPV should also be considered for recurrent apnoea, bradycardia, and desaturation
- Caffeine is known to prevent apnoea of prematurity and facilitate faster weaning from respiratory support. Consider starting caffeine within the first few days of life in all preterm infants <30 weeks gestation. More mature preterm infants should be considered for caffeine on an individual basis
- Consider packed red blood cell transfusion in anaemic preterm babies with significant apnoea. Refer to local guidelines for this as they vary considerably
- Consider prevention and treatment of GOR if this is suspected by ensuring correct NG tube positioning, positioning the baby with a head up tilt, prone or lateral, decreasing feed volume by increasing frequency, and considering milk thickening and anti-GOR medication.

Upper airway problems: cleft lip and palate, choanal atresia, and Pierre–Robin sequence

Cleft lip and palate
- Develop due to failure of fusion of maxillary and pre-maxillary processes
- Unilateral or bilateral, lip or palate, or both
- Incidence approximately 1/700 live births
- Associated with genetic syndromes (e.g. trisomy 13, 22q deletion, Apert's), maternal phenytoin, and Pierre–Robin sequence
- May require early feeding assessment and intervention (e.g. NG feeds, specialized teat, dental plate), but many able to breastfeed normally
- Early (or antenatal) referral to specialized cleft lip and palate multidisciplinary team recommended
- Surgical repair, usually at 3 months for cleft lip, 6–12 months for cleft palate (may be staged surgical approach)
- Prognosis good, but often require long-term SALT (speech and language therapy), orthodontic, and ENT input (chronic otitis media).

Choanal atresia
- Failure of completion of bucconasal membrane breakdown in early fetal life
- Incidence ~1 in 8000 (more common in females)
- Unilateral or bilateral, bony or membranous
- 60% associated with other congenital malformations (e.g. CHARGE— Coloboma, Heart defects, choanal Atresia, Retardation of growth and/or development, Genital abnormalities, and Ear abnormalities)
- Presents immediately after birth with respiratory distress and inability to pass NG tube
- Diagnosis confirmed with computed tomography (CT) scan or contrast study
- Surgical treatment by perforating or drilling atretic segment +/− short-term nasal stents.

Pierre–Robin sequence
- Micrognathia, cleft palate, and glossoptosis. May be isolated or part of syndrome (22q, Stickler, etc.)
- May present with obstructive apnoea
- Manage initially with prone positioning. May require intervention with oral or nasopharyngeal airway, or nCPAP, and in severe cases intubation with later tracheostomy
- Long-term resolution due to catch-up mandibular growth occurs over months and years.

Upper airway problems: CHAOS, EXIT, and laryngeal obstruction

Congenital high airway obstruction syndrome (CHAOS) and ex utero intrapartum treatment (EXIT)

Antenatal diagnosis (US and MRI) of high airway obstruction (external compression due to cystic hygromas and other masses compressing the upper airway, or laryngeal abnormalities) has made immediate airway management possible using the EXIT procedure.

EXIT is carried out by delivering the baby's upper body by Caesarean section and establishing the airway, usually by tracheostomy, prior to the remainder of the delivery and cutting of the umbilical cord.

Laryngeal obstruction

- Most commonly due to laryngomalacia, but may be due to cysts or webs or vocal cord paralysis (congenital or acquired)
- **Laryngomalacia ('floppiness' of the supraglottic airway)**—commonest cause of stridor in the 1st year of life, usually resolving by 2 years of age
  - Presents with inspiratory stridor, worse with crying, activity, supine position, and URTIs
  - May be exacerbated by GOR
  - Referral to ENT should be considered if associated with apnoea, significant accessory muscle use or failure to thrive
  - Upper airway endoscopy and aryepiglottoplasty may be required in severe cases.

Upper airway problems: subglottic stenosis and tracheobronchomalacia

Subglottic stenosis (SGS)

- Acquired in 95% cases, presenting with failure of extubation and post-extubation stridor
- Risk factors:
  - extreme prematurity
  - prolonged, recurrent, and/or traumatic intubation
  - keloid scarring (racial predisposition)
  - GOR
  - infection
- Severity graded using Cotton classification, according to reduction in airway lumen:
  - *Grade 1*: <50%
  - *Grade 2*: 50–70%
  - *Grade 3*: 70–90%
  - *Grade 4*: 100%
- Management:
  - conservative with mild cases; time +/− short course of systemic steroids
  - some mild cases may require upper airway endoscopy and laser or cryotherapy to granulomatous tissue
  - more severe grade 1/2 cases require surgical intervention with anterior cricoid split or single stage laryngotracheal reconstruction
  - Grade 2–4 SGS may require a staged laryngotracheal reconstruction with initial tracheostomy.

Airway vascular compression

- Occurs secondary to congenital anomalies of the great vessels (e.g. double aortic arch, aberrant pulmonary artery)
- Presents with stridor +/− swallowing/feeding difficulty
- Upper airway endoscopy shows pulsatile external airway compression often with secondary tracheo- or bronchomalacia
- Echocardiography, cardiac MRI, and upper GI contrast studies may be necessary prior to cardiac surgical correction of anatomy. Further surgical management of the airway may also be required (tracheostomy, stent insertion, etc.).

Tracheobronchomalacia

- May be primary or secondary
- Tracheomalacia presents with expiratory stridor and is most commonly secondary to vascular ring and/or tracheo-oesophageal fistula
- Assessed with upper airway endoscopy +/− contrast bronchography
- Surgical correction of underlying cause, tracheostomy, and stenting may be required.

Chronic lung disease

CLD is also known as bronchopulmonary dysplasia (BPD).

Definition

- Requirement for respiratory support with supplementary oxygen +/−
  mechanical ventilation >28 days, with typical CXR changes (see Fig. 7.5)
- Alternative definition often used in VLBW babies. Requirement for
  respiratory support with supplementary oxygen +/− mechanical
  ventilation >36 weeks corrected gestational age, with typical CXR
  changes.

Incidence

Incidence varies due to distribution of gestational ages in the populations
studied, as well as differences in levels of oxygenation accepted in different neonatal units. Regional studies suggest incidence may be rising due to
improving survival after extreme preterm birth.

Risk factors

- Preterm birth
- Maternal chorioamnionitis
- Severe RDS
- Prolonged PPV
- Lung over-inflation ('volutrauma')
- Hyperoxia
- Pulmonary air leak (pneumothorax and PIE)
- PDA
- postnatal sepsis
- GOR.

Presentation

- Chronic ventilator/oxygen dependence
- CXR changes: often generalized opacification of lung fields initially; then
  streaky areas of opacification; later changes in severe cases include areas
  of patchy opacification and over-inflation (see Fig. 7.5)
- Increased work of breathing
- Often have increased respiratory secretions and/or bronchospasm
- Frequent apnoea, bradycardia, and desaturation episodes
- Often have feeding difficulties and growth failure
- Other problems of extreme prematurity common (e.g.
  osteopenia, GOR)
- Severe cases at risk of developing pulmonary hypertension.

Management

- Minimize ventilator settings to avoid lung over-inflation in babies at
  risk of CLD
- Early nCPAP may reduce risk of CLD
- Avoid hyperoxia in babies at risk of developing CLD. Therefore, suggest
  aiming for oxygen saturations 90–95% and transcutaneous/arterial PO_2
  6–8 kPa, unless there is established CLD with evidence of pulmonary
  hypertension

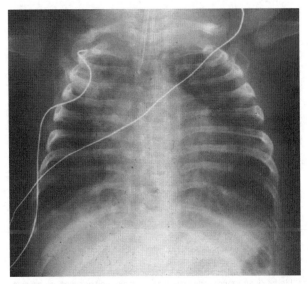

Fig. 7.5 CXR showing severe chronic lung disease with patchy areas of collapse/consolidation and lower lobe hyperinflation. Note the horizontal, poorly mineralized ribs.

- Suggest echocardiographic assessment in all oxygen dependent babies at 36 weeks gestation and maintaining oxygen saturations >95% in babies with evidence of pulmonary hypertension
- Optimize nutrition. Increased alveolar growth accompanies general growth, particularly during the 1st 1–2 years. Calorie requirement is likely to be as high as 120–150 kcal/kg/day
- Monitor for and treat metabolic bone disease of prematurity
- Treat GOR
- Start caffeine early
- Consider nebulized bronchodilators for infants with clinical evidence of lower airway obstruction. Salbutamol 2.5 mg 4–6 hourly; ipratropium bromide 62.5 µg 4–6 hourly
- Consider diuretics, particularly if evidence of excessive weight gain, or peripheral or pulmonary oedema. Results of RCTs suggest some short term benefits, but long-term benefit uncertain.

Systemic steroids (dexamethasone):
- May facilitate weaning off ventilator and reduce risk of CLD, but concern due to increased risk of adverse neurological outcomes, particularly cerebral palsy

- Consider dexamethasone in babies with severe or worsening CLD after:
  - exclusion of significant infection
  - exclusion or treatment of a significant PDA
  - consideration of treatment with diuretics
  - excluding CMV infection (urine CMV DEAFF test)
  - fully discussing possible side effects and uncertainty of benefit with parents
- A low-dose, short-course regimen may have same benefits but reduced risks, although evidence from RCTs is limited. Suggest either: dexamethasone 0.3 mg/kg/day for 3 days, then 0.2 mg/kg/day for 3 days, then 0.1 mg/kg for 3 days, then stop. Give as 2 or 3 divided doses *or* 'minidex' regime of 0.05 mg/kg/day for 10 days, then same dose on alternate days for 6 days
- Blood sugar and blood pressure should be checked at least twice daily whilst babies are receiving systemic steroids. Consider oral fungal prophylaxis during systemic steroid use.

Respiratory syncytial virus prophylaxis with monoclonal antibodies (palivizumab) reduces the risk of hospitalization in high risk cases, but is controversial because of high drug costs and need for monthly IM injections throughout the RSV season.

Discharge home on supplementary oxygen is possible for babies if:
- Oxygen requirements are stable
- There are no other acute medical concerns
- Home circumstances adequate (space for oxygen concentrator, parents able to cope, etc.)
- Equipment installed (usually after completing Home Oxygen Order Form, 'HOOF')
- Parents prepared (equipment/resuscitation training, etc.)
- Community support and follow-up arranged.

Prognosis
- Most babies discharged home on oxygen are weaned off within a few weeks. Few require oxygen beyond 1 year of age
- Readmission to hospital is common—average of two admissions in 1st 2 years
- Higher risk of adverse neurodevelopmental outcome
- Risk of recurrent cough and wheeze is increased over 1st few years
- Most have normal exercise tolerance at school age, although this may be reduced in the most severe cases.

Congenital diaphragmatic hernia

Incidence
1 in 3000 (M:F ratio 2:1).

Anatomy and pathophysiology
- 85–90% occur as a defect of the posterolateral segment (Bochdalek hernia)
- Others include anterior or Morgagni hernias, usually right-sided
- 80% of Bochdalek hernias are left-sided and the hemithorax contains herniated bowel, spleen, stomach, and often part of the left lobe of the liver (see Fig. 7.6)
- Right-sided hernias usually contain the right lobe of the liver (see Fig. 7.7)
- Significant pulmonary hypoplasia in most cases—ipsilateral > contralateral
- PPHN is common and pulmonary vasculature is hyper-responsive to hypoxia, acidosis, and hypercarbia
- Up to 50% of affected fetuses will have other associated anomalies (up to 30% in liveborn):
  - karyotype abnormalities in 30%
  - abnormalities in other systems in 40% (malrotation 20%).

Clinical features
- Usually diagnosed on routine antenatal US
- May present antenatally with polyhydramnios
- Postnatal presentation:
  - severe respiratory distress immediately after birth
  - heart sounds on right side of chest
  - absence of left-sided breath sounds
  - scaphoid abdomen
  - bowel sounds on left side of chest
- *CXR*: air-filled loops of bowel in the hemithorax with mediastinal displacement
- *Differential diagnosis*: CCAM.

Management
- *In utero* surgical repair, and tracheal plugging or ligation have been attempted. Outcomes are variable so far
- Resuscitation after birth/pre-operative management
  - intubate and commence PPV immediately after birth (avoid mask PPV)
  - pass wide-bore NG tube (8 Fr), aspirate, and then leave on free drainage
  - establish IV access, and consider early sedation and muscle relaxation
  - consider HFOV and exogenous surfactant if respiratory failure severe
  - PPHN is common and may require iNO (see ➲ Persistent pulmonary hypertension of the newborn, pp. 122–3)

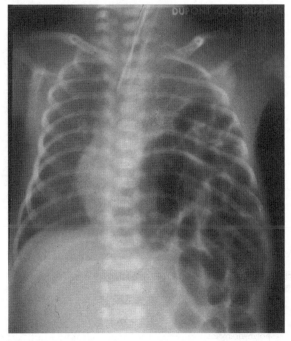

Fig. 7.6 CXR of left-sided congenital diaphragmatic hernia. This baby also had oesophageal atresia and tracheo-oesophageal fistula. Note the feeding tube coiled in the upper oesophagus.

- Surgical management:
  - surgery should be delayed until after baby stabilized
  - diaphragmatic defect closed with primary repair or synthetic patch
  - malrotation corrected if present
  - post-operative respiratory support may include HFOV, iNO, and ECMO, but no evidence for routine use of any of these.

Prognosis
- Overall mortality approximately 40%
- Survival close to 100% in cases with normal antenatal scans presenting after 1st 24 hours of life

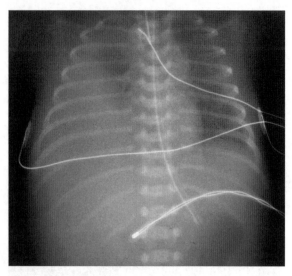

Fig. 7.7 CXR of right-sided congenital diaphragmatic hernia with liver in the right hemithorax.

- Poor prognostic indicators:
  - polyhydramnios
  - preterm birth
  - low Apgar scores
  - associated cardiac or other severe congenital abnormalities
  - poor blood gases/ventilation indices
  - large diaphragmatic defect.

Pulmonary agenesis and pulmonary hypoplasia

Pulmonary agenesis

- **Bilateral:** rare, not compatible with postnatal life
- **Unilateral:**
  - associated with other congenital abnormalities (congenital heart disease, oesophageal atresia, vertebral anomalies, etc.)
  - presents with early respiratory distress, CXR shows absent lung with compensatory hyperinflation of contralateral lung.

Pulmonary hypoplasia

Primary pulmonary hypoplasia

- Rare
- Presents soon after birth with persistent tachypnoea
- Resolves after months due to 'catch-up' lung growth.

Secondary pulmonary hypoplasia

May be due to:
- ↓ Amniotic fluid volume:
  - congenital renal abnormalities (renal agenesis, bilateral cystic dysplastic kidneys, polycystic kidney disease, posterior urethral valves)
  - preterm ROM before 26 weeks gestation; outcome usually poor if ROM <24 weeks
  - mid-trimester amniocentesis increases risk of respiratory distress in newborn and respiratory symptoms in 1st year
- Lung compression:
  - CDH
  - CCAM
  - congenital chylothorax
  - small chest syndromes (e.g. thanatophoric dwarfism, asphyxiating thoracic dystrophy)
- **Congenital neuromuscular disease:** fetal movements essential for *in utero* lung growth (e.g. congenital myotonic dystrophy, spinal muscular atrophy, congenital myopathies).

Congenital cystic adenomatoid malformation and congenital lung cysts

Congenital cystic adenomatoid malformation

- Abnormal proliferation of bronchial epithelium containing cystic and adenomatoid areas
- Three types described:
  - *type 1*: single or small number of large cysts, symptoms from compression, good prognosis
  - *type 2*: multiple small cysts, prognosis variable
  - *type 3*: solid mass, often associated with hydrops, poor prognosis
- More common in left lung and lower lobe
- May involute partially or fully either antenatally or postnatally
- Often diagnosed on antenatal US, 30% with hydrops +/− polyhydramnios
- 20% associated with other congenital anomalies
- **Variable postnatally presentation:** 50% asymptomatic, but may have severe respiratory distress requiring extensive respiratory support
- Symptomatic cases require early surgical resection
- Recurrent lower respiratory tract infection may occur in babies who initially had no symptoms; there are also reported cases of later malignant change. Therefore, surgical resection usually recommended in asymptomatic cases also.

Congenital lung cysts

- Extrapulmonary (from trachea or bronchi): commonest around carina, or
- Intrapulmonary (from alveoli)
- Usually single
- Only 10% present with neonatal respiratory symptoms, others present later in life
- Diagnosis with CXR, US, CT, MRI, or bronchoscopy.

Chylothorax and non-chylous pleural effusions

Chylothorax

- Effusion of lymph into pleural space
- Fluid contains lymphocytes and also triglycerides after milk feeds initiated. May be:
  - **primary**: congenital abnormality of pulmonary lymphatics (see Fig. 7.8). May be part of generalized lymphatic abnormality (as in Turner's syndrome and Noonan's syndrome). Diagnosis often on antenatal US scan, ↑ risk pulmonary hypoplasia
  - **secondary**: iatrogenic from cardiothoracic surgery, SVC obstruction following central venous catheter insertion, or rarely from birth trauma.

Management

- Antenatal drainage may facilitate better lung growth and easier post-natal resuscitation. Remember to seal, clamp, or remove drains immediately after birth to prevent pneumothorax
- Long-term ventilatory support and pleural drainage may be required
- Complications also occur due to chronic protein and lymphocyte loss

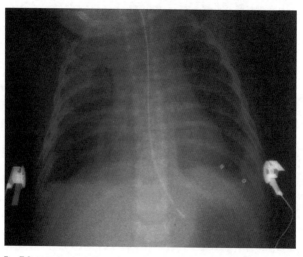

Fig. 7.8 CXR showing bilateral pleural effusions due to congenital chylothorax.

- Chyle volume may be reduced by delaying enteral feeds and using medium-chain triglyceride formula (e.g. Monogen®)
- Persistent chylous effusion may only respond to pleurodesis or ligation of thoracic duct.

Prognosis
- Variable, with mortality higher than 50% if bilateral.

Non-chylous pleural effusions

Associated with:
- Chromosomal or other congenital anomalies (e.g. CDH)
- Congenital infection (e.g. CMV, toxoplasmosis)
- As part of generalized hydrops (see ➲ Hydrops fetalis, pp. 84–6)
- Iatrogenic, associated with central venous catheter.

Management
- Antenatal intercostal drainage (as above)
- Needle thoracocentesis (send fluid for cytology, culture, and viral studies)
- Intercostal drainage if reaccumulates
- Treat underlying cause.

Prognosis
- Depends on underlying cause.

Pulmonary sequestration and congenital pulmonary lymphangiectasis

Pulmonary sequestration

- Area of lung tissue with non-pulmonary blood supply. Blood supply usually from aorta
- Usually intrathoracic (left lower lobe most common), but may be abdominal
- Usually no connection to airways
- May present antenatally as echogenic mass on US +/– polyhydramnios and/or hydrops. Antenatal regression may occur
- Only 20% present with neonatal respiratory symptoms. Others often present later with recurrent respiratory tract infection
- Other congenital malformations common (e.g. congenital heart disease, CDH)
- Postnatal diagnosis with CXR, US + Doppler studies, MRI, and angiography
- **Management**: surgical resection or catheter embolization.

Congenital pulmonary lymphangiectasis

- Cystic dilatation of pulmonary lymphatics with lymphatic obstruction
- Usually bilateral and generalized, associated with severe neonatal respiratory failure
- Three subtypes:
  - associated with generalized lymphangiectasis, with hydrops
  - associated with congenital heart disease
  - confined to lung only (occurs in Turner's, Noonan's, and Down syndromes)
- CXR appearance with generalized opacification of lung fields with prominent lymphatics +/– pleural effusions
- Confirmation only possible histologically on lung biopsy or post-mortem specimen
- **Prognosis** poor.

Congenital abnormalities of surfactant, congenital lobar emphysema, and ciliary dyskinesia

Congenital abnormalities of surfactant

- Rare presentation of severe respiratory distress in term babies, associated with abnormalities of surfactant proteins (B or C) or production and secretion of surfactant (ABCA3 mutations)
- Treatment with exogenous surfactant usually leads to temporary improvement
- CXR appearance similar to severe RDS
- Diagnosis confirmed with:
  - *lung biopsy*: electron microscopy shows abnormality of lamellar bodies in type 2 pneumocytes
  - *genetic studies*: various mutations described, associated with:
    —surfactant protein B deficiency—autosomal recessive
    —surfactant protein C deficiency—autosomal dominant or sporadic
    —ABCA3 mutations—autosomal recessive.

Management
- Ventilatory support until diagnosis confirmed
- Lung transplantation has been successful in limited number of patients when this has been available
- Genetic counselling for parents.

Prognosis
- Very poor in most cases
- 50% 5-year survival reported following lung transplantation.

Congenital lobar emphysema
- Over-inflation of affected lobe
- Usually affects upper lobes (L > R)
- 15–20% cases associated with vascular abnormalities → compression of large airways
- Presents with respiratory distress, chest asymmetry, and absence of breath sounds in affected area
- **CXR:** hyperinflation of affected lobe with compression of adjacent lobes and contralateral lung with mediastinal shift
- CT/MRI scan, ventilation-perfusion scan, and bronchoscopy may be useful.

Management
- Surgical correction of vascular abnormalities, if present, lobectomy in some cases. Bronchoscopy may relieve symptoms.

Ciliary dyskinesia

- Incidence 1 in 15,000
- Various abnormalities of ciliary structure and function occur (commonest—absence of dynein arms of outer microtubular doublets)
- Neonatal respiratory symptoms occur in >60% cases—persistent respiratory distress, pneumonia, ↑ nasal secretions +/− dextrocardia
- Diagnosis confirmed from nasal epithelium brush biopsy sample.

Prognosis

- Recurrent respiratory tract infections, sinusitis, and otitis media in childhood; bronchiectasis common by late childhood.

Bronchiolitis on the neonatal unit

- Bronchiolitis (viral lower respiratory tract infection of the terminal bronchioles) may cause severe illness in neonates. Ex-preterm infants with chronic lung disease are particularly at risk
- Seasonal occurrence (October–March), but may occur any time of year
- Infection transmitted via droplets from the respiratory tract (usually from sibling, parent, or staff member) either in the air or on hands
- Caused by RSV (most common), adenovirus, influenza A and B, parainfluenza 1, 2, and 3, and human meta-pneumovirus
- Once infected, likelihood of hospitalization due to bronchiolitis and pneumonia due to RSV is 25% for premature infants (<33 weeks) without CLD and higher for those with CLD.

Clinical features

- Coryza
- Pyrexia
- Respiratory distress or ↑ O_2 requirement in CLD
- Cough
- Apnoea
- Inspiratory crackles +/− expiratory wheeze
- Hyperinflation on CXR.

Diagnosis

Confirmed with nasopharyngeal aspirate or ETT secretion immunofluorescence (most virology laboratories only test for RSV, influenza A & B, parainfluenza, and adenovirus).

Management

- Isolate or cohort affected patients
- Respiratory support as required
- Fluid/nutritional support as required
- No evidence to support routine use of antiviral therapy.

Prevention

- Avoid contact with individuals with coryzal symptoms (staff and family members)
- Strict hand hygiene probably the most important preventive measure— staff, visitors, family
- Isolation/cohorting of affected patients.

Prophylaxis with palivizumab

- Recombinant humanized mouse monoclonal antibody against the RSV F protein (neutralizing antibody that prevents RSV fusing with cell membranes)
- RCT evidence (IMpact trial) suggests 55% reduction in hospital admissions in high risk babies (preterm <36 weeks or CLD), but:
  - number needed to treat to prevent each hospital admission = 17
  - no evidence of ↓ mortality or less severe disease in patients requiring ventilatory support

- requires monthly IM injections during RSV season
- very expensive and probably not cost effective if same group of patients treated as in IMpact trial
- UK Department of Health recommends giving palivizumab for babies with moderate or severe BPD with compatible CXR changes who had required supplementary oxygen or respiratory support at 36 weeks corrected gestational age, according to their age and gestational age at birth as shown in Table 7.1. Policy in most other European countries and North America is to recommend more liberal use of palivizumab.
- RSV prophylaxis should also be considered for other 'high risk' babies (e.g. congenital heart disease, cystic fibrosis, immune deficiency) if discharged from hospital during the RSV season.

Table 7.1 UK Department of Health recommended chronological age and gestational age at birth for babies with moderate or severe bronchopulmonary dysplasia requiring palivizumab. Shaded areas in table indicate babies that should receive palivizumab

Chronological age (months)	Gestational age at birth (weeks)						
	≤24	24^{+1}–26	26^{+1}–28	28^{+1}–30	30^{+1}–32	32^{+1}–34	≥34^{+1}
< 1.5							
1.5–3							
3–6							
6–9							
>9							

Further information

Rennie JM (ed.). Congenital malformations of the respiratory tract. In: Rennie JM. (ed.) *Rennie & Roberton's Textbook of Neonatology*, 5th ed. pp. 1259–1292. Churchill Livingstone, London, 2012.

Rojas-Reyes MX, Morley CJ, Soll R. Prophylactic versus selective use of surfactant in preventing morbidity and mortality in preterm infants. Cochrane Library, 2012. DOI: 10.1002/14651858. CD000510.pub2

RSV. Green Book, Chapter 27a v2.0. (2015) ℜ www.gov.uk/government/uploads/system/uploads/attachment_data/file/458469/Green_Book_Chapter_27a_v2_0W.PDF

Respiratory support

Aims of respiratory support in neonates

- Maintain adequate gas exchange
- Minimize risk of lung injury (ventilator-induced lung injury (VILI))
- Minimize haemodynamic impairment
- Avoid injury to other organs (brain, kidneys, gut)
- Reduce work of breathing.

Oxygen

- Supplementary oxygen may be delivered to unventilated babies via:
  - incubator (if FiO_2 <0.25)
  - headbox
  - nasal cannulae (either low- or high-flow oxygen). **NB** Use correct sized cannulae for babies of different weight
- Results of randomized controlled trials (RCTs) comparing maintenance of oxygen saturations (SpO_2) of 85–89% (low) to 90–95% (high) in oxygen-dependent babies <28 weeks gestation suggest that:
  - mortality and necrotizing enterocolitis are significantly *increased* in low compared to high SpO_2 targets
  - severe retinopathy of prematurity (ROP) is significantly *reduced* in low compared to high SpO_2 targets
  - there were no differences for bronchopulmonary dysplasia (BPD)/ chronic lung disease (CLD), brain injury, or PDA between the groups
  - based on these results, it is suggested that SpO_2 should be targeted to 90–95% in babies <28 weeks at birth and up to 36 weeks corrected gestational age
- Fluctuations in SpO_2 are associated with ↑ risk of ROP, therefore should be avoided
- Optimal levels of oxygenation for ventilated or unventilated oxygen dependent babies >28 weeks at birth are uncertain
- SpO_2 levels >95% should probably be avoided in babies at risk of ROP or CLD.

Low-flow oxygen

- Oxygen delivered by nasal cannualae with flow rate <1 l/min.

High-flow oxygen

- Also known as heated humidified high-flow (HHHF) or high-flow nasal cannula (HFNC) respiratory support
- Devices such as Vapotherm™ and Optiflow™ deliver air or blended oxygen/air with flow rate 2–7 l/min. (**NB** usually start at ~5 l/min and wean as tolerated)
- HFNC can be used to provide high concentrations of oxygen and may deliver positive end-expiratory pressure (PEEP), ↓ nasal resistance, 'washout' dead space, and ↑ compliance to improve gas exchange
- Gas mixture is warmed and humidified (usually to saturation vapour pressure) →↓ risk of mucosal injury and nosocomial infection and energy expenditure
- HFNC support for babies ≥28 weeks gestation compared to nasal continuous positive airway pressure (nCPAP)
  - → no difference in intubation rates, time in oxygen, airleak, or BPD/ CLD when used for post-extubation or early initial noninvasive support
  - may →↓ risk of nasal trauma
  - may facilitate suck feeding and kangaroo care and be better tolerated
  - evidence for weaning strategy from HFNC support is limited but usually → low-flow oxygen when flow weaned → 2–3 l/min.

Continuous positive airways pressure and nasal intermittent positive pressure ventilation

Benefits of continuous positive airways pressure (CPAP)

- Maintains functional residual capacity by preventing alveolar collapse during expiration
- Stabilizes chest wall
- Maintains upper airway and prevents mixed and obstructive apnoea.

CPAP and intermittent positive pressure ventilation (IPPV) delivery

- **Endotracheal tube (ETT) CPAP**: not usually recommended due to significant work of breathing to overcome resistance of tube. If ever used should only be in bigger babies with ETT size >3–3.5 mm
- **Facemask CPAP**: not usually recommended in small preterm babies due to practical difficulties maintaining seal around mask and risk of peri/intra-ventricular and cerebellar haemorrhage
- **Single nasopharyngeal prong (npCPAP/nplPPV)**: via a shortened ETT placed in the naso-pharynx
- **Short bi-nasal prongs or nasal mask (nCPAP/nIPPV)**: This is the most commonly used method of CPAP/IPPV delivery in small, preterm babies and is more effective than npCPAP/nplPPV. One recently published study suggests that nasal masks may ↓ reintubation rates further
- **Nasal injury**: particularly to the nasal septum of extremely preterm babies is a relatively common concern. The risk of this can be reduced with softer, better fitting patient interfaces and appropriate skin care.

CPAP/IPPV generation

- **Ventilator**: may not deliver constant level of distending pressure due to leakage around attachment and via the baby's mouth
- **Underwater seal 'bubble' circuit**: may increase efficiency of gas exchange due to bubbles causing vibrations of baby's chest
- **Flow driver device**: limits variations in distending pressure by changing direction of high-pressure jet with changes in nasal airway pressure according to phase of baby's respiratory cycle ('Choanda' effect).

Evidence from RCTs comparing different CPAP/IPPV systems is limited, but suggests that a flow driver or bubble circuit attached to bi-nasal prongs or nasal mask is likely to be more efficient.

nCPAP pressure levels

- Pressure required varies according to the size of the baby and underlying lung pathology—a term baby or baby with respiratory distress syndrome (RDS) may require 6–8 cmH_2O, whereas a preterm baby with minimal lung disease needing nCPAP for apnoea may require 5–6 cmH_2O
- nCPAP pressure too low→↑risk of atelectasis and need for reintubation
- nCPAP pressure too high→CO_2 retention, ↑ risk of pneumothorax and CLD.

Nasal intermittent positive pressure ventilation (nIPPV)

- nIPPV = nCPAP + intermittent positive pressure 'breaths' via short bi-nasal prongs or nasal mask
- Used as an intermediate level of respiratory support between mechanical ventilation and nCPAP
- May enhance the level of respiratory support by:
  - ↑ minute ventilation (→↓ $PaCO_2$)
  - ↑ mean airway pressure (→↑ PaO_2)
  - 'washout' of upper airway anatomical dead space (→↓ $PaCO_2$)
  - ↓ work of breathing
  - ↓ inspiratory chest wall distortion
  - ↑ respiratory drive (→↓ $PaCO_2$ and ↑ PaO_2)
- Nasal bi-level positive airway pressure (nBiPAP) is a form of nIPPV with intermittent positive pressure 'breaths' 2–3 cmH_2O above the level of CPAP
- nIPPV with patient-triggered modes may provide further clinical advantages. These include new technologies such as neurally adjusted ventilator assist (NAVA), where a diaphragmatic electromyography (EMG) signal determines the timing of supported breaths and peak inspiratory pressure (PIP).

Early nCPAP in preterm babies

- In non-randomized, cohort studies with historical controls, nCPAP immediately after birth is associated with:
  - ↓need for intubation
  - ↓use of surfactant
  - ↓incidence of CLD
- Recent RCT evidence (COIN trial) suggests that early nCPAP (started within 5 minutes of birth) in babies 25–28 weeks gestation →
  - no difference in mortality or CLD at 36 weeks corrected gestational age
  - 46% of babies initially on nCPAP requiring intubation over first 5 days
  - halving of surfactant use
  - significant ↑ incidence of pneumothorax (9% vs. 3%). Long-term outcomes from the COIN trial are awaited.

nCPAP and nIPPV following mechanical ventilation in preterm babies

- nCPAP → ↓ reintubation rates in preterm babies following mechanical ventilation
- CPAP pressure should be ≥5 cmH_2O
- Evidence regarding the best weaning strategy is limited but there appears to be no advantage to 'cycling' on and off CPAP or nIPPV prior to discontinuation
- nIPPV is likely to be more effective than nCPAP with:
  - ↓ apnoea
  - ↓ reintubation
  - ↓ BPD/CLD.

Conventional ventilation

Indications

- Respiratory disease
- For circulatory support
- Peri- or post-operative
- Failure of central respiratory drive (e.g. apnoea, convulsions, iatrogenic).

Ventilatory strategy

May be determined by:
- Indication for ventilatory support
- Underlying lung condition
- Gestation/size of baby
- Need to minimize the risk of VILI
- Need to minimize risk of other organ damage (e.g. avoid hyperoxia in babies at risk of ROP; avoid hypocarbia due to risk of PVL)
- Therefore, guidelines for ventilating babies are not necessarily absolute indications and are likely to vary locally
- Most babies require intubation and ventilatory support if:
  - arterial PaO_2 <6.0 kPa, with FiO_2 >0.5–0.6
  - $PaCO_2$ >7.5 kPa (not applicable in a baby with CLD who is compensating)
  - arterial pH <7.20 if mainly respiratory
  - insufficient respiratory drive for any reason
  - significant circulatory failure (e.g. baby with hypoplastic left heart with poor perfusion and worsening acidosis).

Once intubated and ventilated

Oxygenation is dependent on mean airway pressure (MAP), which can be derived from:

$$MAP = PEEP + \{(PIP - PEEP) \times [Ti/(Ti + Te)]\}$$

Thus, MAP (and oxygenation) can be improved by:
- ↑ PIP
- ↑ PEEP
- ↑ Inspiratory time (Ti).

Carbon dioxide clearance is dependent on alveolar ventilation, which is proportional to:
- Tidal volume (VT)—increased by:
  - ↑ PIP
  - ↓PEEP
  - ↑ Ti
- Minute volume (MV)—increased by:
  - ↑ ventilator rate.

Suggested initial ventilator settings

- PIP should be just great enough to produce adequate chest inflation or VT >5–6 ml/kg.
- PEEP 4–6 cmH$_2$O
- Ti 0.35–0.4 s
- Rate initially 60/min in preterm infant with surfactant deficiency (**NB** Ventilator rate should usually be decreased after administration of surfactant)
- FiO$_2$: adjust to maintain O$_2$ saturation. 90–95% in preterm infants <28 at birth and up to 36 weeks corrected gestational age; >90% in more mature infants with saturations in upper 90s if there is known to be pulmonary hypertension (see ⮕ Persistent pulmonary hypertension of the newborn, pp. 122–3).

Subsequent modifications to ventilator settings

To improve oxygenation

- ↑ FiO$_2$ (**NB** At high concentrations O$_2$ is likely to be toxic and may increase atelectasis)
- ↑ PEEP to 6–8 cmH$_2$O (**NB** This may also →↑PaCO$_2$)
- ↑ PIP (may increase risk of baro-/volutrauma)
- Increase Ti
- Consider surfactant
- Synchronize ventilator inspiration with baby's own spontaneous inspiratory effort (patient-triggered ventilation)
- Increase sedation if 'fighting' ventilator or baby looks uncomfortable
- Consider muscle relaxant (e.g. pancuronium or vecuronium)
- Consider high frequency oscillatory ventilation (HFOV) (see ⮕ High frequency oscillatory ventilation, pp. 160–1).

To ↑ CO$_2$ clearance

- Consider suction or change ETT if possibly blocked/coated with secretions
- ↑ Ventilator rate
- ↓PEEP
- ↑ PIP
- ↓System dead space (shorten ETT)
- Consider HFOV.

Other considerations in ventilated babies

- Ensure adequate monitoring (transcutaneous and blood gases, etc., see ⮕ Routine monitoring, p. 54)
- Ensure adequate sedation/analgesia
- Ensure adequate humidification of ventilator circuit.

Patient-triggered ventilation

- Ventilator senses patient's inspiratory effort and delivers a positive pressure breath, thereby synchronizing patient and ventilator inspiration
- Airway flow or pressure, or abdominal movement may be used by different ventilators to detect patient inspiratory effort and trigger positive pressure breath
- Critical trigger level (trigger threshold) must be reached in order for each positive pressure breath to be delivered
- A 'back-up' ventilator rate is set so that positive pressure breaths continue to be delivered if the baby is apnoeic or has insufficient inspiratory effort to exceed trigger threshold.

Advantages of PTV

- Better synchrony with patient breaths may help to ↓patient discomfort
- Oxygenation may improve
- Possible ↓ risk of air leak
- ↓ work of breathing
- ↓ duration of ventilation

There are two basic types of PTV (see also ⊃ Pressure support ventilation, p. 157):
- *Assist-control (A/C)*: also called synchronized intermittent positive pressure ventilation (SIPPV) or PTV depending on ventilator manufacturer. A positive pressure breath is delivered each time the patient's own inspiratory effort exceeds the trigger threshold
- *Synchronized intermittent mandatory ventilation (SIMV)*: the number of positive pressure breaths are preset. Any spontaneous breaths above the set rate will not be ventilator assisted.

There is no evidence that weaning from ventilation is better with A/C compared with SIMV unless ventilator rate is <20/min.

Ventilator settings on PTV

- ↓Ti to <0.4 s (but not <0.2 s)
- ↑Trigger sensitivity so that the baby's inspiratory efforts trigger ventilator positive pressure breaths (**NB** If trigger sensitivity is set too high, 'autotriggering' may occur)
- Set back-up rate (rate of positive pressure breaths on SIMV). This should be >20/min. A back-up rate significantly >40/min will not allow sufficient time between back-up ventilator breaths for the baby to generate triggered breaths
- If hypocapnia occurs on A/C, consider reducing PIP or, if already on low PIP, consider switching to low rate SIMV (not <20/min) or extubation.

Proportional assist ventilation (PAV)

- PAV is a newer mode of PTV where the ventilator pressure is servo-controlled during spontaneous breaths
- PIP is servo-controlled according to the baby's lung physiology by:
  - VT change (compliance load) → elastic unloading
  - flow change (resistance load) → resistive unloading
- Early trials suggest that PAV may improve oxygenation and ↓ work of breathing.

Pressure support ventilation

PSV is a form of patient-triggered ventilation.
- Positive-pressure breaths (at preset PIP) are triggered by the baby's inspiratory effort
- Inspiratory time limited by end of spontaneous breath
- Operator can control when positive pressure ventilator breath is terminated by adjusting percentage of maximum inspiratory flow (as inspiratory flow reduces, having already reached maximum) before this can occur. This is usually when inspiratory flow decreases to <25% maximum, towards the end of spontaneous inspiratory effort
- Long-term outcomes for preterm babies on PSV have not yet been assessed.

Volume-targeted ventilation

- With conventional ventilation—pressure-limited, time-cycled (PLTC):
  - PIP is constant, unless adjusted by operator
  - tidal volume (VT) varies from breath to breath as lung physiology (compliance and resistance) changes
- This may increase the risk of ventilator-induced lung injury by leading to:
  - hyperinflation ('volutrauma')
  - atelectasis ('atelectotrauma')
- With volume-targeted ventilation, VT is controlled by the operator by selecting desired VT
- PIP is automatically adjusted so that set VT is delivered
- In the past, volume-targeted ventilation was technically more difficult in small, preterm babies due to:
  - loss of gas volume in ventilator circuit and humidifier due to compression and compliance of ventilator tubing
  - loss of gas volume due to leak around uncuffed ETT
  - inability to deliver extremely small volumes.

Advances in ventilator technology have resulted in new modes enabling more accurate delivery of 'targeted' volumes.

Clinical trials have suggested that volume-targeted ventilation may:
- Produce effective gas exchange with lower ventilator pressures
- ↓Hypocarbia
- ↓Excessive VT
- ↓Pneumothorax
- ↓Severe intraventricular haemorrhage (IVH)
- ↓Ventilator days
- ↓BPD
- ↓Mortality in babies <1000 g.

Ventilator settings on volume-targeted ventilation

- Suggest starting with VT ~5 ml/kg
- Adjust VT in 0.5 ml/kg steps according to $PaCO_2$
- Higher VT (up to 6–8 ml/kg) may be required in babies <750 g (due to dead space, mainly because of the relative size of the flow sensor) and babies with CLD (due to dead space because of airway stretching and ventilation/perfusion (V/Q) mismatching)
- Adjust PIP_{max} (i.e. PIP that will not be exceeded even if desired VT is not reached) to approximately 20% of working PIP
- Use with A/C, rather than SIMV.

High frequency oscillatory ventilation

HFOV = Ventilator rates >150/min (usually 10–15 Hz).
  Differs from conventional ventilation as:
- Tidal volumes very small (may be <50% dead space)
- Gas exchange enhanced by facilitated diffusion and ↓ turbulence
- Active expiratory phase may occur. This may improve CO_2 clearance further and help reduce risk of gas trapping
- There is no strong evidence to support the use of HFOV routinely (i.e. 'prophylactically' in all ventilated preterm babies)
- HFOV usually used as a 'rescue' method in babies with severe respiratory failure
- Consider using HFOV if:
  - blood gases/oxygenation poor on optimal conventional ventilation
  - severe lung disease (severe RDS, pulmonary hypoplasia (including diaphragmatic hernia), persistent pulmonary hypertension of the newborn (PPHN), or other bilateral homogeneous changes on chest X-ray (CXR).

Starting a baby on HFOV

- Check ventilator and circuit before attaching to patient
- Set bias flow to level recommended by ventilator manufacturer (e.g. 20 l/min for SensorMedics 3100A®). This setting rarely needs to be changed
- Set frequency. This should usually be 10 Hz and rarely needs to be changed
- Set inspiratory time/I:E ratio. This may vary according to local guidelines. Recommended I:E ratio is usually between 1:1 and 1:2
- Set MAP:
  - ↑ MAP →↑lung volume ('recruitment')→ improved oxygenation
  - ↓MAP if lungs hyperinflated on CXR
  - usually start with 'high volume strategy' (unless lungs already hyperinflated or pulmonary interstitial emphysema on CXR) by setting MAP to 2 cmH_2O above that used on conventional ventilation. Start MAP at 6–8 cmH_2O for babies being oscillated from the outset
  - ↑ MAP in 1–2 cmH_2O steps to improve oxygenation if CXR suggests low lung volumes or until FiO_2 stabilizes
  - check degree of lung inflation on CXR. This should normally be done within 1 hour of starting baby on HFOV and may be required up to 6-hourly subsequently in unstable patients
  - worsening oxygenation may indicate lung hyperinflation, or pneumothorax (cold light examination may not be reliable on HFOV)—urgent CXR required
  - hyperinflation should be managed by disconnecting ETT from ventilator for 1–2 s and then restarting HFOV after decreasing MAP by 2–4 cmH_2O
  - set amplitude (also called delta pressure or ΔP) to a level that produces visible vibration/oscillation of the baby's chest wall
  - ΔP controls CO_2 removal. Increase ΔP to decrease PCO_2 and vice versa

- usually start with ΔP 20–30 cmH_2O depending on the size of the baby and severity of lung disease
- adjust ΔP in 5 cmH_2O steps according to the degree of chest wall vibration, arterial gas PCO_2, or $TcPCO_2$.
- occasionally in severe lung disease, PCO_2 may remain high despite high ΔP. Decreasing frequency to 8 Hz may then be beneficial ($\rightarrow\uparrow$ tidal exchange)
- ensure adequate humidification of ventilator circuit
- avoid disconnection of the ventilator circuit (unless done to manage hyperinflation. Use of 'in-line' suction system usually recommended
- ensure adequate monitoring:
  —pulse oximetry
  —$TcPO_2$ and $TcPCO_2$
  —arterial line for continuous BP monitoring and frequent blood gases.

Weaning from HFOV

- Wean FiO_2 first. When FiO_2 is down to 0.3–0.4, wean MAP in steps of 1–2 cmH_2O
- Wean ΔP by steps of 5 cmH_2O according to PCO_2. Occasionally, even at very low ΔP, the PCO_2 is still too low. In this case increase frequency to 12–15 Hz, which will reduce tidal volume, or consider changing to conventional ventilation or even extubation
- Once MAP is <10–12 cmH_2O, with low amplitude (<20–25 cmH_2O), consider changing to conventional ventilation or wean further on HFOV
- If MAP is <6–8 cmH_2O and low amplitude (<15–20 cmH_2O) consider extubation.

Extracorporeal membrane oxygenation

- Extracorporeal membrane oxygenation (ECMO) is a form of cardiopulmonary bypass used in neonates with severe respiratory and/or circulatory failure. Venous blood is removed from circulation, oxygenated via a silicone membrane, then returned to circulation
- ECMO may be either:
    - *veno-arterial (VA)*—blood removed from superior vena cava (SVC), oxygenated, then pumped into right carotid artery. Used if circulatory as well as respiratory support required
    - *veno-venous (VV)*—blood removed and replaced via SVC. Used if respiratory support only is required
    - both VV and VA ECMO require large surgically-placed neck catheters. These are connected to a heparinized circuit as shown in Fig. 8.1
- Indications for ECMO in neonates include recoverable, severe respiratory failure that is refractory to other conventional management, and severe heart disease, either pre- or post-operatively, for example:
    - meconium aspiration syndrome (MAS)
    - PPHN
    - congenital pneumonia
    - myocardial failure associated with sepsis
    - pre- or post-operative congenital heart disease surgery
    - pre-cardiac transplantation (very unusual in neonates)
- Referral for ECMO should be considered early in severe respiratory or circulatory failure if:
    - OI >40
    - OI = mean airway pressure × FiO$_2$ (as %)/PO$_2$ (in kPa) × 7.6
    - >34 weeks corrected gestational age
    - >2 kg—due to technical difficulties (line insertion, clotting problems, etc.) small, preterm babies are not usually considered for ECMO

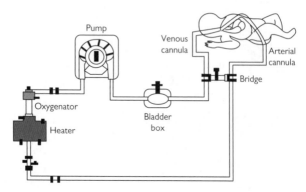

Fig. 8.1 VA ECMO circuit.

- reversible underlying cardiorespiratory disease (e.g. MAS, PPHN, severe surfactant deficiency, congenital pneumonia, CDH)
  - <10 days high-pressure ventilation
  - no lethal congenital abnormalities
  - no significant intracranial haemorrhage (i.e. > grade 1 IVH)
- The best outcomes with ECMO in patients with single organ failure, early in the disease (e.g. term infants with MAS or PPHN). Worse outcomes have been experienced with babies with pulmonary hypoplasia (e.g. secondary to congenital diaphragmatic hernia).

Possible complications of ECMO

- Haemodynamic:
  - hypotension
  - hypertension
  - haemorrhage (e.g. IVH, from wound sites, from circuit)
  - circuit failure
- Haematological:
  - coagulopathy
  - thrombocytopenia
  - RBC fragmentation
- Sepsis
- Vascular (e.g. damage to the right carotid artery)—surprisingly this is usually well tolerated
- ECMO circuit malfunction (e.g. oxygenator failure, clots/air bubbles in circuit, leaks).

Tracheostomy

Indications for tracheostomy in neonates

- Congenital anomalies
    - Pierre–Robin sequence
    - laryngomalacia (severe)
    - vascular 'rings'
    - large airway/extrinsic haemangiomas
    - cystic hygroma
    - airway papillomata
    - congenital tracheomalacia
    - tracheal stenosis
    - long-term ventilation for congenital neuromuscular or lower respiratory tract disease
- Acquired
    - subglottic stenosis
    - tracheobronchomalacia
    - bilateral vocal cord palsy
    - laryngeal trauma from long-term ventilation.

Care of baby with tracheostomy

- Immediately post-operatively use CXR to check tracheostomy tube position, and exclude pneumothorax, atelectasis, and assess lung inflation (if ventilated). Ensure stay sutures are taped securely to chest
- If ventilated, higher ventilator pressures may be required if large leak around tracheostomy tube
- Adequately humidify ventilator gases or use 'Swedish nose' in self-ventilating babies in order to decrease risk of tube blockage with dried secretions. Change air filter/humidifier as necessary
- Airway suction as required. Use suction pressure of 8–10 cmH$_2$O via a suction catheter 2× tracheostomy tube size (e.g. for a 3.5 mm tracheostomy tube, use a size 7 FG suction catheter). Record length of the tracheostomy tube and avoid advancing suction catheter beyond this
- Ensure equipment available (including spare appropriate-sized tracheostomy tubes) and staff adequately trained to manage airway in an emergency
- In a newly-formed tracheostomy, for emergency recannulation, pull stay sutures forward and down to open stoma, and re-insert new tracheostomy tube
- Check tracheostomy tapes twice daily for neck swelling, tightness and security
- Delay first tube change until 1 week (if possible) to facilitate tracheostomy 'tract' development (should be carried out by experienced neonatal unit medical staff or ENT team)
- Subsequent tracheostomy tube changes should usually be weekly
- Ensure at least two experienced members of staff are present for any tracheostomy tube change.

Complications related to tracheostomy

- Accidental tube displacement
- Tube occlusion
- Large leak around tube
- False passage formation due to failed recannulation
- Massive haemorrhage (rare)
- Surgical emphysema
- Wound infection (meticillin-resistant *Staphylococcus aureus*, etc.)
- Respiratory tract infection
- Respiratory tract trauma.

Prognosis in babies with tracheostomy

- Decannulation should be as early as possible following resolution of airway/lung/neurological condition or corrective surgery, following endoscopic assessment
- Mortality due to tracheostomy-related complications approximately 3%
- Speech and language delay relatively common (worse with prolonged tracheostomy placement).

Home oxygen

Indications for neonatal long-term/home oxygen therapy

- Chronic lung disease of prematurity/bronchopulmonary dysplasia (commonest indication)
- Other neonatal lung disease (e.g. pulmonary hypoplasia)
- Pulmonary hypertension secondary to lung or heart disease
- Sleep-related disorders of breathing
- Neuromuscular disease
- Chest wall deformities.

Discharge home on supplementary oxygen is possible if
- Oxygen requirements are stable and usually <0.5 l/min flow rate
- There are no other acute medical concerns (e.g. apnoea, frequent desaturations, temperature instability, sepsis)
- Home circumstances adequate (space for oxygen concentrator, parents able to cope, etc.)
- Equipment installed (usually after completing Home Oxygen Order Form (HOOF) in UK)
- Parents prepared (equipment/resuscitation training, etc.)
- Community nursing support and medical/multidisciplinary follow-up arranged.

Aims of long-term/home oxygen
- Prevention of hypoxaemia
- Prevention of hypoxia induced pulmonary hypertension
- Increase potential for normal growth and development
- May reduce risk of SIDS.

Equipment required
- Large (static) oxygen cylinders
- Lightweight ambulatory oxygen cylinders
- Low-flow nasal cannula tubing.

Prior to discontinuing continuous oxygen saturation (SpO_2) monitoring and arranging discharge, objective assessment of oxygen requirement is made by analysis of download from 12-hour (usually overnight) SpO_2 study:
- Trace should be relatively artefact free
- Mean SpO_2 should be ≥95%
- <5% of trace should have SpO_2 <90%
- Repeat study after discharge home (usually within 48 hours), then at regular intervals (usually weekly) to wean oxygen.

Further information

De Paoli AG, Davis PG, Faber B, Morley CJ. Devices and pressure sources for administration of nasal continuous positive airway pressure (NCPAP) in preterm neonates. *Cochrane Database Syst Rev* 2002: CD002977.

Greenough A, Dimitriou G, Prendergast M, Milner AD. Synchronized mechanical ventilation for respiratory support in newborn infants. *Cochrane Database Syst Rev* 2008; **1**: CD000456.

Johnson AH, Peacock JL, Greenough A, et al. High frequency oscillatory ventilation for the prevention of chronic lung disease of prematurity. *N Engl J Med* 2002; **347**: 633–642.

Morley CJ, Davis PG, Doyle LW, Brion LP, Hascoet JM, Carlin JB. COIN Trial Investigators. Nasal CPAP or intubation at birth for very preterm infants. *N Engl J Med* 2008; **358**: 700–708.

Peng W1, Zhu H, Shi H, Liu E. Volume-targeted ventilation is more suitable than pressure-limited ventilation for preterm infants: a systematic review and meta-analysis. *Arch Dis Child Fetal Neonatal Ed* 2014; **99**: F158–165.

Saugstad OD, Aune D. Optimal oxygenation of extremely low birth weight infants: A meta-analysis and systematic review of the oxygen saturation target studies. *Neonatology* 2014; **105**: 55–63.

Sweet DG, Carnielli V, Greisen G, et al. European Consensus Guidelines on the Management of Neonatal Respiratory Distress Syndrome in Preterm Infants: 2013 Update. *Neonatology* 2013; **103**: 353–368.

UK Collaborative ECMO Trial Group. UK collaborative randomized trial of neonatal extracorporeal membrane oxygenation. *Lancet* 1996; **384**: 75–82.

Wilkinson D, Andersen C, O'Donnell CP, De Paoli AG. High flow nasal cannula for respiratory support in preterm infants. *Cochrane Database Syst Rev.* 2011: CD006405.

Cardiovascular problems

Fetal circulation and changes at birth

A basic understanding of the fetal circulation and the changes that occur following birth are valuable when considering the consequences of congenital heart defects and their management (see Figs. 9.1 and 9.2).

Fetal circulation

The fetal circulation differs from the postnatal circulation in three important ways (Fig. 9.1):

- Oxygenated blood enters the circulation from the placenta
- Pulmonary blood flow accounts for less than 20% of total cardiac output due to high pulmonary vascular resistance
- Five fetal vascular structures exist to direct blood flow:
  - *ductus arteriosus* connects the pulmonary artery to the aorta and shunts blood right to left, thereby diverting flow away from the fetal lungs that are filled with fluid
  - *foramen ovale* is a communication that directs blood flow returning to the right atrium through the septal wall into the left atrium thus bypassing the lungs
  - *ductus venosus* receives oxygenated blood from the umbilical vein, and directs it to the inferior vena cava and right atrium, thus bypassing the liver
  - *two umbilical arteries* carry deoxygenated blood to the placenta and the *umbilical vein* carries oxygenated blood from the placenta.

Circulatory changes following birth

Starting from birth and continuing over the first few days of life, the circulation undergoes several physiological changes:

- The lungs inflate and lung fluid is absorbed and expelled leading to increased oxygen tension and decreased pulmonary vascular resistance allowing *increased pulmonary blood flow*
- Increased pulmonary blood flow and increased pulmonary venous return causes increased right atrial pressure, and the flap valve of the *foramen ovale closes* thus separating the right and left atria
- The *ductus arteriosus closes* soon after birth as the surrounding smooth muscle constricts in response to increased oxygen tension and fall in prostaglandins. Functional closure is complete within 60 hours in the vast majority of term newborns
- The *ductus venosus closes* as blood flow dwindles in the umbilical vein following umbilical cord clamping.

Physiological closure of fetal structures in certain types of congenital heart disease (CHD) may lead to deterioration in the infant's clinical condition (e.g. closure of the ductus arteriosus leading to collapse in a duct dependent circulation).

Clinical problems are also seen when fetal structures remain patent beyond the immediate postnatal period (e.g. persistent ductus arteriosus leading to heart failure).

Duct dependent circulation: structural or functional CHD where the pulmonary or systemic circulation is supplied solely by flow through the ductus arteriosus and not the corresponding ventricular outflow tract.

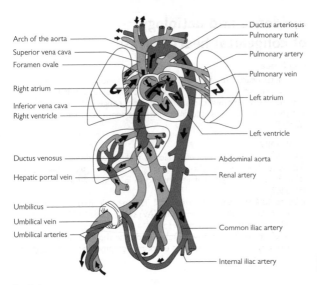

Fig. 9.1 Fetal circulation.

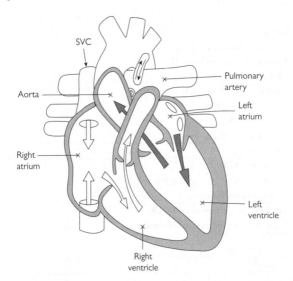

Fig. 9.2 Normal heart structure. Dark arrows: oxygenated blood flow; white arrows: deoxygenated blood flow.

Incidence and aetiology of congenital heart disease

Incidence

Congenital heart disease is relatively common, with an incidence around 8/1000 live births, and accounts for 10–30% of all congenital anomalies. CHD is the commonest cause of death from congenital anomalies in the first year of life. There is little difference in incidence between racial groups (Table 9.1).

Aetiology

Many genetic and environmental factors make heart disease more likely and these should be sought when taking the history (see Table 9.2 and Table 9.3). Specific gene defects are known in almost all the conditions in Table 9.2.

- Up to 40% of infants with trisomy 21 (Down syndrome) will have a cardiac defect, with atrioventricular (AV) septal defects (45%) and VSDs (35%) accounting for 80% of these.
- Therefore, all newborns with Down syndrome should undergo a full cardiology assessment, including echocardiography, even if they appear asymptomatic

Table 9.1 Types of CHD

Lesion	% of all CHD cases
Acyanotic lesions	71
Ventricular septal defect (VSD)	32
Persistent ductus arteriosus (PDA)	12
Pulmonary stenosis (PS)	8
Coarctation of the aorta (CoA)	6
Atrial septal defect (ASD)	6
Aortic stenosis (AS)	5
Atrioventricular septal defect (AVSD)	2
Cyanotic lesions	20
Tetralogy of Fallot (ToF)	6
Transposition of the great arteries (TGA)	5
Physiologically single ventricle	4
Hypoplastic left heart syndrome (HLHS)	3
Total anomalous pulmonary venous connections (TAPVC)	1
Truncus arteriosus	1
Complex lesions	9

Table 9.2 Genetic factors and associated defects

Genetic factors	Associated defects
Parent or previous infant with CHD	Any, especially isomerism
Trisomy 21 (Down syndrome)	AVSD, VSD, ToF
Trisomy 18 (Edward syndrome)	VSD
Trisomy 13 (Patau syndrome)	VSD
Turner syndrome (45 XO)	CoA, AS, MS, PAPVC
22q11.2 deletion (DiGeorge syndrome)	Truncus, IAA, ToF
Williams syndrome	Supravalvar AS, PS
Noonan syndrome	PS, ASD, HCM
VACTERL association	VSD
Holt–Oram syndrome	ASD

AS: aortic stenosis; ASD: atrial septal defect; AVSD: atrioventricular septal defect;
CoA: coarctation of the aorta; HCM: hypertrophic cardiomyopathy; IAA: interrupted aortic
arch; MS: mitral stenosis; PAPVC: partial anomalous pulmonary vein connection; PS: pulmonary
stenosis; ToF: tetralogy of Fallot; VSD: ventricular septal defect.

Table 9.3 Maternal factors and associated defects

Maternal factors	Associated defects
Diabetes mellitus	VSD, HCM
Rubella, congenital infection	CoA, PS, VSD, PDA
Phenytoin	ASD
SLE	Congenital heart block
Alcohol	VSD
Warfarin	ASD/VSD, ToF
Lithium	Ebstein's anomaly

ASD: atrial septal defect; CoA: coarctation of the aorta; HCM: hypertrophic cardiomyopathy;
PDA: persistent ductus arteriosus; PS: pulmonary stenosis; ToF: tetralogy of Fallot;
VSD: ventricular septal defect.

- Newborns with trisomy 18 (Edward syndrome) and trisomy 13 (Patau syndrome) will often have multiple cardiac defects. Surgical intervention is usually considered inappropriate because of the bleak prognosis.

Outcome

- Outcome depends on the type and severity of the defect, as well as the presence of extra-cardiac malformations, which occur in 10%
- Complex, cyanotic defects carry a poorer prognosis. Without surgical treatment many of these are associated with death in infancy. Those who have successfully undergone surgery usually remain well into childhood, but the prognosis for adult life remains unclear.

Sequential segmental analysis

A standardized system used to accurately describe cardiac anatomy in complex defects.

Situs

Situs solitus describes the normal situation, where the atrial and lung arrangement is usual.

- *Situs inversus* describes the mirror image of the usual situation. Often the heart is in the right chest (dextrocardia), but not always
- *Situs ambiguus* describes an atrial arrangement where both atria have the same morphology (either they are both right atria, or both left atria) with failure to lateralize properly (laterality disorder). Lung morphology is the same on both sides, the liver is midline, the stomach position is variable, and there is abnormality of the spleen. There is a strong association with extra-cardiac abnormalities.

Right atrial isomerism
- Two morphological right atria, two morphological right lungs
- Asplenia
- May have severe cyanotic CHD including TAPVC, complete AVSD, pulmonary atresia, transposition of great arteries (TGA)
- Bleak prognosis.

Left atrial isomerism
- Two morphological left atria, two morphological left lungs
- Polysplenia (may be functionally asplenic)
- May have partial anomalous pulmonary venous connection and may not be cyanotic.

Atrioventricular connections

- **Concordant**: right atrium (RA) connects to right ventricle (RV), left atrium (LA) to left ventricle (LV)
- **Discordant**: RA connects to LV, LA to RV
- **Double inlet**: both atria connect to the same ventricle (usually left)
- **Absent**: no connection from a particular atrium to a particular ventricle.

Ventriculo-arterial connections

- **Concordant**: RV connects to pulmonary artery, LV to aorta
- **Discordant**: RV connects to aorta, LV to pulmonary artery
- **Single outlet**: single great artery
- **Double outlet**: both arteries arise from one ventricle (usually right).

Cardiac position

- **Levocardia**: heart on left side of chest with apex pointing to left
- **Dextrocardia**: heart on right side with apex pointing right
- **Mesocardia**: heart in the centre of thorax
- **Dextro-position**: heart on right side, but apex points left.

Additional defects

Septal defects, valve stenoses, coarctation.

Presentation and general management of congenital heart disease

Antenatal diagnosis

Antenatal screening in the UK includes ultrasound of the heart with a four-chamber view and detects around 70% of major cases of CHD. Parents can be counselled and delivery planned in a tertiary centre as appropriate. Certain defects, such as coarctation and transposition can be difficult to detect antenataly.

Postnatal presentation

- CHD may present at any time from birth to adult life. It may require intervention immediately or not at all
- About a third of children with CHD have severe defects and become symptomatic in infancy.

CHD presents in five main ways:
- Cyanosis
- Heart failure
- Collapse
- Murmur
- Oxygen saturation screening.

It is often difficult to differentiate CHD from *pulmonary disease* or *sepsis* in the newborn. Always consider CHD in the differential diagnosis of a critically ill newborn.

History

- Maternal illnesses, infections, medications, substance abuse
- Family history of CHD
- Poor feeding
- Sweating
- Excessive weight gain.

Symptoms and signs

General
- Dysmorphic features
- Grunting
- Respiratory distress
- Hepatomegaly
- Oedema
- Metabolic acidosis
- Raised lactate.

Cardiovascular
- Cyanosis
- Tachycardia
- Poor perfusion
- Clammy, mottled skin
- Pulses decreased/unequal/bounding

- Hyperactive precordium
- Hypotension
- Shock
- Gallop rhythm
- Murmurs and thrills
- Ejection click
- Second heart sound single/widely split/loud.

General management of suspected CHD

Resuscitation (if appropriate)
- Careful use of *oxygen*—may stimulate ductal closure and decrease pulmonary vascular resistance—and accept SpO_2 75–85% in cyanotic heart disease
- Consider *ventilatory support* if there are signs of respiratory failure (see ➲ Conventional ventilation, pp. 154–5)
- Consider *inotropes* if shocked (see ➲ Treatment of CHD: inotropes, p. 190)
- Consider *prostaglandin* infusion if a duct dependent lesion is suspected and monitor for apnoea (see ➲ Treatment of CHD: prostaglandin, p. 192)
- Treat hypoglycaemia, hypocalcaemia, and metabolic acidosis (see ➲ Metabolic acidosis: management, p. 380).

History and examination
- Take a comprehensive history searching for possible aetiological factors
- Thorough examination for signs of CHD.

Investigations
- **Pulse oximetry**: pre-ductal (right arm) and post-ductal (left arm or lower limb, a difference of >10% is significant)
- **Blood gas**: assess ventilation, lactate, and venous saturations
- **Blood tests**: FBC, U&Es, CRP, blood culture, coagulation, and consider genetic testing (e.g. chromosomes, 22q11.2del)
- **Hyperoxia test**: if cyanotic CHD is suspected
- **Chest X-ray**
- **ECG**
- **Echocardiogram**.

Treatment
- Consider *antibiotics* if there is any suspicion of sepsis (see ➲ Investigation of suspected sepsis, p. 325)
- Consider *diuretics* if there are signs of heart failure (furosemide IV 1 mg/kg every 6–12 hours) (see ➲ Heart failure, pp. 180–2)
- Early discussion with *cardiologist*
- *Stabilization* and *transfer* for cardiac assessment if necessary.

Differential diagnosis of CHD
- Sepsis
- Respiratory disease
- Persistent pulmonary hypertension of the newborn (PPHN)
- Metabolic disease.

Investigation of suspected congenital heart disease

The investigation of suspected CHD is summarized in Box 9.1.

> **Box 9.1 Investigation of suspected CHD**
> - Palpate femoral pulses
> - BP (non-invasively in both arms and one leg, invasively if the infant is unwell). Be aware that false diagnosis of normality can occur
> - Oxygen saturations—pre-ductal (R hand) and post-ductal (foot)
> - Blood gas (assess hypoxaemia, metabolic acidosis, and lactate +/− hyperoxia test)
> - Careful search for dysmorphic features and extra-cardiac abnormalities
> - ECG
> - CXR
> - Echocardiography (assess structure and function)
> - Consider genetic testing (not usually for simple ASD and VSD)
> - Consider immunological tests (if 22q11.2 del suspected)
> - Cardiac catheterization and MRI (for complex cases).

Chest X-ray

Most often performed to exclude respiratory disease, rather than to diagnose heart disease.

Assess for:
- Position of heart
- Size of heart (cardiomegaly = cardiothoracic ratio >0.6)
- Side of aortic arch
- Pulmonary vascularity
- Other lung pathology
- Vertebral or rib abnormalities
- Bronchial situs
- Abdominal situs.

Electrocardiogram

See **⊃** Interpreting the electrocardiogram in neonates, p. 228.

Hyperoxia (nitrogen washout) test

- May help differentiate between cardiac and respiratory causes of cyanosis. Its formal use has declined but remains useful when cardiology assessment is not readily available.
  - measure arterial partial pressure of oxygen (PaO_2) before and after giving 10 minutes of >85% inspired oxygen
  - PaO_2 >20 kPa (150 mmHg) suggests respiratory disease (the gradient for oxygen transfer is increased to overcome hypoxaemia)
  - PaO_2 <20 kPa or increase <4 kPa (30 mmHg) suggests possible cardiac disease (mixing of pulmonary and systemic circulations cannot be overcome using oxygen) but may still be extremely severe respiratory disease (e.g. PPHN).

In addition, a low $PaCO_2$ suggests cardiac disease, whereas a high $PaCO_2$ suggests respiratory disease.

The exceptions are cardiac defects with high pulmonary blood flow that will 'pass' the test (e.g. unobstructed TAPVC, but these are never severely cyanosed).

Arterial blood is the most accurate measure but transcutaneous oxygen tension monitors can be used. Pulse oximetry is not reliable since 100% saturation can equate with PaO_2 much below 20 kPa.

Echocardiography

Echocardiography has revolutionized the management of CHD in new-borns and has become the definitive diagnostic tool. It is rapid, non-invasive, and uses ultrasound to gain information about the structure and function of the heart. The three main modalities are:

- *Two-dimensional echocardiography* provides tomographic slices through the heart and vessels. Standardized views illustrate different elements of cardiac anatomy and function (left parasternal long and short axis, four-chamber, subcostal sagittal, abdominal, and suprasternal notch views)
- *M mode* illustrates movement in a very narrow part of the ultrasound beam against time. This is especially useful for examining motion in a valve or ventricular wall
- *Doppler echocardiography* uses the change in frequency of sound waves striking moving blood cells to illustrate the direction and velocity of blood flow. Doppler allows estimation of pressure differences across valves and septa. Colour flow can be superimposed upon the two-dimensional echocardiogram. *Red* represents flow *towards* the transducer, *blue away* from the transducer and a mixture of red and blue represents high velocity flow.

Cardiac catheterization

The role of catheterization in newborns is largely *interventional* since most diagnostic information can be gained through transthoracic echocardiography. The most common procedures are *balloon atrial septostomy* and *balloon dilatation* of stenotic valves. Stenting of vessels and device closure of defects are less common. Access is either through the umbilical vessels or percutaneously (femoral or axillary). Mortality for interventional catheterization is less than 1% and largely restricted to high-risk cases.

Magnetic resonance imaging

Cardiac MRI is an evolving modality that provides excellent anatomical information. However, echocardiography remains adequate for the purposes of diagnosis and management in the vast majority of cases.

Heart failure

- Heart failure is a clinical syndrome resulting from cardiac output insufficient to meet the metabolic demands of the body
- Tachypnoea is the major feature of heart failure in neonates
- Up to 7 days of age, most infants presenting with heart failure have an obstructed left heart, commonly with duct dependent lesions
- After 7 days, heart failure is most likely due to left to right shunt.

Symptoms and signs of heart failure

General

- Poor feeding
- Excessive weight gain
- Tachypnoea, breathlessness
- Head bobbing
- Respiratory distress
- Fine crepitations on auscultation
- Hepatomegaly.

Cardiovascular

- Sweating
- Poor peripheral perfusion
- Mottled, clammy, cool skin
- Tachycardia
- Hyperdynamic precordium
- Gallop rhythm
- Cardiomegaly and increased pulmonary vascularity on chest X-ray) (Fig. 9.3)
- Specific signs due to underlying cause.

Cardiac causes of heart failure

Less than one week of age

- Coarctation of aorta (CoA)
- Interrupted aortic arch
- Critical aortic stenosis (AS)—duct dependent/aortic atresia
- Total anomalous pulmonary venous connection (TAPVC)
- Hypoplastic left heart syndrome (HLHS)
- Myocardial disease (ischaemia, myocarditis, cardiomyopathy)
- Arrhythmias
- Arteriovenous malformation.

2–4 weeks of age

- Ventricular septal defect (left to right shunts rarely cause signs or symptoms in first few days of life, but usually present after 1 week, when the pulmonary vascular resistance falls and the shunt becomes manifest)
- Atrioventricular septal defect
- Common mixing: TGA + VSD, and truncus arteriosus.

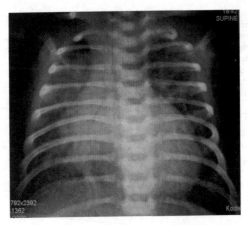

Fig. 9.3 Heart failure. CXR showing increased heart size and increased vascular markings.

Management

- The principles of managing heart failure in the first week are to give prostaglandin with or without inotropes
- The principles of managing heart failure presenting at 2–4 weeks of age are to *reduce preload* with diuretics and *reduce afterload* with angiotensin converting enzyme (ACE) inhibitors
- *Optimizing nutritional intake* is vital to counteract fluid restriction in the face of increased metabolic demand.

Acute heart failure
- Resuscitate as appropriate
- Maintain *adequate oxygenation*
- *Correct anaemia* if present
- Consider a *prostaglandin infusion* even before an exact diagnosis has been made if there is suspicion of a duct dependent lesion
- Early discussion with *cardiologist* if cause unclear
- *Furosemide* IV (1 mg/kg every 6–12 hours)
- Consider *fluid restriction* (e.g. two thirds maintenance)
- Consider *inotropes* if there is evidence of myocardial dysfunction.

Chronic heart failure
- Discuss with a cardiologist
- Avoid fluid restriction as far as possible
- Maximize calorie intake and involve a dietician
- NG feeding is sometimes useful to provide adequate calorie intake
- Furosemide (0.5–1 mg/kg from od to tds)

- Consider a potassium-sparing diuretic (e.g. spironolactone)—monitor potassium level
- Consider an ACE inhibitor (e.g. captopril), starting with a test dose of 0.1 mg/kg, monitoring BP for hypotension, before increasing further—monitor potassium level
- Use of furosemide may lead to hyponatraemia and/or hypokalaemia, which should be managed by reducing the dose and fluid restriction, rather than supplements that will exacerbate fluid retention
- ACE inhibitors should not be used if there is left ventricular outflow tract obstruction.

Cyanosis

- Cyanosis is the clinical description of bluish discolouration of the skin and mucous membranes that is caused by greater than 5 g/dl of deoxygenated haemoglobin in arterial blood
- Mild degrees may not be observed and a saturation monitor should be used to confirm normality
- Cyanosis with little or no respiratory distress and lack of X-ray evidence of lung disease suggests underlying CHD.

Causes of cyanosis

- Sepsis
- Respiratory disease
- Cardiac disease
- Metabolic disease.

Look for central cyanosis in the *tongue and mucous membranes*.

- Peripheral cyanosis or acrocyanosis is normal in the first few days of life and cyanosis only present whilst crying is rarely significant
- Polycythaemia or methaemoglobinaemia may cause a baby to appear blue, but are not associated with structural cardiac defects
- Anaemia and dark skin tones make it more difficult to detect cyanosis
- Some babies with cyanotic heart disease may appear pink due to the high affinity for oxygen of fetal haemoglobin.

Symptoms and signs of cyanotic heart disease

- *Family history* of CHD
- *Mild respiratory distress* in relation to degree of cyanosis
- Normocapnoea
- Specific signs of cardiovascular disease (e.g. dextrocardia, murmurs, signs of heart failure, strength and symmetry of pulses)
- *Abnormal heart shadow on CXR* with lack of signs of lung disease
- ECG sometimes *abnormal*.

Cardiac causes of cyanosis

- Tetralogy of Fallot (common)
- Transposition of great arteries (common)
- Pulmonary atresia (less common)
- Total anomalous pulmonary venous connection (less common)
- Truncus arteriosus (rare)
- Ebstein's anomaly (rare)
- Double inlet LV (rare).

Cardiac causes of common mixing (both cyanosis and heart failure)

- Transposition of great arteries + VSD
- Hypoplastic left heart syndrome
- Total anomalous pulmonary venous connections
- Truncus arteriosus
- Tricuspid atresia + VSD
- Double inlet LV
- Arteriovenous malformation.

Collapse and shock

Collapse is an acute deterioration due to circulatory failure (shock).

Shock is an acute state where the circulation is inadequate to meet the metabolic demands of tissues.
- All the conditions listed below may present with heart failure before worsening to a shocked state
- Collapse due to structural heart disease is usually associated with left-sided obstructive lesions leading to inadequate systemic blood flow
- Sepsis and inborn errors of metabolism must be considered in the differential diagnosis of a baby presenting with collapse and a metabolic acidosis.

Cardiac causes of shock
- Arrhythmias
- Myocardial disease
- Duct dependent CHD:
  - cyanotic
    - —transposition of great arteries (TGA)
    - —pulmonary atresia (PA)
    - —tricuspid atresia
  - obstructed
    - —coarctation of the aorta (CoA)
    - —hypoplastic left heart syndrome (HLHS)
    - —interrupted aortic arch
    - —critical aortic stenosis.
- Not duct dependent CHD: total anomalous pulmonary venous connections (TAPVC).

Non-cardiac causes of shock
- Hypovolaemia (blood loss, third space loss in sepsis or acute abdomen, feto-maternal transfusion, dehydration from diuresis, or insensible losses)
- PPHN
- Asphyxia (respiratory failure, anaemia, polycythaemia)
- Obstruction of venous return (tension pneumothorax, cardiac tamponade, excessive ventilation pressures, abdominal distension)
- Distributive (sepsis, extreme prematurity, vasodilation).

Specific symptoms and signs of shock
Neurological
- Irritability
- Reduced spontaneous movements
- Coma.

Peripheral
- Tachycardia
- Mottled skin
- Prolonged capillary refill time
- Decreased pulses or narrow pulse pressure
- Hypothermia and widening of toe-core temperature difference.

End organ
- Hypotension
- Tachypnoea and respiratory distress
- Oliguria/anuria
- Lactic acidosis.

Management
- General principles of *resuscitation* are crucial, in particular, airway, breathing, then circulation
- Maintain *adequate oxygenation*
- Consider commencing a *prostaglandin infusion,* even before an exact diagnosis has been made
- Invasive BP monitoring
- Consider central venous pressure monitoring
- Correct metabolic acidosis
- Discuss with a cardiologist early
- Consider volume expansion, but only repeat if there is an improvement or evidence of hypovolaemia
- Consider inotropes
- Use markers of tissue perfusion to decide threshold for intervention
- Assess *effects of intervention* using HR, BP, acid base status, and capillary refill time.

Volume expansion
- Only give fluid if there is good evidence of hypovolaemia
- Follow local policy on whether to use colloid or crystalloid, but consider:
  - *normal saline* 10 ml/kg
  - *plasma expander* (e.g. 4.5% human albumin solution) 15ml/kg
  - *packed red cells* 15 ml/kg if there is evidence of recent blood loss or PCV <0.35
- Give fluid volume cautiously in increments
- Larger or faster boluses may be required for rapid intravascular expansion.

Inotropes
- Ideally administer through a *central venous line*
- Increase in a step-wise fashion using BP and markers of tissue perfusion to assess response
- Cardiology assessment with echocardiography
- Generally, wean incrementally one at a time, in reverse order that they were started.

(See ➲ Treatment of CHD: inotropes, p. 190).

Heart murmurs

Heart murmurs can be a normal finding in newborns or a sign of underlying structural heart disease. The presence or intensity of a murmur is not necessarily linked with the severity of a heart defect. Murmurs are often detected incidentally on routine newborn examination. It is important to distinguish the features of murmurs likely to be clinically significant.

- Most innocent heart murmurs in newborns are the result of turbulent flow through the branch pulmonary arteries that resolve within 6 months in most cases
- Obstructive cardiac defects (e.g. AS usually produces a murmur from birth)
- Left to right shunts (e.g. VSD usually does not produce a murmur until after the first week when pulmonary vascular resistance falls and allows turbulent flow across the defect).

Cardiac defects causing murmurs

Present in the first 24 hours of age
- Pulmonary stenosis (PS)
- Atrial stenosis (AS)
- Tetralogy of Fallot (ToF)
- Tricuspid regurgitation.

Present after 24 hours of age
- Patent or persistent ductus arteriosus (PDA)
- Ventricular septal defect (VSD)
- Atrial septal defect (ASD)
- Atrioventricular septal defect (AVSD).

Management

- Ask about a *family history* of CHD or other congenital malformations
- Review *antenatal details*, especially antenatal ultrasound or echocardiogram, and maternal medical history
- Complete a thorough *clinical examination* looking for signs of cardiovascular disease, dysmorphism, and other congenital malformations. Pay particular attention to femoral pulses
- See Fig. 9.4.

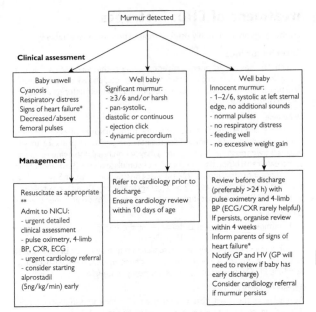

*Signs of heart failure in the newborn — poor feeding, lethargy, pallor, sweatiness, cyanosis, apnoea, breathlessness, failure to gain weight.

**As detailed in ➲ Heart failure, p. 180-2; ➲ Cyanosis, p. 184; and ➲ Collapse and shock, pp. 186-7

Fig. 9.4 Management of babies presenting with cardiac murmur.

Treatment of CHD: inotropes

Several drugs are commonly used to treat hypotension. See Table 9.4.

Catecholamines

Catecholamines are adrenergic receptor agonists that increase cardiac output by increasing myocardial *contractility, heart rate*, and *AV conduction velocity*. Their potency and other actions depend upon their differing affinity for α- and β-adrenoceptors.

Dopamine

Dopamine is often the first-line inotrope in the majority of cases because it increases cardiac function whilst maintaining perfusion pressure to vital organs. Lower doses (<4 µg/kg/min) may act on renal dopamine receptors to increase renal blood flow. Higher doses stimulate α- and β-adrenoceptors to increase inotropy and peripheral vasoconstriction. Start at 5 µg/kg/min and increase in increments of 2.5–5 µg/kg/min every 15 minutes until there is response. Be aware that it may reduce tissue perfusion at higher doses.

Dobutamine

Dobutamine can be added to dopamine if there is inadequate response at infusion rates between 10 and 15 µg/kg/min.

Dobutamine causes *peripheral vasodilation* that may lower BP and is used as a first-line inotrope where there is evidence of peripheral vasoconstriction (e.g. PPHN, or certain types of cardiomyopathy).

Adrenaline (epinephrine)

Adrenaline is the most potent inotrope and is indicated in *life-threatening hypotension*, or when there is inadequate response to dopamine and dobutamine. It has marked *peripheral vasoconstrictor effects* that may cause myocardial ischaemia by increasing afterload and should be used concomitantly with a peripheral vasodilator, such as dobutamine or enoximone.

Noradrenaline (norepinephrine)

Noradrenaline acts similarly to adrenaline by increasing contractility and systemic vascular resistance. It should be considered as an alternative to adrenaline if there is *marked peripheral vasoconstriction* (e.g. PPHN) or as an adjunct when using vasodilators, such as phosphodiesterase inhibitors.

Hydrocortisone

Hydrocortisone increases blood pressure through several mechanisms. It should be considered when there is inadequate response to dopamine and dobutamine, particularly in preterm infants where relative adrenocortical insufficiency may contribute to hypotension.

Phosphodiesterase inhibitors

Milrinone

Milrinone is a phosphodiesterase inhibitor that has positive inotropic, and pulmonary and systemic vasodilator properties. It also has a positive lusitropic effect by improving diastolic relaxation and filling of the LV. It reduces afterload and thereby increases cardiac output when systemic vascular resistance is high or when using inotropes that cause peripheral vasoconstriction (see Table 9.4).

Table 9.4 Inotropic agents, indication, and dosing

Drug	Indication	Loading	Range	Increments
Dopamine	First-line	None	2.5–20 µg/ kg/min	2.5–5 µg/kg/ min
Dobutamine	Second-line or high SVR or PHTN	None	2.5–20 µg/ kg/min	2.5–5 µg/kg/ min
Hydrocortisone	Third-line	2.5 mg/kg every 4h for 2 doses	2.5 mg/kg every 6h	
Adrenaline (epinephrine)	Life-threatening hypotension	None	0.1–1.0 µg/ kg/min	0.1 µg/kg/min
Noradrenaline (norepinephrine)	Alternative to adrenaline in PHTN and high SVR	None	0.02–0.1 µg/ kg/min	0.02 µg/kg/min
Milrinone	High SVR	None	0.25–0.75 µg/kg/min	0.25 µg/kg/min

PHTN: pulmonary hypertension; SVR: systemic vascular resistance.

Treatment of CHD: prostaglandin

The ductus arteriosus can be manipulated to allow mixing of pulmonary and systemic circulations by administering prostaglandins. Prostaglandin (PG) E_1 and E_2 both maintain patency and may dilate the ductus arteriosus.

- There is little to lose by starting a prostaglandin infusion in a baby that is unwell when heart disease is suspected, but not yet confirmed
  - PGE_1 IVI 5–100 ng/kg/min
  - PGE_2 IVI 5–50 ng/kg/min
- Discuss with a cardiologist if prostaglandin is being considered
- Start at 5–10 ng/kg/min and increase at 15–30 min intervals until there is improvement
- Can be increased to 50 ng/kg/min to reopen the ductus.

Side effects

- **Apnoea:** most common adverse effect due to central action of prostaglandins, monitor the need for respiratory support
- **Hypotension:** usually with higher doses causing systemic vasodilation, consider invasive BP monitoring in unwell babies
- **Flushing and hyperthermia:** complicates the assessment of sepsis
- **Irritability, abnormal electroencephalogram (EEG), and seizures:** restricted to higher doses
- **Loose stools**
- **Long-term side effects:** include hypertrophy of gastric mucosa and periosteitis, but are rarely seen at the doses currently used
- Side effects are dose dependent and usually respond to stopping the infusion briefly and restarting at a lower dose.

Oral PGE_2: Used occasionally when long-term administration is indicated. Most commonly, in small babies until they reach an optimal weight before surgical intervention. PGE_2 po 25–40 µg/kg hourly; start with 1 hour between doses, which can gradually be increased to 4 or 6 hours.

Treatment of CHD: surgery

Open heart surgery is necessary for intracardiac procedures (e.g. arterial switch, Norwood, and VSD closure) and involves a median sternotomy, cardioplegia, and cardiopulmonary bypass.

Closed heart surgery for extra-cardiac procedures is often performed through a lateral thoracotomy (e.g. ductus arteriosus ligation, pulmonary artery banding, Blalock–Taussig shunt, and coarctation repair).

Arterial switch

Performed within the first 2 weeks of age to correct transposition of the great arteries. It involves restoring ventriculo-arterial concordance by connecting the LV to the distal ascending aorta and the RV to the distal main pulmonary artery. The coronary arteries are transplanted to the neo-aorta, which was the pulmonary trunk, along with a button of tissue. Any ASDs or VSDs are closed and the ductus arteriosus ligated at the same time.

Blalock–Taussig shunt

The modified Blalock–Taussig shunt is used to provide an adequate, but *controlled pulmonary blood flow at low pressure*. A *tube graft* connects the innominate or *subclavian artery*, to the right or left *pulmonary artery*, usually placed on the opposite side to the aortic arch. It can be performed using a median sternotomy or lateral thoracotomy. (The 'classical' Blalock–Taussig shunt is no longer commonly performed and employs a direct end-to-side anastomosis of the subclavian artery to the right or left pulmonary artery.)

Coarctation repair

There are two surgical approaches to aortic coarctation in the neonate:
- Coarctation excision and end-to-end anastomosis is used when the coarctation coexists with hypoplasia of the aortic arch
- The subclavian flap repair is performed less often and involves suturing part of the subclavian artery to the aorta as a patch to augment the vessel diameter around the coarctation. This interrupts the left subclavian artery, but is tolerated well in infants.

Norwood procedure

This is the first of three, palliative stages for heart disease with single ventricle physiology (e.g. hypoplastic left heart syndrome). The aim is to convert the single functional ventricle into the pumping chamber for both systemic and pulmonary circulations. The pulmonary artery is connected side-to-side with the aorta to provide systemic flow; the aortic arch is repaired and widened, usually with homograft material; a modified Blalock–Taussig shunt provides controlled pulmonary flow; and an atrial septectomy allows complete mixing. The Sano modification involves using a conduit between the RV and pulmonary artery, instead of a Blalock–Taussig shunt to provide pulmonary flow.

Left to right shunts: atrial septal defect

Atrial septal defects are common. The commonest type is a secundum ASD in the middle of the atrial septum. They are not to be confused with patent foramen ovale, which are a normal finding in neonates and mostly close spontaneously. They are rarely symptomatic. Defects can cause atrial arrhythmias in adult life and should be closed at about 4 years old using a transcatheter approach.

Other types of ASD exist, including partial atrioventricular septal defects, and sinus venosus ASDs that should all be repaired surgically before school age.

Left to right shunts: persistent ductus arteriosus

Account for 10% of CHD cases. It only becomes abnormal if it persists beyond 4 weeks after the due date of delivery.

Anatomy

The ductus arteriosus connects the main pulmonary artery to the descending aorta, and is patent in all newborns at the time of delivery but almost always closes by 48 hours in newborns born at term. As pulmonary vascular resistance decreases after birth, blood can shunt from left to right through a PDA and, if large, can cause heart failure.

Clinical features

- PDA may present with signs of *heart failure* (see ➲ pp. 180–2) from 3 weeks of age when the pulmonary vascular resistance falls and allows increased pulmonary blood flow
- Full or bounding pulses, hyperdynamic precordium
- Heart sounds: continuous murmur at the left sternal edge
- ECG: left ventricular hypertrophy (LVH), sometimes right ventricular hypertrophy (RVH)
- Usually a clinical diagnosis and confirmed by echocardiography.

Management

If symptomatic, *surgical closure* should be undertaken. Closure in asymptomatic cases is delayed until large enough for *catheter device closure at 1 year old*. Long-term outcome is excellent.

Left to right shunts: ventricular septal defect

Ventricular septal defects are the most common congenital heart defect, accounting for 30% of CHD cases. They can be single or multiple, and lie in a variety of different locations within the ventricular septum.

Anatomy

Allows blood to flow from the LV into the RV through the interventricular septum (see Fig. 9.5).

Clinical features

Clinical symptoms of heart failure (see ➲ Heart failure, pp. 180–2) may not present until the pulmonary vascular resistance drops after the first week of age when the shunt becomes haemodynamically significant. A large left to right shunt results in increased pulmonary blood flow leading to pulmonary oedema and tachypnoea. Diagnosis is usually on clinical grounds and confirmed by echocardiography.

Large VSD
- Normal pulses, active precordium
- Heart sounds: loud P2, soft pan-systolic murmur at the left lower sternal edge or no murmur
- CXR: cardiomegaly, increased pulmonary vascularity
- ECG: LVH and RVH.

Small VSD
- Normal pulses, normal precordium
- Heart sounds: soft P2, loud pan-systolic murmur at the left lower sternal edge only audible after the first day of life
- CXR: normal
- ECG: normal.

Management

Heart failure should be managed using diuretics and high calorie intake to meet increased metabolic demands of heart failure. About two-thirds, especially small defects, close spontaneously over the first few years of age. Infants may remain symptomatic with poor growth if the defect is large necessitating surgical correction at around 3 months of age.

Surgical repair

Defects may be closed using a patch, either autologous (pericardium) or synthetic (Dacron®). Surgery has a mortality of less than 2%. Occasionally, defects can be closed with a device during cardiac catheterization or during cardiac surgery. Multiple VSDs may be technically difficult to close and are sometimes managed by pulmonary artery banding.

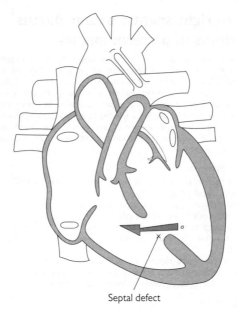

Septal defect

Fig. 9.5 Ventricular septal defect.

Left to right shunts: patent ductus arteriosus in preterm infants

Common in preterm babies and incidence is inversely related to gestational age and birth weight. 70% of newborns with weight <1000 g have a PDA and up to 70% are treated. PDA is more common in preterm babies with moderate to severe respiratory distress syndrome (RDS) due to the presence of acidosis, persistently elevated prostaglandins, and low oxygen tension acting on ductal tissue. An untreated PDA may prolong the need for O_2 therapy, delay the establishment of feeding, and may contribute to the development of pulmonary haemorrhage, intraventricular haemorrhage, and necrotizing enterocolitis.

Clinical features

The typical clinical picture is an infant failing to improve from RDS or deteriorating at 1 week of age.

- *Increasing oxygen requirement*, apnoeas, increasing dyspnoea, or increasing support in ventilated infants
- *Poor perfusion*, tachycardia, hyperactive precordium, *bounding pulses*, *low diastolic pressure*, and wide pulse pressure (>20 mmHg), *metabolic acidosis*
- Heart sounds: gallop rhythm, *systolic murmur* that may extend into diastole, loudest at the pulmonary area/left sternal border
- CXR: cardiomegaly, increased pulmonary vascularity.

Management

- *Optimize oxygenation* (sats limits appropriate to gestation), higher positive end expiratory pressure (PEEP) may be beneficial and *treat anaemia*
- If there are signs of heart failure, consider *fluid restriction* to 2/3 maintenance and using *diuretics*, although furosemide may promote ductal patency
- Assess *feeding carefully*, if the PDA causes haemodynamic instability then perfusion of the gut will be compromised, increasing the risk of NEC
- Consider involving a *cardiologist*
- *Echocardiogram* to rule out structural heart disease, visualize the ductus, measure flow across the duct, assess left atrial size/overloading, and assess haemodynamic significance. Echocardiography is not always necessary before starting treatment if there is a strong clinical suspicion.

Pharmacological closure

Ibuprofen (a non-steroidal anti-inflammatory drug (NSAID)) may be used if PDA is *haemodynamically significant*. Commencing *treatment early*, within the first week of age improves closure rates.

- Up to a third will relapse and a second course of treatment further improves closure rates. Giving more than two courses of treatment becomes progressively less effective. At present, there is insufficient evidence that prophylactic use of NSAID has greater benefit than symptomatic treatment of PDA and, although NSAIDs improve the respiratory condition in the short-term, there is no evidence for improvement in long-term outcome

- Consider decreasing or not increasing feeds, and check platelets (>50) and *renal function* (urine output >1 ml/kg/h and creatinine <120) before each dose with strict monitoring of fluid balance
- **Ibuprofen**: IV, one dose of 10 mg/kg, then two doses 5 mg/kg, 24 hours apart.

Side effects
NSAID may cause renal impairment, decrease urine output, decrease GI blood flow, cause gastrointestinal haemorrhage and perforation, have anti-platelet activity, and decrease cerebral blood flow.

Contraindications to NSAID
- Active bleeding (e.g. intraventricular haemorrhage or thrombocytopenia)—may choose to transfuse platelets prior to starting treatment
- Active or suspected NEC
- Poor or rapidly deteriorating renal function
- Suspected duct dependent CHD
- Gastrointestinal or renal anomaly.

Surgical closure
Surgical PDA ligation is tolerated well with low morbidity and mortality even in preterm babies.

Indications for surgical closure
- PDA remains haemodynamically significant:
  - despite two courses of NSAID
  - *or* contraindications to using NSAID for pharmacological closure.

Post-operative care:
- Routine care (e.g. fluid restriction, monitoring fluid balance, and analgesia)
- May need more respiratory support immediately following surgery
- CXR to assess air leak (radio-opaque clip may be visible)
- Echocardiogram to confirm closure.

Right to left shunts (cyanotic CHD): transposition of the great arteries

Transposition of the great arteries accounts for approximately 5% of CHD in children with an incidence of 1 in 3000 live births. It is the most common cyanotic lesion presenting in the newborn period. It is more common in term babies and rarely associated with extra-cardiac abnormalities.

Anatomy

Ventriculo-arterial discordant connection: the aorta arises from the RV, and lies anterior and usually to the right of the pulmonary artery. The pulmonary artery arises from the LV. Pulmonary and systemic circulations are in parallel and not in series with no mixing. Oxygenated blood flow to the systemic circulation is dependent on mixing via the ductus arteriosus, and any septal defects. There is an association with ASD, VSD, coarctation of the aorta, and pulmonary stenosis. See Figs. 9.6 and 9.7.

Clinical features

- Usually a duct dependent lesion that presents in the first 2 days after birth with cyanosis, hypoxia, tachypnoea, acidosis, and eventually collapse. Severity depends upon the degree of mixing between the systemic and pulmonary circulations through coexisting shunts, such as a patent ductus arteriosus, patent foramen ovale, or VSD. The smaller these shunts, the more cyanosed and unwell the baby will become
- Mild respiratory distress, normal pulses, RV impulse
- Heart sounds: single S2, systolic murmur, but may be absent
- ECG: initially normal evolving right axis deviation (RAD), RVH, and upright T waves in V1
- CXR: large RV, normal or plethoric lung fields, classical 'egg on side' appearance develops later.

Management

- Start intravenous *prostaglandin* to maintain ductal patency and increase mixing and systemic oxygenation
- *Balloon atrial septostomy* (Rashkind procedure) can be performed if the patent foramen ovale is restrictive to increase the size of the shunt and allow greater atrial mixing. Performed by a cardiologist under US guidance through the umbilical or femoral vein. Ensure baby is ventilated, sedated, and muscle relaxed
- It is important to identify the coronary anatomy before surgical repair.

Surgical repair

The *arterial switch* procedure (see ⊃ Treatment of CHD: surgery, p. 193) is usually performed in the first week and surgical mortality is less than 5%. The switch should be performed within 3 weeks—before the left ventricular wall involutes in response to the lower pulmonary pressures and eventually becomes unable to sustain higher systemic pressures following correction. The outcome is determined by the arrangement of the coronary arteries and also by the presence of associated anomalies.

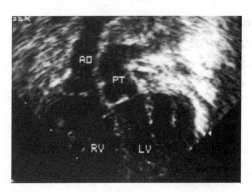

Fig. 9.6 Transposition of great arteries—echocardiogram showing the connection of the aorta (AO) to the right ventricle (RV), and of the pulmonary trunk (PT) to the left ventricle (LV).

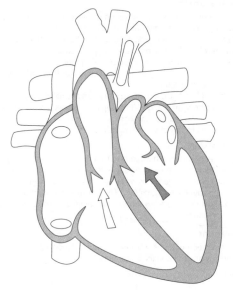

Fig. 9.7 Transposition of the great arteries.

Right to left shunts (cyanotic CHD): tetralogy of Fallot

Tetralogy of Fallot is the most common cyanotic heart defect presenting beyond the neonatal period and accounts for 10% of CHD cases. Although one fifth present in the newborn period with cyanosis, most will have a loud heart murmur on the first day of age, with little cyanosis. This is often mistaken for a VSD, which would not be heard within the first few hours of birth.

Anatomy

It consists of four elements (see Fig. 9.8):
- Large outlet subaortic VSD
- Right ventricular outflow tract stenosis sometimes with associated pulmonary valve stenosis
- Enlarged aorta that overrides the VSD
- Consequently right ventricular hypertrophy

There may be an ASD associated. Rarely there may be pulmonary atresia.

Clinical features

- The degree of cyanosis depends upon the severity of pulmonary stenosis. Infants with a tight pulmonary stenosis will be severely cyanosed with a duct dependent circulation. Infants with minimal stenosis may have little or no cyanosis ('pink tetralogy')
- No respiratory distress, normal pulses, RV impulse
- Heart sounds: single S2, ejection systolic murmur from right ventricular outflow tract obstruction
- CXR: normal heart size, pulmonary oligaemia, small PA leaving a pulmonary artery 'bay' and RVH giving an upturned apex and the classical 'boot shaped' appearance
- ECG: RAD, RVH, upright T waves in V1.

Hypercyanotic spells

Although rare, infants may have intermittent episodes of severe cyanosis or collapse, known as hypercyanotic spells that can be fatal. They result from infundibular spasm triggered by stress (crying, dehydration, fever) leading to right to left shunt across the VSD. The murmur may disappear as pulmonary blood flow decreases. Hypercyanotic spells are a relative indication for surgical intervention.

Management

Severely cyanotic neonates will need a *prostaglandin* infusion to maintain ductal patency and pulmonary blood flow.

Management of hypercyanotic spells

- Oxygen
- Repeated, full flexion of hip and knees
- Morphine (50–100 µg/kg SC/IM/IV)
- Propranolol (20 µg/kg slow IV)

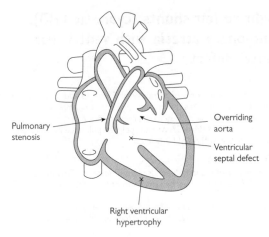

Fig. 9.8 Tetralogy of Fallot.

- Sedation and ventilation rarely needed
- Regular oral propranolol (1–2 mg/kg tds) is sometimes used to prevent recurrent spells until surgery can be performed.

Surgical repair

In severe cases, a modified Blalock–Taussig shunt is used as a palliative procedure to provide adequate pulmonary blood flow before definitive repair. Complete surgical repair is performed between 4 and 6 months to allow for growth of the pulmonary arteries.

Right to left shunts (cyanotic CHD): pulmonary atresia with ventricular septal defect

Anatomy

This is an extreme form of tetralogy of Fallot. In addition to pulmonary valve abnormalities, the pulmonary arteries are small and often non-confluent. There may be varying degrees of major aorto-pulmonary communicating arteries (MAPCAs) that supply the pulmonary circulation. There is an association with 22q11.2 deletion.

Clinical features

- The degree of *cyanosis* depends upon the size and flow through MAPCAs and there may be symptoms of *heart failure* if the MAPCAs are large
- Mild respiratory distress, normal pulses, sometimes RV impulse
- Heart sounds: single S2, continuous *murmur* throughout the chest from MAPCAs
- ECG: upright T waves in V1
- CXR: normal heart or cardiomegaly, pulmonary oligaemia (plethora if large MAPCAs), small PA.

Management

Initially with *prostaglandin* to maintain ductal patency (if present) and adequate pulmonary blood flow.

Surgical repair

Approach and outcome depend on size and continuity of the pulmonary arteries. In cases with adequate branch pulmonary arteries supplied by the ductus, surgical repair is with an RV–PA conduit and VSD closure. In cases with hypoplastic and discontinuous pulmonary arteries, surgery is difficult and palliative procedures are sometimes recommended.

Right to left shunts (cyanotic CHD): Ebstein's anomaly

Anatomy

This rare anomaly describes an abnormal tricuspid valve (septal leaflet) that is apically displaced causing atrialization of part of the RV. The valve is usually regurgitant leading to right atrial dilatation. If there is an atrial communication, then right to left shunt causes cyanosis. Atrial enlargement impinges upon lung development and can lead to tracheobronchomalacia or pulmonary hypoplasia.

Clinical features

- Mild cases may be asymptomatic. Severe cases present at birth with *cyanosis* and cardiomegaly. In its most severe form, the RV cannot pump effectively leading to *functional pulmonary atresia* and a *duct dependent circulation*
- Ebstein's anomaly is associated with *arrhythmias* either through an accessory pathway causing Wolff–Parkinson–White (WPW) syndrome or atrial wall stretching and fibrosis leading to atrial flutter. Some mild cases present with an arrhythmia
- CXR: massively dilated RA, massive cardiomegaly, rarely a 'wall-to-wall' heart appearance, pulmonary oligaemia
- ECG: weak RV forces, S wave in V1, delta wave of WPW.

Management

- Start a *prostaglandin infusion* to maintain ductal patency and pulmonary blood flow. Over the first few weeks, pulmonary vascular resistance falls and, consequently, pulmonary blood flow improves.

Surgical repair

In cases where there is little or no forward flow from the RV and pulmonary vascular resistance remains high, surgical palliation with a *Blalock–Taussig shunt* is used to improve pulmonary blood flow. Overall survival is 60% at 10 years.

Common mixing: complete atrioventricular septal defect

Associated with trisomy 21, tetralogy of Fallot, double outlet RV, and sub-AS. 80% of babies with complete AVSD will have Down syndrome and it accounts for a third of all heart defects in babies with Down syndrome.

Anatomy

There is abnormal formation of the endocardial cushions (which give rise to the atrial septum primum, AV valves, and the inlet segment of the ventricular septum). In complete AVSD, there is a common AV valve that straddles the ventricular septum, which tends to leak even after surgery. Balance refers to the size of the left and right ventricular inlets relative to each other. See Fig. 9.9.

Clinical features

- Symptoms depend on the size of the left to right shunt. They may present with severe cyanosis due to a right to left shunt associated with high pulmonary vascular resistance at birth, especially in Down syndrome. Resistance then falls and the resulting increase in pulmonary blood flow leads to congestive cardiac failure over the next few weeks.
- Heart sounds: loud P2, soft pan-systolic murmur at the lower left sternal edge
- ECG: superior QRS axis, RVH, and RA enlargement.

Management

In complete AVSD, *surgical correction* is required in infancy with optimal timing at 3 months. Mortality is less than 10%. The post-operative course is often difficult, due to increased pulmonary vascular resistance from high pulmonary blood flow, which often persists following correction.

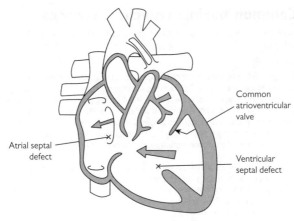

Fig. 9.9 Atrioventricular septal defect.

Common mixing: truncus arteriosus

Accounts for less than 1% of CHD cases. One third will have 22q11.2 deletion.

Anatomy

The left and right ventricular outflow tracts form a common trunk known as the truncus arteriosus. The truncus overrides a large VSD and often has a single, abnormal truncal valve with multiple leaflets, that can be both stenotic and regurgitant. There is intracardiac mixing of the pulmonary and systemic circulations. There may be a right-sided aortic arch or an interrupted arch. The left and right pulmonary arteries may arise either directly from the truncus or from a short main pulmonary artery (Fig. 9.10).

Clinical features:
- Presentation is usually in the *second or third week* with signs of *heart failure* due to increased blood flow through the lower resistance pulmonary circuit. Mild *cyanosis* is due to intracardiac mixing
- Normal or full pulses, active precordium
- Heart sounds: loud, single S2, ejection click, systolic murmur at upper left sternal edge, early diastolic murmur from truncal valve insufficiency
- ECG: RVH, sometimes LVH, ST depression, T wave inversion in V5/6.

Management

Heart failure (see ⮱ Heart failure, pp. 180–2) should be managed in the conventional way with *diuretics* and ACE inhibitor (e.g. captopril) until repair is appropriate. Look for associated defects of 22q11.2 deletion (dysmorphism, hypocalcaemia, thymic dysplasia, cleft palate).

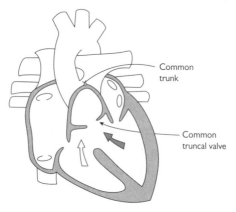

Common
trunk

Common
truncal valve

Fig. 9.10 Truncus arteriosus.

Surgical repair

Surgical repair is performed in the neonatal period to protect the pulmonary vasculature from higher systemic pressures. Surgery consists of detaching the pulmonary arteries from the common trunk and providing pulmonary blood flow through an RV to pulmonary artery conduit. The VSD is closed and a prosthetic valve may be required in later childhood. The overall mortality is less than 10%.

Common mixing: pulmonary atresia with intact ventricular septum

Accounts for less than 1% of CHD, but always presents in the neonatal period with cyanosis.

Anatomy

The pulmonary valve is dysplastic and immobile or completely atretic, and usually associated with a small RV and small tricuspid valve or Ebstein's malformation. The pulmonary artery and branches are usually reasonably developed and confluent. Pulmonary blood flow depends on a patent ductus arteriosus (duct dependent) and a patent foramen ovale to decompress the RA. There is an association with abnormal coronary anatomy.

Clinical features

- Presentation is on the first day with cyanosis and metabolic acidosis
- Mild respiratory distress, normal pulses, and marked hepatomegaly if the RA becomes obstructed
- Heart sounds: single S2, ductal murmur, sometimes TR
- ECG: QRS axis 0–90°, RA enlargement, small RV forces, S wave in V1
- CXR: normal heart size or cardiomegaly, pulmonary oligaemia, small PA leaving a pulmonary artery 'bay'.

Management

Initially with prostaglandin to maintain ductal patency and pulmonary blood flow. Atrial septostomy is sometimes needed if the foramen ovale is restrictive.

Surgical repair

Palliation in the newborn period is with an arterio-pulmonary shunt (e.g. modified Blalock–Taussig shunt). Choice of subsequent surgical intervention depends upon the size of the RV and outflow tract, and some cases proceed to uni-ventricular repair.

Common mixing: tricuspid atresia

Anatomy

Accounts for 2% of CHD cases. The tricuspid valve is absent therefore blood cannot leave the RA through the atretic valve but instead must pass through a patent foramen ovale or ASD to enter the LA. The RV is usually small and there is sometimes an atretic pulmonary valve. It is sometimes associated with VSD, TGA, and aortic coarctation.

Clinical features

- If there is a restrictive VSD or pulmonary stenosis, then pulmonary blood flow will be duct dependent, and the baby will present with cyanosis. If the VSD is large or there is transposition of the great arteries, the baby will present with signs of heart failure and mild cyanosis
- Minimal respiratory distress, normal pulses, normal precordium, hepatomegaly due to increased RA pressure
- Heart sounds: single S2, systolic murmur of VSD or PS
- ECG: RA enlargement, superior QRS axis, small RV forces
- CXR: square-shaped heart, RA enlargement, and pulmonary oligaemia.

Management

- Start *prostaglandin infusion* to maintain ductal patency and pulmonary blood flow
- *Balloon atrial septostomy* may be required if the atrial communication is restrictive.

Surgical repair

Surgical intervention involves a palliative procedure such as a systemic–pulmonary shunt or pulmonary artery banding depending on whether pulmonary blood flow is insufficient or excessive. Most proceed to uni-ventricular repair.

Common mixing: congenitally corrected transposition of the great arteries

Anatomy

This rare condition has both AV and ventriculo-arterial discordance. Oxygenated pulmonary venous blood enters the LA before passing through the tricuspid valve into a morphologically RV and leaves the heart via the aorta. It is sometimes associated with dextrocardia, situs inversus, and various other cardiac defects.

Clinical features

- The presentation depends upon the presence of associated cardiac defects
- If there are no associated defects, then there is no cyanosis and presentation is later
- Some will have a VSD and present with signs of *heart failure* in the first year
- Some will have pulmonary stenosis and present earlier with *cyanosis*, and occasionally there may be *Ebstein's anomaly*
- There is a strong association with *arrhythmias*, mainly complete heart block, and there is a risk of sudden cardiac death in later life.

Surgical repair

Surgical intervention involves palliative procedures, such as pulmonary artery banding if there is a large VSD or systemic to pulmonary anastomosis if there is significant pulmonary stenosis.

Well babies with an obstruction: aortic stenosis

There is a spectrum of severity from mild defects that are asymptomatic to critical AS that presents with collapse in the neonatal period. It is commoner in males and there is an association with Turner syndrome in females.

Anatomy

The aortic valve is thickened and dysplastic with a variable number of cusps and can be both stenotic and regurgitant. The ascending aorta is usually small, but does not normally cause a functional problem. There is often post-stenotic dilatation of the aorta.

Clinical features

- Symptomatic babies present with loss of pulses, acidosis, and shock when the ductus arteriosus closes. Usually they are asymptomatic
- Heart sounds: ejection systolic murmur in the aortic area (right upper sternal edge) radiating into the carotids with a carotid thrill
- CXR: normal
- ECG: LVH.

Management

In severe cases start a *prostaglandin infusion* to maintain ductal patency and systemic blood flow. Most children are well, present with a heart murmur, and can be followed in the outpatient clinic.

Treatment is with transcatheter balloon *valvuloplasty* in most cases. The outcome depends on the need for subsequent procedures for recurrence or regurgitation. All will eventually require aortic valve replacement.

Well babies with an obstruction: pulmonary stenosis

There is a spectrum of severity from mild defects that are *asymptomatic* to critical pulmonary stenosis that presents with *collapse*. It is commoner in females and there is an association with Noonan syndrome.

Anatomy

The pulmonary valve is thickened and dysplastic with a variable number of cusps, and can be both stenotic and regurgitant. There is often post-stenotic dilatation of the pulmonary artery.

Clinical features

- Usually they are asymptomatic. Symptomatic babies will present with cyanosis, acidosis, and shock when the ductus arteriosus closes
- Heart sounds: ejection systolic murmur in the pulmonary area
- CXR: normal
- ECG: RV hypertrophy.

Management

Start a *prostaglandin infusion* to maintain ductal patency and pulmonary blood flow in severe cases. Well children can be followed as an outpatient after the diagnosis is made.

Surgical repair

Treatment is with transcatheter balloon *valvuloplasty* and usually the only treatment that children will need.

Sick babies with an obstruction: coarctation of the aorta

Aortic coarctation is common and accounts for 10% of CHD cases; additional cardiac defects are common. It is more common in males and is strongly associated with Turner syndrome in females.

Anatomy

There is a spectrum from narrowing of the lumen of the aorta usually at the arterial duct to a posterior shelf in the juxtaductal region to hypoplasia of a segment of the aorta. Coarctation can affect the transverse aortic arch or rarely, the abdominal aorta. Coarctation is frequently associated with a bicuspid aortic valve and VSD, as well as other left-sided defects. There is a rare association with an aberrant right subclavian artery arising distal to the coarctation.

Clinical features

- Symptoms manifest when the duct begins to close in the *first week of age*. The degree of coarctation together with patency of the ductus arteriosus determines the severity of symptoms
- Aortic obstruction causes increased left ventricular afterload that results in *poor distal perfusion* and left ventricular failure (*tachypnoea*), and the right to left shunt across the duct leads to *lower limb cyanosis and right heart failure (hepatomegaly)*. There is a discrepancy in blood pressure between upper and lower limbs (>20 mmHg difference), higher proximal to the obstruction and *lower distally*. *Femoral pulses* become *weak* or *absent* when the ductus closes and *brachial pulses* are *bounding* This may progress to *shock*, metabolic *acidosis*, and eventually *collapse*.
- There is an active precordium. Unequal upper limb pulses indicate an aberrant origin of the subclavian artery
- Heart sounds: gallop rhythm and systolic murmur
- ECG: RA enlargement and RVH +/– LVH, T wave inversion in the left chest leads
- CXR: cardiomegaly, increased pulmonary vasculature
- Echocardiography: can be inconclusive whilst the ductus arteriosus remains open; may require serial scans as the ductus closes
- With mild coarctation, infants may be asymptomatic and present in childhood or as adults. They may present with abnormal pulses, a murmur, or hypertension and its complications.

Management

In severe cases, start *prostaglandin infusion* early to maintain ductal patency and systemic blood flow.

Heart failure should be managed by reopening the duct and may need inotropic support. Severe cases need surgical repair.

Surgical repair

Surgical repair involves resection of the coarctation and ductal tissue with an *end-to-end anastomosis*. Alternative approaches are to use a subclavian flap (which results in an absent left brachial pulse, but is well tolerated) or reverse subclavian flap in hypoplastic arches. Mortality is less than 1%, and results have improved over the years in terms of the late complications of recurrence and aneurysms, although recurrence can still be as high as 10% following neonatal repair.

Sick babies with an obstruction: interrupted aortic arch

Accounts for 1% of CHD cases and usually associated with VSD and AS. There is a strong association with chromosome 22q11.2 deletion.

Anatomy

There is *no connection between the ascending and descending aorta*. They can be classified according to the site of the interruption:
- Type A: distal to left subclavian (30%)
- Type B: between left carotid and subclavian (45%)
- Type C: between innominate and left carotid (25%).

Clinical features

- This is a *duct dependent circulation*. It presents in a similar but more severe fashion to coarctation with *shock, acidosis,* and *collapse*
- Stronger pulses proximal to interruption and *weaker distal* to the interruption, active precordium
- Heart sounds: gallop rhythm and systolic murmur
- CXR: cardiomegaly, increased pulmonary vascularity
- ECG: LVH and RVH and T wave inversion in left chest leads.

Management

- Start a *prostaglandin infusion* to maintain ductal patency and systemic blood flow
- Look for associated features of 22q11.2 deletion (dysmorphism, hypocalcaemia, thymic dysplasia, cleft palate)
- Surgical repair is performed once stabilized a few days after presentation. Surgery comprises end-to-end anastomosis of the interrupted segments.

Sick babies with an obstruction: hypoplastic left heart syndrome

Anatomy

Accounts for 1% of CHD cases. HLHS represents a spectrum of defects characterized by hypoplasia/atresia of the mitral valve, hypoplasia of the LV, AS/atresia, hypoplasia of the ascending aorta, and coarctation with endocardial fibroelastosis. In addition, the RV is dilated and hypertrophied with a large pulmonary artery. Extra-cardiac abnormalities are unusual (Fig. 9.11).

Clinical features

This is a duct dependent circulation and presents within the first week when the duct closes. The LV contributes little to cardiac output and the systemic and coronary blood flow is supplied by the RV through the patent ductus arteriosus. There is inter-atrial mixing and decompression of the LA through a patent foramen ovale. The pulmonary circuit has a lower resistance and, therefore, becomes over-perfused at the cost of systemic perfusion. Babies are both cyanosed and have signs of heart failure to varying degrees depending upon the interplay between systemic and pulmonary blood flow at any one time.

- Poor perfusion, metabolic acidosis, weak femoral pulses, active precordium
- Heart sounds: loud single S2, gallop rhythm
- CXR: cardiomegaly, increased pulmonary vascularity
- ECG: small LV forces, RAD, RA enlargement, RVH.

Management

Start a prostaglandin infusion to maintain ductal patency and systemic blood flow. Inotropic support may be required if right ventricular function is impaired. Intubation and ventilation may be required if pulmonary blood flow becomes excessive. If appropriate, infants need transfer shortly after birth to one of the few centres that perform surgery for this condition.

Surgical repair

Surgery comprises three stages, which aim to convert the RV into the systemic ventricle. The first stage is the Norwood procedure, followed by the Glenn or Hemi-Fontan procedures in infancy, and finally the Fontan procedure in early childhood. Mortality is highest for the first stage and decreases thereafter. The long-term outcome remains uncertain.

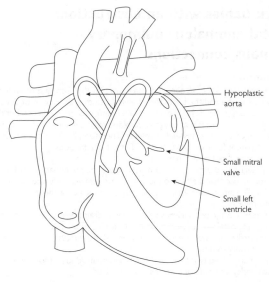

Fig. 9.11 Hypoplastic left heart syndrome.

Sick babies with an obstruction: total anomalous pulmonary venous connections

Anatomy

All *pulmonary veins have abnormal connections to the heart* and often form a confluence behind the LA before draining into the RA via one of several possible routes (Fig. 9.12). There are different forms of this defect, but the underlying problem is that oxygenated blood from the lungs arrives on the right side of the heart instead of the LA. Therefore, blood in the RA must cross a patent foramen ovale or an ASD to reach the body.

There are three main types:

- **Supracardiac:** the most common type where the pulmonary veins form a confluence that drains into the innominate vein via a left-sided vena cava. The innominate joins the right superior vena cava and drains into the RA
- **Infracardiac:** the pulmonary vein confluence drains below the diaphragm into the portal venous system before returning to the RA
- **Intracardiac:** the pulmonary veins connect directly to the RA often via the coronary sinus
- There are mixed types where the left- and right-sided pulmonary veins have different drainage patterns to each other.

Clinical features

Present with varying degrees of *cyanosis* due to mixing in the RA and right to left shunt across the ASD. The severity of symptoms and timing of presentation depend upon the degree of obstruction to pulmonary venous return.

Obstruction to pulmonary venous drainage can occur at the diaphragm, the liver, the confluence with systemic veins, or at the atrial septum. This may be mild with the supracardiac type that is typically unobstructed, presenting beyond the first week and into infancy with heart failure, and failure to thrive, or recurrent chest infections. Infracardiac types are frequently obstructed leading to severe cyanosis shortly after birth. Obstructed babies will also be dyspnoeic and have severe cyanosis. This presentation can easily be confused with respiratory disease:

- Marked respiratory distress, normal or weak pulses if obstructed, RV impulse, enlarged liver
- Heart sounds: loud P2, no murmur
- ECG: normal in first few days progressing to upright T waves in V1, RSR in V1
- CXR: small or normal heart, pulmonary plethora, classically 'snowman in snowstorm' appearance in obstructed supracardiac TAPVC.

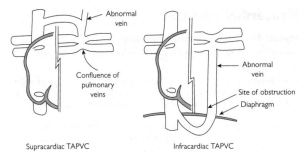

Supracardiac TAPVC

Infracardiac TAPVC

Fig. 9.12 Total anomalous pulmonary venous connection (TAPVC).

Management

Obstructed TAPVC is a surgical emergency since the situation will not be alleviated by prostaglandin infusion.

Surgical correction is carried out as soon as possible and has mortality less than 10% with a good long-term prognosis.

NB TAPVC is one of the few cyanotic heart lesions that does not respond to prostaglandin.

Surgical repair

Unobstructed TAPVC requires surgical repair by reconnecting the pulmonary veins to the RA. The exact approach and long-term outcome depends upon the specific anatomy.

Myocardial disease

Myocardial ischaemia and infarction

The commonest cause of myocardial ischaemia is *perinatal asphyxia*.

Clinical features

- Ischaemia is usually sub-clinical, but some infants develop signs of heart failure. Severe cases may proceed to myocardial infarction, and present with signs of failure or collapse and associated neurological and organ injury
- ECG: ST depression and T wave inversion in the left chest leads, persistent deep Q waves, ST elevation that resolves over a week, and T wave inversion that resolves more slowly.

Management

- *Measure cardiac troponins* and discuss with a *cardiologist*
- Severe cases need *inotropic support*. Those with myocardial ischaemia tend to make a *full recovery*—the outcome following infarction is less clear.

Myocarditis

The aetiology is thought to be *viral* in most cases but often a specific pathogen is not isolated.

Clinical features

Myocarditis is often part of a generalized, multi-system infective illness. Presentation is with signs of heart failure associated with arrhythmias and pericardial effusions, and sometimes tamponade.

Management

Management of heart failure should be initiated after discussion with a cardiologist. Symptomatic pericardial effusions should be drained percutaneously by a cardiologist. Outcome is variable ranging from complete recovery to chronic dilated cardiomyopathy eventually needing transplantation.

Dilated cardiomyopathy

Unusual to present in the neonatal period.

Management

The aetiology is usually ischaemic. Other causes include infection, inborn errors of metabolism, tachyarrhythmia, and ALCAPA (anomalous origin of left coronary artery from pulmonary artery). If there are any positive results from metabolic studies then consider enzymology on leucocytes and fibroblasts, as well as tissue biopsies. A trial of empirical therapy should be started if a metabolic cause is suspected such as carnitine supplements. First degree relatives should be assessed for disease by examination, ECG, and echocardiography.

Hypertrophic cardiomyopathy

- **Primary disease** is an *autosomal dominant* inherited condition
- Management should avoid digoxin and inotropes that will worsen left ventricular outflow tract obstruction. *Propranolol* can be used with careful monitoring for hypoglycaemia and after discussion with a cardiologist
- **Secondary disease** is most commonly associated with hyperinsulinism as a result of *maternal diabetes mellitus* or *corticosteroid* therapy. Infants are usually *asymptomatic,* although some may have a left ventricular outflow tract murmur. Symptomatic babies need *echocardiography* to rule out associated structural heart disease. Hypertrophy *resolves spontaneously* within the first six months of age
- Rarer causes include *Noonan syndrome* and *inborn errors of metabolism.*

Cardiomyopathy screen

- Blood:
  - lactate and pyruvate (fasting)
  - virology (entero-, adeno-, parvoviruses)
  - carnitines and acylcarnitines
  - thyroid function
  - amino acids
  - creatine kinase (MM isoenzyme)
  - vacuolated lymphocytes
  - autoimmune screen
- Urine:
  - amino and organic acids
  - glycosaminoglycans
- Virology:
  - nasopharyngeal aspirates
- ECG (look for tachyarrhythmia)
- Echocardiography (define coronary artery anatomy and look for structural heart disease).

Hypertension

Hypertension is rarely problematic in newborns with an incidence of less than 1%.

Definition

Systolic or mean arterial BP >*95th percentile* for BW, gestational age, and postnatal age (but remember that by definition, 5% of newborns have a BP above the 95th percentile). BP increases with gestational age and postnatal age.

Clinical features

- Cardiovascular compromise due to increased afterload with signs of *heart failure* or *shock*
- Neurological features, such as lethargy, *irritability* progressing to *seizures*, and *intracranial haemorrhage*
- Respiratory signs, such as *apnoea* and *tachypnoea*.

Causes

Renal pathology is the most common cause of hypertension in the newborn.

- *Renal* ('high' umbilical artery catheter, renal artery thromboembolism, renal artery stenosis, renal vein thrombosis, renal anomalies, polycystic, or dysplastic kidneys, acute tubular necrosis, urinary tract obstruction, renal infection)
- *Cardiovascular* (aortic coarctation)
- *Iatrogenic* (glucocorticoids, inotropes, caffeine, phenylephrine, pain, electrolyte disturbances, maternal cocaine abuse)
- *Neurological* (raised intracranial pressure, seizures)
- *Endocrine* (congenital adrenal hyperplasia, hyperthyroidism, hyperaldosteronism, phaeochromocytoma, neuroblastoma)
- *Pulmonary* (hypercarbia, chronic lung disease, early pneumothorax).

Management

- *Multiple BP measurements* on different limbs using correct size cuff and invasive monitoring if unwell
- *First-line tests:* FBC, U&Es, Ca, PO_4, urinalysis, CXR, ECG, cranial US and renal US with Doppler flow studies, echocardiography
- *Second-line tests:* TFT (thyroid function tests), urinary VMA (vanillylmandelic acid) and HVA (homovanillic acid), cortisol, renin, aldosterone, 17-OH progesterone
- Discuss with *nephrology, cardiology,* and *endocrinology* teams
- *Treat the underlying cause* if possible and use anti-hypertensives if symptomatic
- Consider *anticonvulsants* and *sedation* if encephalopathic.

Emergency treatment
- Furosemide 1–2 mg/kg IV bd
- Hydralazine 0.1–0.3 mg/kg IV hourly, then maintenance 0.2–0.5 mg/kg tds
- Nitroprusside 0.5–8 µg/kg/min IVI
- Use invasive BP monitoring, and beware hypotension and shock. Aim to reduce BP slowly to below the 95th centile over 24 hours.

Maintenance treatment or if clinically stable
- Furosemide and spironolactone 1 mg/kg po qds
- Nifedipine 0.2 mg/kg po; maintenance 0.1–0.5 mg/kg tds
- Captopril 0.1–1.0 mg/kg po tds
- Propranolol 1–2 mg/kg po tds.

Interpreting the electrocardiogram in neonates

Obtaining a good quality ECG recording can be challenging in the newborn, but is essential to investigate suspected heart disease.

Assess for:
- **Rate**: 80–160 bpm (term), mean 120; 100–180 bpm (preterm)
- **Sinus rhythm**: every QRS complex preceded by a normal P wave. Atrial or ventricular extrasystoles may occur and resolve spontaneously over the first week
- **P wave axis**: 0 to +90°, P waves upright in leads V1 and V6. Abnormal if there is a 'low atrial' focus other than the sinoatrial node or in atrial isomerism
- **P wave morphology**: <2.5 mm and <120 ms. Peaked P waves, >3 mm indicate right atrial enlargement. Bifid P waves, >120 ms indicate left atrial enlargement
- **PR interval**: 0.09–0.12 s. Lengthened in first degree heart block and decreased in nodal rhythms
- **QRS axis**: +110–180°, mean +135° changing to +75° over the first month:
  - calculate the vector of the QRS axis using lead I and aVF
  - calculate height of R wave in lead I and plot on x axis, calculate height of maximum amplitude in aVF and plot on y axis
  - superior axis seen in tricuspid atresia, AVSD, WPW, and Noonan's syndrome
- **QRS duration**: <80 ms. Wide QRS complex >80 ms indicates a ventricular conduction defect
- **QRS progression**: dominant R wave in V1 to dominant S wave in V6 at birth, progressing to dominant R wave in V6 by 1 month
- **Q wave**: small Q waves in left chest leads can be normal. Large Q waves >4 mm indicate septal hypertrophy. Q waves in V1 indicate RVH
- **Right ventricular hypertrophy**: R wave in V1 >20 mm, S wave in V6 >10 mm, upright T waves in V1 after 7 days, Q wave in V1
- **Left ventricular hypertrophy**: S wave in V1 >20 mm, R wave in V6 >20 mm, Q wave in V6 >4 mm
- **ST segment**: elevation seen in acute ischaemia and myocarditis. Depression seen in strain, ischaemia, electrolyte disturbances, and digoxin toxicity
- **Corrected QT interval**: normally <0.45 ms, QT interval divided by square root of RR interval preceding the measured complex. Prolonged in long QT syndrome and hypocalcaemia
- **T wave inversion**: can be due to perinatal stress and resolves over a week.

Arrhythmias

Primary arrhythmias are rare in the newborn period. Most arrhythmias are secondary to a non-cardiac cause. Identification of arrhythmias in newborns is difficult and the natural history differs from that observed in older children.

- Arrhythmias may be asymptomatic or present with signs of heart failure or collapse
- Sinus arrhythmia is the normal phenomenon of increase in heart rate on inspiration, causing a regularly irregular rate that is synchronous with respiration with an otherwise normal ECG.

Arrhythmias: bradyarrhythmias

See Fig. 9.13.

Sinus bradycardia

Heart rate below 80/min (term) or 100/min (preterm). There is a normal P wave (morphology and axis) *preceding each QRS* complex. This can be a normal phenomenon if transient during sleep or when straining. If sustained, it may be secondary to a non-cardiac cause—apnoea, hypoxaemia, raised intracranial pressure, hyperkalaemia, handling of unwell babies, sedation, digoxin, propranolol, or hypothyroidism.

Sinus arrest/pause

Occasional and brief pauses between P waves causing an irregularly irregular heart rate with an otherwise normal ECG.

First-degree heart block

There is a prolonged, but constant PR interval >110 ms and P waves are always conducted (followed by a QRS complex). This is never symptomatic, but may progress to 2nd degree heart block. The condition may be familial or secondary to underlying structural heart disease (e.g. AVSD, myocardial disease) or drugs (e.g. digoxin).

Second-degree heart block

P waves are intermittently not conducted.

Mobitz type I (Wenckebach phenomenon)

The PR interval progressively increases until a P wave is not conducted, resulting in a dropped beat before the cycle repeats. It can occur during sleep or anaesthesia, and is not always associated with underlying heart disease.

Mobitz type II

The PR interval is prolonged and fixed, and P waves are intermittently not conducted, usually in a regular pattern (e.g. every 3rd P wave is conducted = 3:1 block). This is more often associated with underlying heart disease and often progresses to third-degree heart block.

Third-degree heart block (complete heart block)

No P waves are conducted so that P waves and QRS complexes are completely dissociated. There is a normal atrial rate with ventricular rate between 40 and 80/min. When associated with structural heart disease such as AVSD and congenitally corrected TGA there is often heart failure and a poor outcome. When associated with a structurally normal heart, there is often evidence of maternal connective tissue disease, although sometimes mothers are asymptomatic, and only have serological evidence of disease. Anti-Ro or anti-La maternal antibodies cause His bundle fibrosis. These babies usually tolerate low heart rates without symptoms.

Treatment of symptomatic babies involves management of heart failure with diuretics, isoprenaline infusion to maintain adequate heart rate, and oesophageal or transvenous pacing. Permanent epicardial pacing is rarely needed.

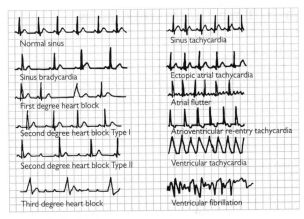

Fig. 9.13 Neonatal arrhythmias.

Arrhythmias: tachyarrhythmias

See Fig. 9.13.

Atrial ectopics

Caused by a focus in the atrium depolarizing before the sinus node. If this occurs immediately after a QRS complex within its refractory period, the ectopic is not conducted. If it occurs after the refractory period a normal, but premature QRS complex is conducted. An ectopic occurring between these two points may cause an aberrantly conducted, broad QRS complex. Atrial ectopics are benign and resolve spontaneously within 3 months in the majority of cases. If in doubt, a 24-hour ECG should be performed before discharge and discussed with a cardiologist.

Sinus tachycardia

There is *a normal P wave* (morphology and axis) *preceding each QRS complex*. The underlying cause should be identified and treated: usually secondary to a systemic cause: fever, sepsis, hypovolaemia, pain, respiratory failure, anaemia, fluid overload, inotropes. Occasionally secondary to structural heart disease or myocardial disease.

Atrial flutter

Not infrequent in preterms and associated with myocardial disease and structural heart disease. Atrial rates are above 300/min with a varying degree of AV block. Flutter waves may not be apparent unless adenosine is administered. Flutter may resolve spontaneously. Sustained flutter will lead to heart failure. If in shock, DC cardioversion is indicated or oesophageal override pacing if available under adequate sedation or anaesthesia. Otherwise, digoxin can be used with the addition of propranolol if required.

Atrioventricular re-entry tachycardia (AVRT)

The commonest supraventricular tachycardia (SVT) in the newborn period and is caused by an accessory AV pathway. ECG shows a short PR interval and a delta wave (slurred upstroke) in the narrow QRS complex in Wolff–Parkinson–White syndrome. There may be additional P waves with abnormal axis. The QRS rate is usually between 180 and 300/min. Cases may be asymptomatic, but if the arrhythmia is sustained, present with signs of heart failure before eventual collapse. One fifth will recur after treatment.

Management of supraventricular tachycardia

Assessment with 12-lead ECG; monitor HR and BP; check blood glucose, U&Es, blood gas; and correct any disturbances. Discuss with a cardiologist.
- Vagal manoeuvres:
  - facial immersion in cold water for up to 10 s (diving reflex) or, more usually, ice pack to the face; use superseded by adenosine
  - adenosine 100–300 µg/kg rapid IV bolus
  - start with a low dose (100 µg/kg), increase in 50–100 µg/kg increments, using a large cannula, as close to heart as possible, with 3-way tap to administer rapid IV bolus followed by saline flush with continuous ECG recording
  - retry vagal manoeuvres and adenosine at intervals

- **Propranolol** (if there are no signs of heart failure): 0.05 mg/kg IV then 1–2 mg/kg every 8 h maintenance after discussion with cardiologist
- **Digoxin** (if there are signs of heart failure or propranolol has failed): ensure not hypokalaemic and no WPW:
  - *loading*: 10 μg/kg IV over 15 min then 5 μg/kg IV after 6 hours, repeat after further 6 h
  - *maintenance*: 4 μg/kg every 12 h (60% of oral dose if giving IV)
- **Amiodarone** (as directed by a cardiologist): 2 mg/kg over 5 hours loading dose. This is very effective and has the least negatively inotropic effect
- **Artificial pacing** (transvenous or oesophageal): capture then override pacing if there is sufficient time and expertise
- **Electrical cardioversion**
  - if the baby is in shock, synchronous DC cardioversion with 0.5, 1, then 2 J/kg is indicated with appropriate sedation and analgesia.

Maintenance therapy for 6–12 months with the agent that successfully converted rhythm.

Ventricular ectopics (VE)

Premature and broad QRS complexes without a preceding P wave and followed by a compensatory pause. Occasional VE in a well baby do not require further investigation, but follow up in 6–8 weeks. If VE are frequent and/or there are any features of cardiac disease, the baby needs to be investigated with echocardiography and 24-hour ECG to look for ventricular tachycardia.

Ventricular tachycardia

Ventricular tachycardia is rare in the newborn period. It consists of more than three in a row or continuous VE at a rate of 150–250/min. If P waves are seen at all, they are dissociated from the QRS complexes and may be abnormal. Usually secondary to a non-cardiac cause, such as hypoxia, acidosis, or electrolyte disturbance, but can occasionally be due to myocardial disease or structural heart disease. Symptomatic cases require an anti-arrhythmic (e.g. lidocaine) infusion. If collapsed then synchronized DC cardioversion is needed, but if pulseless full cardiopulmonary resuscitation (CPR) should be initiated. Most cardiologists advocate prophylactic treatment with propranolol or amiodarone even if asymptomatic.

Ventricular fibrillation (VF)

This is fortunately rare in newborns. QRS complexes are *broad* and *chaotic*. Full *CPR* should be initiated with asynchronous DC shocks of 4 J/kg as per advanced paediatric life support (APLS) algorithm. This is usually a terminal arrhythmia.

Further information

Family support resources at ℗ www.bhf.org.uk/heart-health/conditions/congenital-heart-disease

Malviya MN, Ohlsson A, Shah SS. Surgical versus medical treatment with cyclooxygenase inhibitors for symptomatic patent ductus arteriosus in preterm infants. *Cochrane Database Syst Rev* 2013; **28**:3:CD003951.

Ohlsson A, Walia R, Shah SS. Ibuprofen for the treatment of patent ductus arteriosus in preterm or low birth weight (or both) infants. *Cochrane Database Syst Rev* 2015; **18**:2:CD003481.

Schranz D, Michel-Behnke I. Advances in interventional and hybrid therapy in neonatal congenital heart disease. *Semin Fetal Neonatal Med* 2013; **18**: 311–321.

Sekarski N, Meijboom EJ, Di Bernardo S, Ksontini TB, Mivelaz Y. Perinatal arrhythmias. *Eur J Pediatr* 2014; **173**: 983–996.

Thangaratinam S, Brown K, Zamora J, Khan KS, Ewer AK. Pulse oximetry screening for critical congenital heart defects in asymptomatic newborn babies: a systematic review and meta-analysis. *Lancet* 2012; **379**: 2459–2464.

Gastrointestinal problems

Gastrointestinal signs: vomiting

- Occasional, small amounts of non-bilious vomiting (usually curdled milk) is common and usually normal
- Bilious vomiting in the newborn should be assumed to be a sign of intestinal obstruction until proven otherwise and requires further assessment.

Initial management of persistent or bilious vomiting

- Stop enteral feeds and start IV maintenance fluids
- Insert nasogastric tube (NGT) and aspirate regularly or put on free drainage
- Perform a detailed examination, abdominal X-ray (AXR), U&Es, partial septic screen
- If assessment suggests obstruction then discuss with surgical team
- Gastrointestinal (GI) contrast studies, abdominal ultrasound scan and/or rectal biopsy may be indicated
- If investigations are normal, attempt to reintroduce feeds after 24 hours.

Differential diagnosis of vomiting

Intestinal causes
- Normal posseting
- Gastro-oesophageal reflux
- Mechanical bowel obstruction
  - oesophageal atresia (OA)
  - duodenal atresia
  - Hirschsprung's disease
  - malrotation and volvulus
  - necrotizing enterocolitis
  - meconium ileus
  - meconium plug
  - obstructed inguinal hernia
  - diaphragmatic hernia
  - pyloric stenosis
  - lactobezoar.

Extra-intestinal causes
- Infection (meningitis, UTI, pyelonephritis)
- Neurological (intracranial haemorrhage, hydrocephalus with ↑ ICP)
- Cardiac (cardiac failure)
- Metabolic (galactosaemia, congenital adrenal hyperplasia, thyrotoxicosis).

Clues to the cause
- Low volume regurgitation in a well infant may be posseting or a sign of gastro-oesophageal reflux
- Beware persistent vomiting that may indicate a bowel obstruction. A high obstruction will present shortly after birth, whereas a low obstruction usually presents later
- Bile-stained vomiting is a significant sign associated with lower GI obstruction

- Polyhydramnios on antenatal scans may herald a bowel atresia
- Excessive oral mucous secretions combined with inability to pass a NGT necessitates the exclusion of oesophageal atresia
- Delayed passage of meconium (>48 h) and abdominal distension may be due to Hirschsprung's disease
- In the ex-preterm, check for inguinal hernias that may have become obstructed.

Haematemesis/bloody gastric aspirates

- Small amounts of fresh blood or 'coffee grounds' vomit are not uncommon and self-limiting in most infants
- Check FBC and coagulation
- Determine whether there is maternal blood present by sending a sample to check fetal Hb content (Apt's test).

Differential diagnosis of haematemesis

- Swallowed maternal blood at delivery or cracked nipple
- Trauma (following NGT insertion, suctioning, laryngoscopy)
- Stress-induced ulceration (from perinatal asphyxia, intensive care)
- Steroid-induced ulceration.

Rarer causes of haematemesis

- Haemorrhagic disease of the newborn
- Liver disease (acquired vitamin K deficiency)
- Disseminated intravascular coagulation
- Inherited clotting disorders
- Upper GI haemangioma
- Peptic ulcer
- Congenital oesophageal varices.

Gastrointestinal signs: bloody stools and diarrhoea

Bloody stools

Assess for signs of dehydration and anaemia. Check FBC and coagulation.

Differential diagnosis of bloody stools
- Includes causes of haematemesis
- Anorectal fissure
- Necrotizing enterocolitis
- Cow's milk protein intolerance.

Rarer causes
- Hirschsprung's disease
- Meckel's diverticulum
- Malrotation and volvulus
- Intussusception
- Haemangioma/telangiectasia
- Intestinal polyp
- Intestinal duplication.

Diarrhoea

Frequent and loose stools may lead to dehydration and failure to thrive. Initially assess for infection and cow's milk protein intolerance. Investigations for rarer causes need specialist gastroenterology input.

Differential diagnosis of diarrhoea
- Infection (GI or generalized)
- Cow's milk protein intolerance
- Necrotizing enterocolitis
- Hirschsprung's disease.

Rarer causes
- Cystic fibrosis
- Electrolyte transport defects (congenital chloride or sodium diarrhoea)
- GI mucosal disorders (e.g. congenital microvillous atrophy)
- Immunodeficiency (e.g. Shwachman syndrome)
- Autoimmune enterocolitis.

Gastro-oesophageal reflux

Relaxation of the lower oesophageal sphincter allowing gastric contents to ascend the oesophagus.

Aetiology

Reflux of gastric contents into the oesophagus is controlled by the lower oesophageal sphincter. The resting tone of the sphincter is low in preterm babies, predisposing them to reflux. This is exacerbated by slower gastric emptying in preterms, leading to higher residual gastric volumes; and babies with chronic lung disease will also have higher intra-abdominal pressure. In addition, giving caffeine lowers sphincter tone. Gastric emptying is faster in breastfed infants, although breast milk fortifier delays emptying in fully-fed infants. GOR is common following repair of oesophageal atresia and congenital diaphragmatic hernia, and in infants with severe brain injury.

Clinical features

- Vomiting
- Apnoea and desaturations; may occasionally cause severe acute life-threatening events (ALTE).

Complications

- Oesophagitis
- Aspiration into lungs
- Worsening of BPD/CLD
- Failure to thrive.

Investigations

- In practice, trial of therapy is often started based upon a clinical diagnosis
- Investigations are used when diagnosis remains unclear
- Test for acidic oral secretions using litmus
- Upper GI contrast study (to exclude congenital malformations)
- 24-hour oesophageal pH study is the gold standard (but not always performed) and simultaneous impedance study may reveal non-acid reflux.

Management

In preterm infants the benefits of treating reflux with medication need to be balanced with the risk of additives to feeds given the poor evidence base for anti-reflux medications and recognized adverse effects.

- Smaller feed volumes
- Elevated head position to 30° from horizontal
- Prone position (not recommended at home)
- Feed thickener (e.g. Carobel® or Thick and Easy®)
- Antacid (e.g. Gaviscon®, contains 1 mmol sodium per dose)
- Ranitidine and domperidone (associated with arrhythmias)
- Erythromycin (prokinetic dose)

- Surgery (fundoplication) is rarely needed, but is considered when there is recurrent aspiration, or life-threatening events and failure of medical management.

Outcome

- Reflux decreases with age as the lower oesophageal sphincter matures and has nearly always resolved by 1 year of age
- Infants with neurological or anatomical abnormalities are more likely to have persistent and severe reflux.

Pyloric stenosis

Acquired hypertrophy of the circular muscle layer of the stomach pylorus, resulting in upper intestinal obstruction and requiring surgical treatment.

Epidemiology

- Incidence: 3 in 1000 live births
- M:F ratio 4:1
- Genetic predisposition
- Oesophageal atresia and transpyloric feeding both increase risk.

Clinical features

- Presents between 2 and 8 weeks of age
- Episodic, non-bilious, projectile vomiting at the end or following feeds
- Characteristically hungry feeder
- Hypochloraemic alkalosis
- Unconjugated hyperbilirubinaemia
- Remember as a cause for persistent vomiting in ex-preterm infants.

Diagnosis

- Perform a 'test' feed: palpate for the hypertrophied pylorus (feels like an olive) during feeding and observe for gastric peristalsis and projectile vomiting
- U&Es and blood gas
- US scan of the pylorus is the gold standard.

Management

- Stop enteral feeding and start IV fluids
- Correct any electrolyte disturbance before surgery
- Surgical treatment with Ramstedt's pyloromyotomy
- Post-operatively, feeding is reintroduced within 24 hours with transient vomiting being common.

Complications are unusual and long-term outcome is generally good.

Oesophageal atresia/tracheo-oesophageal fistula

A congenital malformation where the oesophagus ends in a pouch and fails to connect to the stomach. Often associated with an abnormal connection between the trachea and oesophagus.

Epidemiology
- Incidence: 1 in 3500 live births
- More than half will have additional malformations including VACTERL association.

Types of OA
See Fig. 10.1.

History
Antenatal US scan often shows polyhydramnios, and/or absent stomach bubble, and/or associated congenital anomalies.

Clinical features
- Preterm birth more common due to polyhydramnios
- Excessive production of frothy saliva
- Episodes of choking and cyanosis exacerbated by attempts to feed
- Failure to pass NGT
- Choking and abdominal distension predominate in infants with an isolated tracheo-oesophageal fistula.

Investigation
- Attempt to pass a large NGT (10 or 12 Fr) that typically halts around 10 cm from the lips (smaller tubes tend to curl in the oesophageal pouch)
- Perform CXR with nasogastric tube (NGT) in situ—reveals the tip in the oesophageal pouch usually at level of T2–T4, presence of gas in the stomach indicates a fistula (see Fig. 10.2)
- Search for features of trisomy 13 and 18, VACTERL association (vertebral anomalies, anal atresia, cardiac malformations, cardiovascular anomalies, tracheo-esophageal fistula, esophageal atresia, renal and/or radial anomalies, limb anomalies) and other congenital malformations using echocardiogram, renal US scan, AXR, spine X-ray.

Management
- Position head up and prone
- Pass a Replogle tube (large bore, double lumen), maintain on low-level suction and may need regular flushing with saline. This prevents build-up of secretions in the oesophageal pouch aspirating into the lungs
- If Replogle tube unavailable—use a wide-bore NGT and aspirate regularly (e.g. every 10 min)
- Transfer to a surgical centre when stable

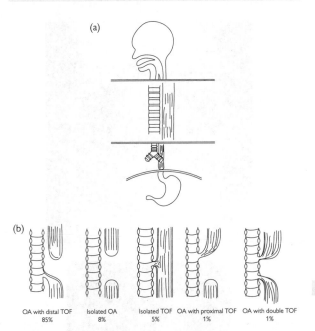

Fig. 10.1(a) and (b) Anatomical types of oesophageal atresia (OA) and tracheo-oesophageal fistula (TOF) with relative frequency. Trachea on left and oesophagus on right showing upper oesophageal pouch, fistula, and lower oesophageal segment.

- Rarely, in babies with severe respiratory disease (e.g. preterms), ventilation may become difficult because respiratory gases will take the path of least resistance (i.e. through the fistula into the stomach). Emergency ligation of the fistula is then indicated. As a temporizing measure, use low-pressure ventilation and position endotracheal tube tip below the fistula.

Surgical treatment
- Ligation of the fistula and primary anastomosis of the oesophageal segments, usually through a right thoracotomy approach
- Post-operative feeding is initially through a transanastomotic feeding tube for the first few days then orally when the surgical team are confident the repair will hold. A contrast study may be helpful if there is concern.

(a)

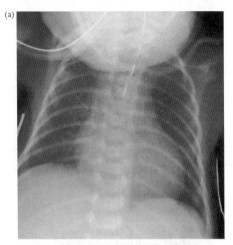

(b)

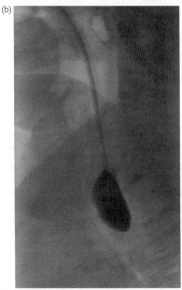

Fig. 10.2 (a) CXR shows a Replogle tube in the upper oesophageal pouch with the tip at the level of T5. Absence of air within the stomach suggests there is no fistula. (b) Contrast study (lateral view) shows collection of contrast in the upper oesophageal pouch.

In cases where there is a large gap between oesophageal segments

- A repair under tension can be attempted. The proximal segment may be extended with a myotomy or using a flap. Post-operatively, muscle relaxation and ventilatory support for 5 days, with head maintained in a flexed position, may be required
- Alternatively, anastomosis can be delayed (e.g. by 3 months) allowing time for oesophageal growth, with gastrostomy for feeding in the interim. Sham feeding before repair may reduce subsequent oral aversion
- In severe cases, a segment of colon may be used to bridge the gap.

Complications

Immediate complications are uncommon, but include anastomotic leak that usually improves with conservative management. Later complications include anastomotic stricture and GOR that respond well to dilatation and medication, respectively. Most infants have a degree of tracheomalacia and a cough ('TOF cough') that usually improves with age.

Outcome

Depends on the presence or absence of associated anomalies. Survival is over 95% with good functional outcome in well-grown infants with isolated OA and TOF, but morbidity is increased in very low birth weight (VLBW) infants with serious cardiac defects.

Malrotation and volvulus

Malrotation is the congenital malposition of bowel resulting from the failure of normal rotation during embryogenesis, and it predisposes to volvulus. Volvulus is the twisting of bowel and its mesentery that obstructs blood flow and results in bowel ischaemia and infarction.

Epidemiology
- M > F
- Associated with congenital diaphragmatic hernia, abdominal wall defects, duodenal atresia, Hirschsprung's disease, situs inversus, and biliary atresia.

Aetiology
Failure of rotation during midgut development results in small bowel mesentery attaching to a narrow pedicle. This predisposes to a volvulus around the axis of the superior mesenteric vessels.

Clinical features
- Commonly presents in the first month of life with bilious vomiting but may present later (may even present in adulthood)
- Initially, vomiting is intermittent then becomes persistent with a volvulus
- Abdominal distension
- Rectal bleeding
- Progressing to hypovolaemic shock in volvulus.

Investigations
- **AXR**: non-specific at first, but progresses to show an abnormal bowel gas distribution, with small bowel on the right, large bowel on the left, and sometimes a 'double bubble' sign
- **US scan**: abnormal relationship of superior mesenteric vessels
- **Upper GI contrast study**: with malrotation the duodenum does not cross the midline, the duodenojejunal flexure lies to the right of the spine, and abnormal position of the caecum in the upper abdomen. With a volvulus, contrast is obstructed and forms a 'corkscrew' pattern.

Management
- Resuscitation as appropriate
- If volvulus is suspected then emergency surgery is indicated to untwist the volvulus, prevent further ischaemia, and resect necrotic non-viable bowel
- Surgery is required electively for malrotation even in well infants because of the risk of volvulus. Surgical treatment (Ladd's procedure) involves division of peritoneal (Ladd's) bands attached to the caecum, broadening the base of small bowel mesentery, placing the small bowel on the left and the large bowel on the right of the abdomen, and appendicectomy.

Duodenal atresia

A congenital discontinuity of the duodenum usually in the region of the ampulla of Vater that leads to bowel obstruction.

Epidemiology
- Incidence: 1 in 6000 live births
- Associated with malrotation, Down syndrome (30%), and prematurity.

Clinical features
- Antenatal history of polyhydramnios and 'double bubble' on US scan
- Bilious vomiting within hours of birth
- Distended stomach/epigastrium
- Visible gastric peristalsis
- Delayed passage and small amounts of meconium
- In around 20% of cases, the obstruction is proximal to the ampulla resulting in non-bilious vomiting, less abdominal distension, and normal meconium that may delay diagnosis.

Investigations
- AXR: 'double bubble' sign of gas distending the stomach and duodenum along with absence of distal intestinal gas (Fig. 10.3)
- U&Es, glucose, blood gas.

Management
- Stop enteral feeds and start IV fluids
- Insert NGT, and leave on free drainage
- Correct any electrolyte or acid-base disturbances
- Examine for signs of trisomy 21 and other congenital anomalies, and check karyotype if suspected
- Early definitive surgical treatment is usually by anastomosis of the duodenal segments
- Post-operatively, parenteral nutrition is required for around a week until intestinal function recovers
- Long-term outcome is good, but depends on associated anomalies.

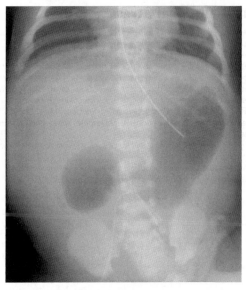

Fig. 10.3 AXR showing 'double bubble' sign of duodenal atresia.

Jejunal and ileal atresia

- Often caused by intrauterine mesenteric infarction and subsequent absorption of a bowel segment leaving small bowel atresia
- Often associated with shortened bowel length and microcolon
- The clinical signs are similar to duodenal atresia. Bilious vomiting starts within 48 hours of age with higher atresias presenting earlier. In jejunal atresia, vomiting is more prominent whereas in ileal atresia, abdominal distension is more prominent. Sometimes meconium is passed
- AXR: dilated bowel loops, multiple fluid levels, peritoneal calcification (due to intrauterine perforation), 'triple bubble' appearance in jejunal atresia
- Perform genetic testing for cystic fibrosis, or a sweat test as 15% will have meconium ileus
- Management is similar to duodenal atresia, but may involve resection of a dilated proximal segment and there may be multiple atresias.

Necrotizing enterocolitis

- A disease with significant morbidity mainly affecting the bowel of preterm infants
- The cardinal features are abdominal distension, bilious aspirates, and bloody stools.

Epidemiology

Incidence: 1–3 per 1000 live births, 2–5% of VLBW infants.

Aetiology

Numerous risk factors for necrotizing enterocolitis (NEC) have been identified and the most significant are hypoxia, prematurity, and enteral nutrition. See Fig. 10.4.

Pathogenesis

Gut ischaemia causes haemorrhage and ulceration predisposing to NEC. Ischaemia may be chronic, such as persistent fetal hypoxia associated with intrauterine growth retardation (IUGR), or acute, from perinatal asphyxia.

Most babies that develop NEC have been enterally fed. Undigested milk acts as a substrate for gas- and toxin-producing bacteria and the preterm gut is more permeable to micro-organisms and relatively deficient in immunoglobulins.

Several bacteria are associated with NEC including *Escherichia coli*, *Klebsiella*, *Enterobacter*, and coagulase negative staphylococci—up to 50% of infants with NEC have a positive blood culture. A minority of cases occur in epidemics associated with a similar range of organisms, but including clostridia and rotavirus.

History

- Presence of any risk factors (see Fig. 10.4)
- Fetal echogenic bowel and abnormal fetal blood flow (e.g. absent or reversed end-diastolic flow in the umbilical arteries).

Clinical features

- Typically presents in the second or third weeks of age in preterms (but may present at any time in the first few weeks until term)
- Presents in the first few days in term infants following perinatal asphyxia, or with congenital heart disease
- Onset may be rapid (hours) or insidious (days)
- Commonest sites affected are the terminal ileum, caecum, and ascending colon, although NEC may affect any part of the gut
- Consider NEC in any unwell preterm infant with abdominal distension.

Staging of NEC

(After Bell et al.) Infants may present at any stage.

Stage I: suspected
- History of perinatal 'stress'
- **Systemic signs:** temperature instability, lethargy, apnoea, desaturations, bradycardias

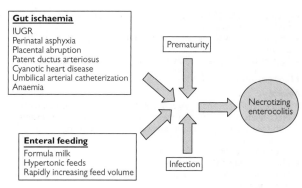

Fig. 10.4 Risk factors for necrotizing enterocolitis.

- **GI signs**: not tolerating feeds, increased gastric aspirates, bilious aspirates, vomiting, mild abdominal distension, faecal occult blood, absent bowel sounds
- **AXR**: distension, mild ileus.

Stage II: confirmed

Features of stage 1 plus:
- **Systemic signs**: metabolic acidosis
- **GI signs**: persistent GI (occult/gross) bleeding, marked abdominal distension and ascites, palpable distended bowel loops, tender abdomen, abdominal discolouration
- **AXR**: significant distension, bowel wall oedema, fixed bowel loops, pneumatosis intestinalis, portal vein gas.

Stage III: advanced

Features of stage 1 and 2 plus:
- **Systemic signs**: deterioration of vital signs, hypotension, shock
- **GI signs**: marked GI haemorrhage
- **AXR**: pneumoperitoneum.

Investigations

- ↑ WCC and CRP, ↓ Hb, platelets initially ↑, but later ↓
- **U&Es**: progressively deranged as fluid is lost into the abdomen and tissues
- **Blood gas**: metabolic (lactic) acidosis
- **AXR**: dilated loops, thickened bowel wall, fixed bowel loops (stays in the same position in serial X-rays), pneumatosis intestinalis (pathognomonic, intramural gas—i.e. within the bowel wall produced by bacteria seen radiologically and histologically), fluid levels, 'white out' from gross ascites, gas in portal venous system, free peritoneal gas from a perforation, Rigler's sign (i.e. air on both sides of bowel wall), football sign, air outlining the falciform ligament

- Lateral decubitus X-ray may aid detection of free gas if bowel perforation is suspected
- US scan: bowel wall thickening, intramural gas, free peritoneal fluid
- Blood culture
- Test for occult blood in aspirates and stool (rule out anal fissure).

Management

Medical

- Stop enteral feeds and medications. If there is only mild suspicion of NEC, feeds can be restarted after a few hours of observation. Infants with stage I disease should be reviewed after ~48 hours regarding restarting feeds
- Insert NGT and leave on free drainage
- Monitor hourly gastric aspirates
- Start antibiotics with broad spectrum cover (e.g. gentamicin, amoxicillin, metronidazole)
- Analgesia is necessary because NEC is painful (e.g. morphine IVI)
- Close monitoring (e.g. bloods and blood gas ~6-hourly, AXR up to 12-hourly in first 48 hours to look for perforation then consider daily until improving)
- Have a low threshold for initiating respiratory support. Abdominal distension may need ventilation using high pressures
- Remove umbilical artery catheter (UAC) in confirmed cases
- Restrict maintenance fluids and provide cardiovascular support using fluid boluses and inotropes to maintain adequate perfusion. Significant fluid volume may be lost into the abdomen
- Transfuse blood products as needed—red cells, platelets, fresh frozen plasma, clotting factors
- Total parenteral nutrition (TPN) probably required if feeds are to be stopped for more than 24 hours. Consider withholding lipid for first 24 hours in the sickest infants
- Insert central venous line (to administer PN) or for inotropic support if required
- Treat with antibiotics and withhold enteral feeds for at least 7 days for confirmed cases (severe cases may need up to 14 days)
- Restart enteral feeds cautiously, when the abdomen is soft; bowel sounds are present; aspirates, AXR, and inflammatory markers have normalized
- Restart feeds at 10–30ml/kg/d using breast milk or term formula for 24 hours
- Thereafter, increase feeds cautiously.

Surgical

- The indications for surgery are perforation or failure to respond to medical management
- Up to 50% of infants with confirmed NEC will require surgery
- Surgery involves laparotomy with resection of necrotic bowel. Anastomosis may be primary if the infant and bowel are in good condition. Otherwise, defunctioning stoma(s) can be formed or multiple

segments can be isolated using the 'clip and drop' method followed by reversal around 2 months later
- Immediate complications include sepsis and wound dehiscence
- Enteral feeds are reintroduced post-operatively after 7–10 days. Re-feeding through a distal mucous fistula may promote gut adaptation
- Rarely, infants have extensive necrosis at laparotomy with insufficient viable bowel to survive. A palliative care approach may then be considered, sometimes with a defunctioning jejunostomy
- Peritoneal drainage can be used in small infants who are too unstable for surgery, but does not usually prevent the need for later surgery.

Outcome

- Overall mortality is 10–20%, but higher in more immature infants and those with extensive disease
- Recurrence rate is 5–10%
- Diarrhoea and malabsorption are transient during recovery and serious long-term problems are uncommon, but include stricture, short gut syndrome, cysts, and fistulae
- Strictures occur in up to 40% and present with intestinal obstruction 2–6 weeks following the acute illness
- Severe NEC is associated with periventricular leucomalacia and neurodevelopmental problems, with a greater risk in those having resection.

Prevention

If there are risk factors for NEC (e.g. prematurity, or absent/reversed end diastolic flow):
- Avoid formula milk with high osmolality and additives
- Trophic feeding (minimal volumes of enteral feed) has not been shown to increase the risk of NEC
- Increase enteral feeds slowly—e.g. start at 10–30 ml/kg/day and increase every 12–24 hours. The optimal rate of increasing feeds remains unclear
- Be guided by gastric aspirates, abdominal distension, and bowel opening when increasing feeds. If there are any concerns consider stopping enteral feeds; do not increase them
- Consider avoiding increasing enteral feeding while UAC in situ (although this is controversial)
- Maintain blood pressure, hydration, and normothermia
- Probiotics and prebiotics are suggested to reduce risk but benefit has not been proven.

Short bowel syndrome

Short bowel syndrome describes the constellation of malabsorption, diarrhoea, and poor growth.

Aetiology

There is loss of bowel absorptive area and the commonest cause is NEC. Up to 10% of infants with NEC surviving surgery develop short gut syndrome. Infants with less than 100 cm or less than 50% of small bowel are at high risk of short bowel syndrome, and infants with less than 40 cm of small bowel will need long-term parenteral nutrition.

Management

- Multidisciplinary management including surgeon, gastroenterologist, dietician, and pharmacist
- Maintain electrolyte balance and adequate caloric intake, as well as nutrients and trace elements
- Enteral feeds promote gut adaptation. A protein hydrosylate (e.g. Pregestimil®) or amino acid formula (e.g. Neocate®) is usually needed. Probiotics may be helpful
- Increase feeds slowly over weeks. Continuous feeding and anti-reflux (e.g. ranitidine), anti-motility medications (e.g. loperamide), and bile acid binders (e.g. colestyramine) may be beneficial
- If the infant is well, PN can be administered at home with appropriate community support
- In severe cases, surgery to increase bowel absorptive area is an option
- Rarely, for infants that remain PN dependent beyond a year, small bowel transplantation has been attempted with mixed results.

Outcome

- A process of gradual gut adaptation occurs over the first few months of age
- An intact ileum and ileocaecal valve increases the chances of adaptation, results in less diarrhoea, and allows vitamin B_{12} and bile acid absorption
- Eventually, most infants are able to feed entirely enterally and more than 90% of infants will survive
- Weight gain is slow, but most reach a normal (above 1st percentile) weight by 3 years.

Hirschsprung's disease

Congenital absence of innervation in the distal bowel leading to obstruction that requires surgical resection.

Pathology

Congenital absence of ganglion cells in the rectal mucosa extending proximally resulting in tonic contraction of the affected segment that leads to distal bowel obstruction.

Length of the affected segment is variable

Often (75%) only the rectum and sigmoid colon are affected, in some cases disease extends to the splenic flexure and transverse colon (15%), or to the entire colon and terminal ileum (8%), and further in rare cases.

Pathogenesis

Failure of migration of neural crest cells along the gut during embryogenesis. There are autosomal dominant and recessive forms. Genes implicated include the RET proto-oncogene and the endothelin-B receptor gene on chromosome 13.

Epidemiology

- Incidence: 1 in 5000 live births
- Ratio M:F of 4:1
- Associated with trisomy 21, congenital central hypoventilation syndrome, Waardenburg syndrome, and multiple endocrine neoplasia.

Clinical features

- Delayed passage of meconium (>48 hours in term babies)
- Progressively worsening abdominal distension
- Poor feeding
- Bilious vomiting
- Rectal examination reveals a contracted ano-rectum, and may provide temporary relief with explosive passage of stool and flatus.

Complications

- Hirschsprung's enterocolitis
- Severe cases may resemble NEC with marked abdominal distension, fever, diarrhoea, and vomiting.

Investigations

- **Suction rectal biopsy:** taken 2 cm above anal canal shows aganglionosis, thickened nerve trunks, and increased acetylcholinesterase activity
- **AXR:** multiple dilated bowel loops, absence of rectal gas, bowel wall thickening and mucosal irregularity in enterocolitis, fluid levels (Fig. 10.5)
- **Contrast enema:** use an isotonic water-soluble contrast medium (e.g. Gastrografin®), proximally dilated colon leading to a triangular transition zone ending in a narrow distal segment (a recent PR examination will make these findings less dramatic; see Fig. 10.6)
- **Anorectal manometry:** raised rectal resting pressure, but rarely performed.

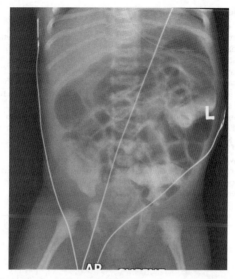

Fig. 10.5 Hirschsprung's disease: AXR showing dilated loops of bowel and absence of air in the rectum.

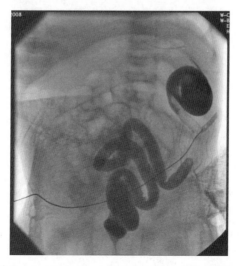

Fig. 10.6 Contrast study showing a transition zone and proximally dilated bowel.

Management
- Liaise with the surgical team for assessment and rectal biopsy
- Decompression by rectal lavage using warm saline twice daily initially then daily as guided by the surgical team
- Antibiotics and PN in severe cases
- Regular dilatation or washouts until feeding well
- **Surgical treatment:** primary pull-through involves resection of the affected segment and primary anastomosis of the healthy colon to the rectal stump
- In severe cases complicated by enterocolitis or perforation, a temporary stoma can be formed and anastomosis delayed until around 6 months.

Outcome
- 75% will achieve good bowel control by adulthood
- Long-term problems include faecal incontinence, constipation, and enterocolitis. These are more common in infants with Down syndrome and those with a difficult post-operative course.

Meconium ileus

Bowel obstruction caused by highly viscid meconium within the lumen.

Epidemiology

- Cystic fibrosis (CF) is almost always the cause
- Around 15% of infants with CF present with meconium ileus.

Clinical features

- Antenatal history of hyperechogenic bowel on US scan
- Family history of CF or parental CF carrier status
- Most common site of obstruction is the distal ileum
- Progressively worsening bilious vomiting
- Failure to pass meconium
- Abdominal distension and rarely perforation
- Palpable and sometimes visible bowel loops
- Sometimes palpable abdominal mass.

Investigations

- **AXR:** dilated bowel loops, bubble appearance of air within meconium, few fluid levels, occasionally free air from perforation
- **Contrast enema:** microcolon, inspissated meconium in ileum, and dilated proximal bowel
- Genetic testing for CF and sweat test.

Management

- Insert NGT
- Stop feeding and start IV fluids
- Therapeutic enema by a radiologist during investigation using contrast (e.g. Gastrografin®) or by a surgeon using saline
- Repeated daily until there is normal bowel opening
- Hyperosmolar solutions draw fluid into the bowel lumen and soften the meconium (and increase fluid requirements)
- Surgery is required if there is no response to medical treatment by enterotomy and irrigation; resection, and primary anastomosis; or resection, and temporary stoma formation
- Survival is >90%, but long-term outcome is related to the underlying disease.

Anterior abdominal wall defects: exomphalos and gastroschisis

Exomphalos (omphalocele)

A congenital umbilical defect with prolapse of gut within an amniotic sac outside the abdominal cavity (Fig. 10.7).

Epidemiology

- Incidence: 1 in 5000 live births
- M = F
- Associated with trisomy 13, 18, and 21, as well as cardiac defects and Beckwith–Wiedemann syndrome. 40% will have another congenital malformation.

Aetiology

Failure of fusion of one of the embryonic components of the anterior abdominal wall (cephalic, caudal, or lateral). As a result, the developing gut fails to complete its return to the abdominal cavity.

Clinical features

- Most cases are identified on antenatal US scan
- Defect is of variable size:
  - **hernia into the cord**: small defect with gut prolapse into the umbilical cord
  - **exomphalos minor**: moderate size defect, <5 cm wide
  - **exomphalos major**: large defect, >5 cm wide, containing gut and often liver. Respiratory insufficiency results from pulmonary hypoplasia.
- There is often some degree of malrotation.

Management

- Respiratory support as indicated
- Insert NGT, aspirate frequently, and leave on free drainage
- Withhold feeds and start IV fluids/TPN
- Monitor blood glucose for hypoglycaemia (due to the association with Beckwith–Wiedemann syndrome)
- Upper GI contrast study
- Karyotype and echocardiography.

Surgical treatment

- Smaller defects can be closed directly
- Larger defects require a delayed repair
- A prosthetic sheath can cover the sac and be tethered to the rim of the defect. Gradually reducing the volume of the silo allows reduction of the sac over 7–10 days before surgical closure of the defect
- Alternatively the sac is allowed to sclerose with epithelialization from the edges. The sac will gradually contract and eventually the defect may be closed. Desiccating agents (e.g. silver sulfadiazine) have been used
- Rupture of the sac at any time needs urgent surgical intervention.

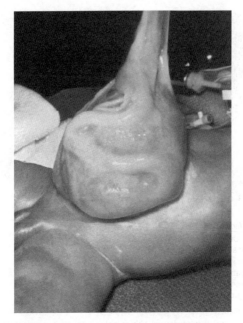

Fig. 10.7 Exomphalos.

Outcome

Good long-term outcome can be expected with repaired exomphalos minor or smaller defects if there are no associated chromosomal abnormalities.

Infants with large defects have a degree of pulmonary hypoplasia and are more likely to have associated anomalies, and mortality ~30%.

Gastroschisis

Abdominal viscera that may include stomach, small bowel, colon, and ovaries/testes prolapse through a congenital defect on the right side of the umbilicus that requires urgent surgical intervention after delivery (Fig. 10.8).

Epidemiology
- Incidence: 1 in 7000 live births
- M = F
- Association with young maternal age and possibly with maternal drugs (e.g. cocaine)
- Pathogenesis remains unclear.

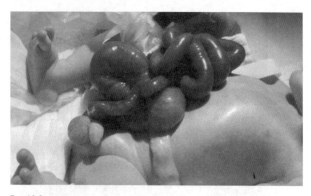

Fig. 10.8 Gastroschisis.

Clinical features
- Most cases are identified on antenatal US scan
- Often small for gestational age
- There is no sac covering the prolapsed abdominal contents
- Appearance of the bowel is variable from normal to covered in a thick fibrin shell
- The gut is unrotated and 10% will have an intestinal atresia.

Management
- Support and wrap the bowel with cellophane or plastic sheath at delivery
- Insert NGT, aspirate frequently, and leave on free drainage
- The exposed bowel is a source of fluid and heat loss. Consider fluid boluses (10–20 ml/kg 0.9% saline or 4.5% human albumin solution). Monitor and correct any electrolyte disturbances
- Withhold feeds, and start IV fluids/PN
- Start IV antibiotics.

Urgent surgical treatment
- Primary closure is possible in some cases. The bowel is reduced and the defect closed along with repair of associated atresias
- Often the bowel is enclosed in a pre-formed plastic silo and gradually reduced over 5–10 days before closure of the defect
- Post-operative care:
  - Monitor for respiratory difficulties, decreased distal perfusion, and abdominal compartment syndrome following reduction
  - PN is needed for around 3 weeks until enteral feeding is established
  - NEC can be a complication.

Outcome
- 90% survival
- Post-operatively problems with absorption and motility are common, with median length of stay around one month.

Inguinal hernia

Herniation of abdominal contents through an area of weakness in the anterior abdominal wall. This is commonly due to failure of closure of the processus vaginalis following descent of the testes in boys. M > F; 1% of boys; more common in preterms.

Clinical features

- 60% right-sided, 30% left-sided, 10% bilateral
- Intermittent swelling in the groin that may involve the scrotum
- Provoked or exacerbated by crying or straining
- A tender, firm lump with vomiting and inconsolable crying may indicate a strangulated hernia.

Management

- Symptomatic hernia:
  - attempt to reduce the hernia using appropriate analgesia
  - this is successful in most cases and surgical closure is undertaken 24–48 hours later
  - irreducible hernias are at risk of strangulating and need urgent surgery
- Asymptomatic hernia:
  - surgery for reducible hernias is undertaken when the baby is fit and just prior to discharge from hospital.

Milk protein intolerance

An allergic reaction to cow's milk that presents with loose stools and poor feeding.

Aetiology

- Antigenic proteins absorbed by the immature gut may provoke an immune reaction
- It may occur in breastfed infants due to small amounts of cow's milk antigen absorbed by the mother and secreted into breast milk
- It is more common in infants with a family history of atopy.

Clinical features

- Diarrhoea, sometimes containing blood and mucus
- Steatorrhoea
- GOR and vomiting
- Abdominal distension
- Weight loss/poor weight gain
- Urticaria.

Investigations

- Guidelines (NICE) have been established in UK for diagnosis, investigation, and management
- Clinical diagnosis: resolution of symptoms after starting an exclusion diet and relapse on reintroduction of feeds
- Radioallergosorbent test (RAST) and skin prick testing
- Intestinal biopsy (only if diagnosis is unclear).

Management

- Hydrolysed protein, hypoallergenic, lactose-free feed (e.g. Pregestimil®, Nutramigen®)
- In severely affected infants with colitis, an elemental feed may be needed (e.g. Neocate®)
- In breastfed infants, excluding maternal ingestion of cow's milk, egg, and soya may lead to resolution of symptoms
- Liaise and follow up with a dietician
- Intolerance resolves by early childhood in most cases.

Anorectal anomalies

There is a wide spectrum of defects of varying severity.

Epidemiology

- Incidence: 1 in 5000 live births
- Around half have another congenital malformation
- There is an association with genito-urinary, skeletal, and gastrointestinal defects, and can be part of the VACTERL association.

Types

See Fig. 10.9.

- 'High' lesions (where the rectum terminates in the pelvis): anal membrane, anal stenosis, perineal fistula, H-type fistula, rectourethral fistula in boys, rectovestibular fistula in girls, rectovesical fistula, cloacal malformations
- 'Low' lesions (where the rectum terminates close to perineal skin): imperforate anus, rectal atresia/stenosis, anterior anus in girls.

Examination

In boys

- Imperforate anus with rectourethral fistula is the most common lesion. There is no patent anal opening but there may be an opening on the perineum or meconium running subcutaneously along the raphe in the midline.

In girls

- An anterior anus or imperforate anus with rectovestibular fistula is the most common lesion
- The normal position of the anus is midway between the posterior fourchette and the tip of the coccyx. If there is no patent anal opening look for a fistula opening just anterior to the posterior fourchette. A single perineal opening suggests a cloacal malformation.

Investigations

- **Lateral prone pelvis XR**: taken after 24 hours of life, with pelvis elevated and radio-opaque marker placed upon the anal dimple, shows the position of rectal gas relative to the marker, gas in the bladder suggests a fistula
- **Look for associated anomalies** using lumbosacral X-ray, CXR, renal US scan, echocardiogram.

Management

Low lesions

- Anal dilation for stenosis to prevent obstruction followed by anoplasty within the newborn period
- Constipation is a common long-term problem.

High lesions

- A temporary colostomy is formed proximal to the defect
- Definitive surgical reconstruction is undertaken a few months later with a posterior sagittal anorectoplasty (PSARP)
- Long-term problems include constipation, faecal incontinence, and psychological problems dependent upon the nature of the defect.

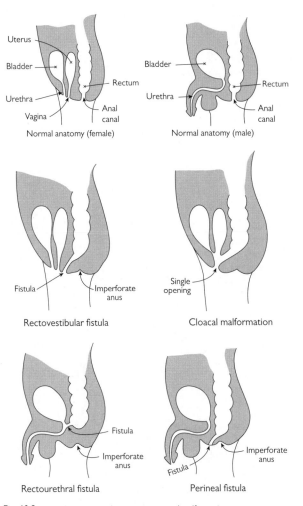

Fig. 10.9 Normal anatomy and common anorectal malformations.

Neurological problems

Neurological examination

A detailed examination is an essential part of the assessment when there is a concern about neurology. It can give diagnostic and prognostic information. Findings change with maturation, for example preterm infants have lower tone than term infants.

Level of consciousness and alertness

Prechtl described five normal behavioural states in term infants:
1. Quiet sleep (eyes closed, regular breathing, no movements)
2. Active sleep (eyes closed, irregular breathing, movements present or absent)
3. Eyes open, regular breathing, no movements
4. Eyes open, gross movements
5. Eyes open or closed, irregular breathing, gross movements, vocalization.

State varies in normal infants depending upon feeding and external stimuli, and is affected by medications (e.g. sedation, anticonvulsants).

Abnormal states include comatose, lethargic, irritable, or hyperexcitable. Listen for a high-pitched or abnormal cry.

General features

- Look for dysmorphic features that may suggest an underlying genetic condition
- Look for skin lesions associated with neurological problems (e.g. port wine stains, café au lait spots)
- Measure and plot head circumference using growth chart
- Assess head shape and anterior fontanelle.

Posture

All four limbs are flexed in term infants.

Movements

Movements vary with state of alertness and are normally smooth, symmetrical, and varied in a writhing manner.

Vision

Term infants fix and follow a face or red ball at 30 cm. Normal pupillary light response and varied eye movements.

Hearing

Response to noise with startle, grimace, head turning.

Face

- Symmetrical facial movements including crying and blinking, particularly palpebral fissures, nasolabial folds, corners of mouth
- Normal suck and rooting (turn to touching corner of mouth)
- Tongue fasciculation can be abnormal.

Tone

- Assess muscle tone by manipulating limbs and using special manoeuvres
- Neck flexor tone (baby pulled to sit from lying)—minimal head lag
- Ventral suspension (baby held up prone)—head extends above body, back extends with limbs flexed
- Vertical suspension (baby held upright under axillae)—takes weight briefly.

Deep tendon reflexes

Depressed with lower motor neuron lesions and increased with upper motor neuron lesions. A few beats of clonus can be normal.

Primitive reflexes

Present at birth and represent intact brainstem. Suppressed by 3–6 months of age and persistence is abnormal.

- Palmar grasp—flexion of fingers when finger placed in palm
- Plantar grasp—flexion of the toes when finger placed on the ball of foot
- Moro—sudden head extension by dropping and catching a short distance causing opening hands, extension and abduction of arms then anterior flexion and cry
- Asymmetric tonic neck reflex—turn head to one side while lying supine causes the fencing posture, extension of arm on that side and flexion of arm on opposite side, and similar but less marked in legs
- Placing/stepping—dorsum of foot touching edge of bed leads to 'walking' motion.

The floppy infant (neonatal hypotonia)

Causes of neonatal hypotonia
See Fig. 11.1.

Assessment
• Preterm infants have reduced tone and power compared to term infants
• Acute causes are often associated with an encephalopathy
• *Difficult delivery* raises the possibility of hypoxic ischaemic injury or rarely spinal cord trauma
• Maternal medications may affect tone (e.g. opiates or substance abuse)
• If there are *dysmorphic* features, consider a chromosomal or genetic disorder (Trisomy 21 or 18, Prader–Willi, or peroxisomal disorders e.g. Zellweger syndrome)
• Is there a *family history* of myasthenia, or myotonic dystrophy, multiple miscarriages, or infant deaths?
• *Good muscle strength* and preservation of/*increased reflexes* may suggest a central cause
• Muscle weakness, more *marked distally* and decreased/*absent reflexes* may suggest a peripheral cause

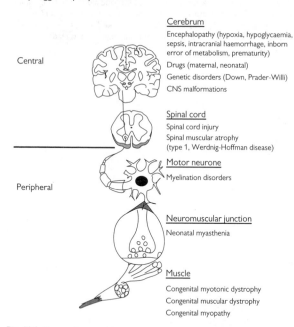

Central

Cerebrum
Encephalopathy (hypoxia, hypoglycaemia, sepsis, intracranial haemorrhage, inborn error of metabolism, prematurity)
Drugs (maternal, neonatal)
Genetic disorders (Down, Prader-Willi)
CNS malformations

Spinal cord
Spinal cord injury
Spinal muscular atrophy
(type 1, Werdnig-Hoffman disease)

Motor neurone
Myelination disorders

Peripheral

Neuromuscular junction
Neonatal myasthenia

Muscle
Congenital myotonic dystrophy
Congenital muscular dystrophy
Congenital myopathy

Fig. 11.1 Causes of neonatal hypotonia.

- Muscle weakness, more *marked proximally* and decreased/*absent reflexes* may suggest a muscular cause
- Ptosis, *bulbar weakness* with *preserved reflexes* may suggest a neuromuscular cause
- Smiling, *alert* but not moving limbs and *tongue fasciculations* may suggest spinal muscular atrophy
- *Contractures* or arthrogryposis may suggest a congenital, rather than acquired cause.

Management of acute hypotonia

- Assess the need for respiratory support as for any other baby
- Quickly exclude acute and life-threatening causes that are reversible (hypoxia, hypoglycaemia, sepsis, electrolyte disturbances)
- Consider starting empirical antibiotics if there is any concern of sepsis
- Cranial ultrasound (CUSS) to investigate intracranial haemorrhage.

Management of persistent hypotonia

Discuss with a paediatric neurologist and keep family informed—investigation and waiting for results in order to establish diagnosis may take weeks.

First-line tests:
- Blood tests (FBC, U&Es, Ca, Mg, glucose, blood gas, thyroid function)
- Septic screen (C-reactive protein (CRP), blood culture, congenital infection screen)
- Creatinine kinase (CPK)
- Metabolic screen (lactate, ammonia, amino acids, acylcarnitines, urine organic acids)
- **Genetics:** karyotype and/or array comparative genomic hybridization (CGH) (LiHep and EDTA samples).

Second-line tests:
- Maternal and baby's acetylcholine receptor (AChR) antibodies (myasthenia)
- Urine toxicology
- Edrophonium test for myasthenia (see ➲ Neuromuscular disease, pp. 316–17)
- **Electrophysiology:** EMG and nerve conduction studies
- **Neuroimaging:** cranial US, MRI brain and spine
- **Muscle biopsy**
- Discuss with metabolic team if any suspicion or results from the screen are abnormal
- Involve a geneticist if there are dysmorphic features or a positive family history.

Neonatal encephalopathy

A clinical syndrome of brain dysfunction in the newborn. The most common cause in newborns is hypoxic ischaemic encephalopathy but there are many other causes of encephalopathy that should not be overlooked.

Causes of neonatal encephalopathy
- Perinatal hypoxic ischaemia
- Septicaemia
- Meningitis
- Maternal substance abuse/neonatal abstinence syndrome
- Maternal anaesthesia and sedation
- Metabolic disease (hypoglycaemia, hypocalcaemia, hyponatraemia, hyperbilirubinaemia, amino acidopathy)
- Cerebral malformation
- Seizure disorder.

Hypoxic ischaemic encephalopathy: incidence, pathophysiology, and clinical features

Acute or chronic impairment of gas exchange causing hypoxia and ischaemia, and consequent damage to the brain (and other organs including kidneys, heart, and liver).

This term more accurately describes the pathophysiology and has replaced the term 'birth asphyxia'.

Incidence

Around 0.5% of term newborns are diagnosed with HIE. Mortality or severe neurodisability due to hypoxic ischaemic injury affects 0.1% of newborns. The incidence is much higher in resource-poor countries.

Pathophysiology

Impaired oxygenation and perfusion may result from:
- Impaired *placental* supply (e.g. uterine contractions, placental abruption, and placental insufficiency)
- Impaired *umbilical* supply (e.g. cord compression/prolapse)
- Impaired *materno*-placental supply (e.g. any cause of maternal hypoxia or hypotension)
- Impaired *neonatal* supply (e.g. difficult delivery and inadequate resuscitation).

Brain injury occurs at the time of the insult (*primary injury*), but a significant injury occurs over the subsequent hours and days (*secondary injury*) due to a cascade of damaging biochemical and cellular processes including free radical production, excitotoxic injury, and apoptosis triggered by the initial insult (see Fig 11.2).

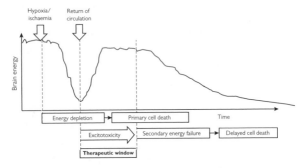

Fig. 11.2 Brain energy failure and injury following hypoxia ischaemia.

Clinical features

- Evidence of a peripartum insult (fetal distress, low Apgar score, depressed condition at birth/need for resuscitation)
- Features of fetal distress are: poor cardiotocograph, acidotic fetal blood sample, meconium-stained liquor, acidotic umbilical blood sample
- **Encephalopathy:** Sarnat staging is often used, see Table 11.1
- Clinical features evolve over the first 72 hours. Milder cases may only become symptomatic after 12 hours whilst on the postnatal ward
- **Respiratory:** apnoeas, PPHN, pulmonary haemorrhage, acute respiratory distress syndrome (ARDS)
- **Renal:** oliguria, haematuria, abnormal urea and creatinine
- **Gastrointestinal:** not tolerating feeds, necrotizing enterocolitis (NEC)
- **Cardiac:** myocardial ischaemia and infarction, ST changes on ECG, hypotension
- **Metabolic:** acidosis, hypoglycaemia, increased AST, ALT, LDH, jaundice, hyponatraemia, fluid overload and SIADH (syndrome of inappropriate antidiuretic hormone secretion), hypocalcaemia, hyperammonaemia
- **Haematological:** disseminated intravascular coagulation (DIC).

Table 11.1 Clinical grading of hypoxic ischaemic encephalopathy (after Sarnat and Sarnat)

Grade	Mild (I)	Moderate (II)	Severe (III)
Conscious level	Hyper-alert	Lethargic	Comatose
Tone	Normal	Mild hypotonia	Flaccid
Posture	Mild distal flexion	Strong distal flexion	Intermittent decerebrate
Reflexes	Increased	Increased	Decreased/absent
Clonus	Present	Present	Absent
Suck	Weak	Weak/absent	Absent
Moro	Strong	Weak, incomplete	Absent
Pupils	Dilated	Pinpoint	Unequal, unreactive
Autonomic	Sympathetic	Parasympathetic	Depressed
HR	Tachycardia	Bradycardia	Variable
GI motility	Normal/decreased	Increased	Variable
Seizures	None	Common, focal	Difficult to control

Hypoxic ischaemic encephalopathy: management I

Management of hypoxic ischaemic encephalopathy: general

- *Resuscitate* effectively following national guidelines using 'ABCD' approach (hyperoxia may be deleterious) (see ➲ Newborn Life Support guidelines in Further information, p. 322).
- Other than therapeutic hypothermia the management is largely supportive (see ➲ Therapeutic hypothermia, pp. 288–9).
- Assess and document severity of encephalopathy—think early about initiating therapeutic hypothermia by passive or active cooling
- Examine for *dysmorphic features*, congenital malformations, or signs of birth trauma
- Detailed documentation of events including resuscitation
- Remain *professional* and do not pass judgement on midwifery or obstetric care.

Ventilation

- Consider respiratory support early. Breathing may be compromised by encephalopathy, meconium aspiration, and seizures
- Ensure *adequate oxygenation*, although hyperoxia may be harmful
- Maintain $PaCO_2$ 4.5–6.0 kPa to preserve cerebral perfusion and limit fluctuations.

Cardiovascular

- Consider invasive BP monitoring and inotropic support early
- Maintain adequate blood pressure (mean arterial BP >40 mmHg in term infants) to ensure adequate organ perfusion. Hypoxic injury to the myocardium may compromise cardiac function
- Start with dobutamine (5–20 µg/kg/min) and dopamine (5–20 µg/kg/min) as needed
- Only give fluid boluses if there is evidence of hypovolaemia
- Monitor Hb, transfuse if low. Acute fall may be a sign of new intracranial haemorrhage
- ECG and echo if there is concern about poor cardiac function.

Fluids

- Initially, *restrict fluids* to 60–80% maintenance (40 ml/kg in first 24 hours), whilst oliguric then liberalize when urine output improves, aiming for a neutral daily fluid balance
- Monitor *urine output* (catheterize if necessary), daily weight, and *U&Es*
- Careful attention to fluid balance to avoid fluid overload, hyponatraemia, and cerebral oedema.

Infection

Look for risk factors and signs of sepsis. If there is any suspicion of sepsis take blood cultures, commence antibiotics, and perform lumbar puncture (LP) when stable.

Hypoxic ischaemic encephalopathy: management II

Neurology

- Observe for *abnormal movements* suggesting seizures
- *EEG*—discontinuous and burst suppression patterns predict poor outcome
- Prompt *treatment of seizures* as detailed in ➔ Neonatal seizures, pp. 290–3. (Seizures in the context of HIE have a particularly detrimental effect by increasing cerebral metabolic demand, hypoxia, and excitation injury, and may worsen neurodevelopmental outcome)
- If muscle relaxants are given then neurology and seizures are difficult to assess and *continuous EEG* should be considered.

Metabolic

- Aim to maintain *normoglycaemia* (2.6–8.0 mmol/l)
- Watch for hypoglycaemia and increase concentration of glucose in maintenance, rather than increasing fluid volume. Start insulin infusion if hyperglycaemic
- Treat hypocalcaemia (corrected Ca <1.7 or ionized Ca <1.0 mmol) with Ca gluconate 10%, 2 ml/kg IV
- Measure LFTs to assess liver injury.

Temperature control

Therapeutic hypothermia is the only treatment proven to be effective (see ➔ Therapeutic hypothermia, pp. 288–9).

Coagulation

Ensure IM phytomenadione (*vitamin K*) is given and monitor *coagulation*; manage any coagulopathy as appropriate using vitamin K, fresh frozen plasma (FFP), cryoprecipitate, or platelets as per local guidelines.

Hypoxic ischaemic encephalopathy: management III

Feeding
- Many withhold enteral feeds for at least 48 hours in babies with moderate or severe encephalopathy due to the *increased risk of NEC*
- Introduce feeds cautiously when clinical condition has improved and increase feed volumes slowly.

Neuroimaging
Cranial ultrasound scan
- Perform early on day 1 and then as guided by clinical condition
- First week: generalized echogenicity, loss of sulci, compressed ventricles (cerebral oedema), bilateral echogenic thalami, discrete periventricular and parenchymal echodensities
- **1–3 weeks:** echolucent cysts
- **>6 weeks:** cortical atrophy and ventriculomegaly
- Initial scan is negative in up to 50% of cases. However, it is important to exclude other causes of encephalopathy, especially intracranial haemorrhage which may need intervention. An abnormal resistance index (<0.55) predicts poor outcome.

MRI brain
- Provides anatomical detail and prognostic information. Conventional MRI shows changes by third day, optimal timing is 5–7 days. Diffusion-weighted imaging (DWI) MRI shows changes in first 24 hours, optimal timing is 2–3 days
- Basal ganglia/thalamus T1 hyperintensity; periventricular white matter T1 hypointensity and T2 hyperintensity; posterior limb of the internal capsule (PLIC) T1 hypointensity; cortical grey–white differentiation lost
- Later there is delayed myelination, cortical atrophy, ventriculomegaly, thinning of the corpus callosum, persistent abnormalities in the basal ganglia and white matter
- DWI: increased signal (decreased diffusion) in injured areas
- Abnormalities in the basal ganglia and PLIC strongly predict motor impairment in childhood.

Redirection towards palliative care
May be appropriate in babies with severe HIE when continuing with intensive care management is likely to be futile. This should be considered carefully using a multidisciplinary approach in conjunction with the family. Review clinical progress and results of EEG and MRI to inform decision-making.

Outcome

Beyond survival, parents are anxious about the risk of long-term disability. Predicting outcome can be difficult and there is no single assessment that is completely accurate.

Severity of encephalopathy can guide outcome:
- **Mild HIE**: no increased risk of death/severe disability
- **Moderate HIE**: 25% risk of death/severe neurodisability
- **Severe HIE**: 75% risk of death/severe neurodisability.

It can useful to consider several predictors and put the infant into a broad group for outcome:
- **Good prognosis** (low risk of disability): mild encephalopathy, no seizures in first 24 hours, no anticonvulsants on discharge, sucking, and feeding on discharge
- **Poor prognosis** (high risk of severe disability): Apgar <5 at 10 minutes, moderate/severe encephalopathy, EEG discontinuous, moderate/severe MRI changes, abnormal neurology and seizures on discharge, not feeding orally on discharge.

The pattern of severe disability is commonly a spastic quadriplegia with severe learning difficulties, visual and hearing loss, and seizures which are difficult to control.

Therapeutic hypothermia

Introduction

Reducing core temperature to 33–34°C for 72 hours instituted within 6 hours of birth followed by gradual rewarming decreases the risk of death and severe disability following moderate to severe HIE. Cooling is recommended as standard care for appropriate infants by the National Institute for Health and Care Excellence and the British Association for Perinatal Medicine. Hypothermia is effective using total body cooling or selective head cooling with a number needed to treat of 7.

Although cooling is relatively easy to institute, there are many physiological and practical considerations. Therefore, cooling can be initiated locally, but should be continued in a specialized centre under the supervision of experienced staff using specialized equipment.

Eligibility for hypothermia

- ≥36 weeks gestation and <6 hours of age
- Infants should meet criteria A, B, and C.

(A) Evidence of perinatal asphyxia

One of the following: Apgar ≤5 at 10 minutes of age; continuing need for respiratory support at 10 minutes of age; pH <7.00 within one hour of birth; base deficit ≥16 within one hour of birth.

(B) Abnormal neurology

Seizures or moderate to severe encephalopathy consisting of: decreased level of consciousness, and hypotonia, and absent/weak suck or Moro response.

(C) Abnormal aEEG

One of the following: seizures; lower margin <5 µV, upper margin <10 µV on aEEG.

- Cooling may be initiated before aEEG is available so that treatment is not delayed. Treatment may be discontinued if neurology and aEEG return to normal within 6 hours of birth.
- Cooling may be considered 'off label' (e.g. infants <36 weeks gestation and initiated >6h after birth) but the benefits and safety are uncertain and should have specific consent from parents.

Initial management

- Cooling should be started as soon as possible ideally in the delivery room
- Continuous rectal and skin temperature monitoring is advisable
- Turn off overhead heating, cot heating, and remove hat and clothing
- 'Passive' cooling can be initiated early and core temperature naturally decreases
- Avoid using fans or ice packs because 'active' cooling is rarely required in the initial period and may lead to overcooling
- Very sick infants may need heating during transport
- Attach aEEG electrodes and begin continuous monitoring
- Discuss with specialized centre and arrange transfer if appropriate.

Physiological effects of cooling
- Bradycardia (HR 80–100 bpm)
- Hypocapnoea (if measured at normothermia and not temperature corrected)
- Increased coagulation times—rarely a problem, treat with blood products if there is active bleeding (e.g. subgaleal haemorrhage)
- Thicker secretions, typically from day 2 (regular suction +/– physiotherapy)
- Discomfort (indicated by HR >110 and facial grimacing)
- Hepatic metabolism reduced (titrate doses of drugs to avoid accumulation)
- Alters the interpretation of prognostic assessments (e.g. clinical examination and aEEG).

Subsequent management
- Target rectal temperature for 72 hours is 33–34°C with whole body cooling and 34–35°C with selective head cooling
- Good neuro-intensive care is vital (strict control of BP, PCO_2, PO_2, electrolytes, glucose) (see ➥ Hypoxic ischaemic encephalopathy: management I, p. 284).
- Maintain PCO_2 45–58 mmHg/6–8 kPa
- Consider withholding feeds during cooling
- Monitor FBC, U&Es, Ca, Mg and coagulation at least daily
- Decrease rates of sedation and muscle relaxants after 12 hours and titrate to clinical signs
- Aggressive treatment of coagulopathy
- Adequate analgesia/sedation (stress may abolish the benefit of hypothermia).

Rewarming
- Rewarm slowly by 0.3°C every hour
- Avoid direct heating of head
- Seizures are more likely to occur during rewarming and should be treated (see ➥ Neonatal seizures, pp. 290–3)
- Hypotension can occur due to systemic vasodilation and should be treated in the usual manner (see ➥ Collapse and shock, pp. 186–7)
- Cease rewarming if there are any adverse effects and restart rewarming at a slower rate when baby has been stabilized (rarely re-cooling is needed)
- Hyperthermia is associated with adverse outcomes.

Neonatal seizures

Seizure: abnormal electrical brain activity causing neurological dysfunction.

Incidence

Seizures affect around 0.1% of all term infants and up to 10% of very low birth weight (VLBW) infants—newborns have a predominance of excitatory synapses relative to adults and alongside other molecular factors are more prone to seizures.

Causes of neonatal seizures

* Hypoxic ischaemic encephalopathy
* Sepsis (meningitis, encephalitis)
* Intracranial haemorrhage (intraventricular, parenchymal, subarachnoid, or subdural)
* Cerebral infarction (stroke, venous sinus thrombosis)
* Congenital brain malformations.

Rarer causes

* Metabolic (hypoglycaemia, hypocalcaemia, hypomagnesaemia, hypo/hypernatraemia, hyperbilirubinaemia/kernicterus, hyperammonaemia, hyperglycinaemia, pyridoxine deficiency)
* Maternal substance abuse/neonatal abstinence syndrome
* Benign non-familial neonatal seizures (5th day fits)
* Benign familial neonatal seizures
* Hypertension.

Clues to aetiology

* *HIE* is the most common cause of seizures in term babies and characteristically presents in the first 24 hours with a history of fetal distress, need for resuscitation at birth, and decreased conscious level
* *Group B streptococci* and *E. coli* are the commonest infective causes, and present from the end of the first week onwards, as does *Herpes simplex*. Intrauterine *toxoplasmosis* and *cytomegalovirus* (CMV) infection present in the first 3 days
* *Cerebral infarction* (stroke) often presents with focal seizures at 24–72 hours of age in an otherwise well infant
* IUGR and preterm infants are at risk of *hypoglycaemia*
* Poor feeding and weight loss may lead to *hypernatraemic* dehydration
* Severe unconjugated jaundice and *kernicterus*—decreased conscious level, abnormal neurology, and typically opisthotonic posture
* Preterm infants may have subtle seizures following intraventricular haemorrhage (IVH) in the first 72 hours, with decreased Hb
* Hyperglycinaemia—increased fetal movements, intractable seizures, hypotonia, burst suppression on EEG, raised plasma and cerebrospinal fluid (CSF) glycine levels
* Neonatal abstinence syndrome—history of maternal substance abuse, presents in first week with other signs of withdrawal

- Pyridoxine deficiency—intractable seizures with dramatic resolution following pyridoxine administration
- Benign familial neonatal seizures—autosomal dominant channelopathy, presents at 3–7 days with clonic seizures
- Benign neonatal sleep myoclonus—presents from 5 days with myoclonic jerks only during sleep.

Clinical features

Seizures in newborns are varied and subtle due to the relative immaturity of the nervous system, and generalized tonic–clonic seizures are rare. Patterns of clinical seizures are:

- *Oculo-orofacial*: eye rolling, eye deviation, staring, nystagmus, chewing, sucking, lip smacking, smiling, and blinking
- *Central/autonomic*: change in breathing, apnoea, desaturation, bradycardia
- *Clonic*: cycling or boxing movements, usually one limb or side, may migrate to other limbs, 2–4 Hz, sharp-slow wave pattern on EEG, may be due to an underlying focal lesion or a metabolic cause
- *Tonic*: stiffening of the limbs or trunk usually symmetrically and sometimes decerebrate or opisthotonic posturing
- *Myoclonic jerks*: fast movement, flexor muscles
- *Multifocal*: more than one site, asynchronous, migratory
- *Generalized*: bilateral, synchronous, non-migratory
- Often electrographic seizures do not have a clinically observable component and vice versa *(electro-clinical dissociation)*
- Seizures must be differentiated from jitters.

Jitteriness is a common, often normal finding, 5 Hz, symmetrical tremor of the limbs, exacerbated by startling, and terminated by holding/flexing the limb, no ocular phenomena, no autonomic changes, normal EEG.

Investigations

- **Bloods**: glucose, blood gas, U&Es, Ca, Mg, FBC + differential WCC, CRP, blood culture, congenital infection screen
- **Urine toxicology**
- **CSF** (delay LP if baby is unstable) glucose, protein, Gram stain, culture, viral PCR
- **EEG** (distinguish from non-seizure activity): newborns often exhibit electro-clinical dissociation, that is poor correlation between EEG changes and clinical events. See Fig. 11.3
- **Neuroimaging**: cranial USS (haemorrhage) and consider CT/MRI (cerebral malformations and infarcts) if aetiology remains unclear. See Fig. 11.4
- **Consider genetic** testing and referral if dysmorphic or family history
- **Consider metabolic** screen if acidotic or family history: ammonia, amino acids, lactate, urine amino and organic acids, +/– CSF glucose, lactate, and amino acids.

Management

- **Monitor breathing**, which may be compromised during seizures and following anticonvulsant administration

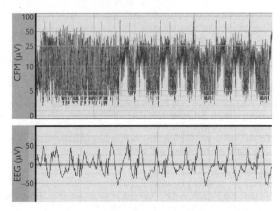

Fig. 11.3 Seizures on cerebral function monitoring (CFM). Characteristic saw tooth pattern of seizures on CFM with electroencephalogram (EEG) showing high amplitude repetitive spikes.

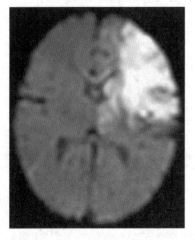

Fig. 11.4 Cerebral infarct. Diffusion-weighted MRI brain scan showing restricted diffusion (bright) corresponding to a large left middle cerebral artery territory infarct involving much of the frontal lobe.

- Rapidly identify and *treat reversible causes* (i.e. dextrose bolus if hypoglycaemic and correct electrolyte disturbances if present)
- Commence *antibiotics* and add *aciclovir* if there is any suspicion of herpes infection (e.g. maternal infection, rash, abnormal LFTs).

Anticonvulsants

The threshold for starting anticonvulsants is based on both clinical condition and seizure duration and frequency. Start an anticonvulsant if there are: prolonged desaturations, haemodynamic instability, seizure lasting >5 minutes, or brief but frequent seizures >3 per hour.

- *First-line:* phenobarbital 'full' loading dose (20 mg/kg IV)
  - *if seizures continue for 30 min:* give a further 'half' loading dose of phenobarbital (i.e. 10mg/kg IV) and take blood for a phenobarbital level
  - *if seizures remain uncontrolled:* either give further 'half' loading dose of phenobarbital if blood levels are low or consider adding another anticonvulsant. Phenobarbital terminates seizures in up to 50% of cases within a few hours
- *Second-line:* phenytoin, loading dose (20 mg/kg IV over 30 min), may cause hypotension and arrhythmias if cardiac function is impaired. Give second dose if seizures not controlled after 20 min. Phenytoin stops a further 15% of seizures
- *Third-line:* clonazepam (10–60 µg/kg/h IVI), midazolam (30–50 µg/kg/h IVI), lidocaine (4–8 mg/kg/h IVI) **NB** should not be used with phenytoin)), or *levetiracetam* (initial dose 7 mg/kg once daily). It remains unclear which is the most effective agent and the management of difficult to control seizures should be discussed with a paediatric neurologist
- *Fourth-line:* consider 1 week trial of pyridoxine (100 mg od, po) if EEG shows a persistent spike and wave pattern and poor response to previous treatment. One week trial of pyridoxal phosphate (30 mg/kg/24 h po) if there is no response to pyridoxine. Trial of creatine (300 mg/kg/24 h) + folinic acid (2.5 mg bd) + biotin (10 mg od) if seizures remain uncontrolled
- Use the *minimum* number of anticonvulsants required to maintain seizure control
- Some anticonvulsants cause *respiratory depression* so breathing must be monitored carefully.

Maintenance treatment is not usually needed unless there is evidence of an underlying seizure disorder:
- If seizures persist use phenobarbital 3–5 mg/kg/24 h IV or po in divided doses
- Most babies can stop anticonvulsants before discharge home. However, those with persistent, abnormal neurology may need to continue.

Outcome

Prognosis depends upon the underlying cause. There is evidence that seizures in themselves and status epilepticus in particular, are associated with adverse neurodevelopmental sequelae.

Brain injury in premature babies: germinal matrix haemorrhage–intraventricular haemorrhage

Definition
The term GMH–IVH describes the spectrum of haemorrhage seen in pre-terms using CUSS and MRI (see Fig 11.5).

Incidence
Increases as gestational age decreases and affects approximately 10% of babies <32 weeks gestation. Incidence decreased in developed countries in the 1990s probably due to the introduction of antenatal steroids, sur-factant, and better regulation of haemodynamics.

Pathophysiology
The commonest site of intracranial bleeding in the premature newborn is the *periventricular area*. Bleeding arises from the fragile and highly vascular subependymal *germinal matrix* that lies between the caudate and thalamus. This area is particularly active during the middle trimester of pregnancy before involuting by term.

Sharp *changes in BP, O_2 and CO_2 levels* cause fluctuating blood flow and predispose to haemorrhage in the germinal matrix.

Haemorrhage may extend into the lateral ventricles and large bleeds may cause *venous obstruction* then *infarction* and secondary *haemorrhage* in the periventricular region known as haemorrhagic periventricular/parenchymal infarction (HPI).

Clinical features
- IVH typically occurs in the first 72 hours (90%) and often within the first 24 hours (50%), but is not usually present at birth so the initial CUSS may be normal
- Presentation varies from an incidental finding in an asymptomatic baby (common) to sudden collapse (rare)
- Most GMH–IVH is asymptomatic and detected on CUSS. Larger bleeds are more likely to be symptomatic
- Bleeding will evolve into haematoma and organize before re-absorption over the next few days or weeks.

Mild
- Reduced spontaneous movements
- Hypotonia
- Anaemia and fall in haematocrit
- Apnoeas
- Abnormal eye movements.

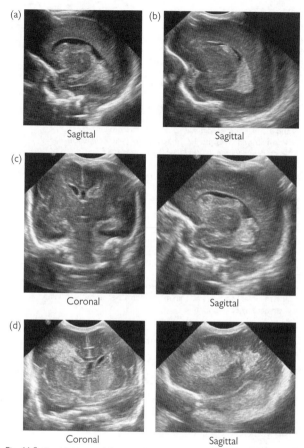

Fig. 11.5 Cranial ultrasound showing: (a) grade I IVH; (b) grade II IVH; (c) grade III IVH; (d) grade IV IVH.

Severe
- Bulging fontanelle
- Decerebrate posturing
- Hypotension
- Coagulopathy
- Hypoxia
- Seizures
- Collapse.

Classification

The Papile system of grades I–IV was based on CT images and describes the pattern and severity of haemorrhage. It is best to describe in appropriate detail the site and extension of each lesion.

- **Germinal matrix haemorrhage (GMH)**: echogenic area between the caudate and ventricle (i.e. confined to the germinal matrix that will evolve into a cystic lesion and eventually resolves—also known as subependymal haemorrhages)
- **Intraventricular haemorrhage (IVH)**: echogenic area within the ventricular system that may or may not cause distension of the walls, and if small may be difficult to distinguish from GMH
  - *small/grade I*: GMH +/− minimal IVH (<10% ventricle)
  - *moderate/grade II*: IVH (10–50% ventricle)
  - *large/grade III*: IVH (>50% ventricle) with distended ventricle
- **Parenchymal lesion**: HPI/grade IV, echogenic lesion that fans out from the ventricular wall in a triangular shape into the brain substance, associated with a large IVH, evolves into cystic lesions that may form a porencephalic cyst.

Prevention

- Reduce the severity of respiratory problems associated with prematurity (antenatal steroids, surfactant)
- Avoid fluctuations in cerebral blood flow by regulating blood pressure and PCO_2
- Reduce infants 'fighting' the ventilator by using synchronized ventilation and minimal handling and minimal endotracheal tube suctioning
- Correct any coagulopathy.

Management

- There is no specific treatment and management is supportive
- Check coagulation is normal
- Treat anaemia if present with blood transfusion
- Consider starting inotropes (e.g. dopamine if hypotension persists)
- Treat seizures (as described in ➔ Neonatal seizures, pp. 290–3)
- Repeat CUSS at intervals to assess the evolution of the haemorrhage and monitor for complications (usually within 3–5 days, then weekly thereafter)
- Update parents and discuss prognosis.

Complications

Post-haemorrhagic ventricular dilatation (PHVD): usually occurs 2–3 weeks after IVH in around 30% of bleeds (↑ risk with larger bleeds). Blood within the ventricles is believed to cause permanent changes in CSF resorption and lead to hydrocephalus that may require neurosurgical intervention.

Porencephalic cyst: large intraparenchymal haemorrhages become organized to leave large cysts in continuity with the ventricle.

Outcomes

- **GMH +/– small IVH**: very good outcome, similar to babies with the same gestational age without haemorrhage
- **Moderate IVH (<50% ventricle)**: good outcome, small risk of severe neurodisability, 10% risk of PHVD
- **Large IVH (>50% ventricle)**: poor outcome, 75% risk of PHVD, 50% risk of severe neurodisability
- **HPI**: poor outcome, up to 90% of babies with cystic change following HPI will have severe neurodisability (commonly spastic hemiplegia)
- **PHVD**: around 30% will require a ventricular shunt, greater risk with larger IVH; up to 50% of babies will have moderate/severe neurodisability (75% of those who have shunt insertions).

Brain injury in premature babies: periventricular leucomalacia

Periventricular leucomalacia (PVL): brain injury in a characteristic distribution (deep white matter) that is seen in premature infants and associated with neurodevelopmental sequelae (commonly spastic diplegia). See Fig 11.6.

Pathophysiology

Remains unclear, but ischaemia in the 'watershed' areas of the brain between arterial territories, where blood supply is vulnerable during periods of low flow, as well as excitoxicity mediated by cytokines in sepsis are involved in the pathogenesis. Injury to oligodendroglia is pivotal.

Clinical features

- Decreased movement and hypotonia are subtle signs at the time of injury
- Abnormal neurology begins to emerge from around 2 months with generalized stiffness, and abnormal posture with flexion of arms, and extension of legs
- Changes are seen bilaterally at the superior and lateral margins of the lateral ventricles. Fronto-parietal in most cases but additionally parieto-occipital in severe cases
- **Periventricular flare:** earliest change seen on cranial ultrasound, increased echogenicity of the periventricular zone (PVZ), seen in up to 20% of babies with BW <1500 g, and frequently resolve spontaneously
- **Cystic change:** periventricular flare may evolve into cysts over the next 10–14 days and sometimes longer. They occur in around 2–3% of babies with BW <1500 g.

Cysts slowly coalesce and resolve, leaving varying degrees of cortical atrophy and ventriculomegaly.

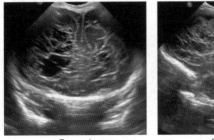
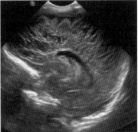

Coronal   Sagittal

Fig. 11.6 Cranial ultrasound showing cystic periventricular leucomalacia.

- Non-cystic damage: diffuse, non-cystic white matter injury seen with MRI affects up to 50% of babies with BW <1500g and described as Diffuse Excessive High Signal Intensity (DEHSI). Associated with decreased volume of specific brain regions and decreased structural organization (fractional anisotropy).

MRI will reveal cysts that are not seen on CUSS and define white matter damage more clearly, particularly in non-cystic PVL.

Outcomes

Outcome depends upon the number and size of cystic changes. There is no effective, specific treatment or preventative measure.

Small anterior cysts have a good outcome with little or no neuro-developmental sequelae. Widespread or large cysts, especially occipital ones, are associated with severe neurodisability with the development of *spastic diplegia* (a form of cerebral palsy), learning difficulties, and visual impairment. Outcome for persistent periventricular flare/echogenicity on CUSS and mild white matter hyperintensity on MRI remain unclear.

There is also a small group of babies who have normal CUSS appearances, but go on to develop cerebral palsy.

Brain injury in term babies

Intracranial haemorrhage
Up to 5% of all term babies will have an intracranial haemorrhage.

Clinical features
Small bleeds may be asymptomatic.

Neurological
- Drowsiness
- Seizures
- Signs of raised intracranial pressure (vomiting, drowsiness, apnoeas, stiffness, seizures)
- Abnormal neurology (bulging fontanelle, hypotonia, hypertonia, facial palsy, pupil changes).

General/non-specific
- Fever
- Signs of birth trauma (moulding, caput, haematomas, fractures)
- Petechiae/bruises, coagulopathy
- Anaemia, hypotension, shock
- Cutaneous haemangioma raising suspicion of an intracranial haemangioma.

Management
- CUSS
- CT/MRI
- Coagulation screen
- If LP is performed to exclude sepsis, CSF may be blood-stained, with low glucose and white cells
- Discuss with neurosurgical team if unwell, evacuation considered if there are signs of raised intracranial pressure, but is rarely undertaken.

Subarachnoid haemorrhage
Usually, the result of disruption of bridging veins, but can also be secondary to an intraventricular bleed. Blood-stained CSF. Blood collects in the posterior interhemispheric fissure that is hyperintense on CT scan. Good prognosis unless associated with a coagulopathy.

Subdural haemorrhage
Caused by trauma most commonly during instrumental delivery. Distortion of the dura leads to rupture of venous sinuses. Diagnosis confirmed on CT, characteristically convex haematoma.

Intraventricular haemorrhage
Originates from the choroid plexus, rather than the germinal matrix as in preterms. Blood-stained CSF. Visualized with CUSS. May be complicated by post-haemorrhagic hydrocephalus.

Intraparenchymal haemorrhage

Causes are varied including coagulopathy, trauma, hypoxia ischaemia, infarction, vascular malformation, tumour, ECMO. Severe neurological impairment with poor prognosis.

Cerebellar haemorrhage

Often caused by difficult breech extraction and sometimes germinal matrix bleed from the fourth ventricle. Difficult to visualize using CUSS. Large bleeds may rapidly cause catastrophic brainstem compression.

Cerebral infarction

Arterial infarction most commonly involves thromboembolic occlusion of the middle cerebral artery. Seizures are common, usually presenting after 24 hours but infants are alert between episodes. CUSS can be normal but may show a wedge-shaped echodensity in the arterial distribution and sometimes midline shift. MRI is helpful to make the diagnosis. Treatment is supportive with treatment of seizures (see ➔ Neonatal seizures, pp. 290–3). An underlying thrombophilic tendency should be investigated (e.g. protein C and protein S deficiency, factor V Leiden mutation). Outcome is usually good due to the plasticity of the newborn brain.

Cerebral venous thrombosis

Dehydration, infection, and inherited thrombophilia may be complicated by thrombosis of the cerebral veins. Diagnosed using MRI or CT, and treatment is supportive.

Hydrocephalus and post-haemorrhagic ventricular dilatation

Hydrocephalus: increased head circumference for gestational age due to CSF accumulation (>2 cm greater than 97th centile).

PHVD: increased size of cerebral ventricles following intraventricular haemorrhage (see Fig.11.7).

Causes

Congenital
- Aqueduct stenosis
- Arnold–Chiari malformation
- Dandy–Walker malformation
- Other cerebral malformations (e.g. encephalocele)
- Congenital infection (e.g. CMV, toxoplasmosis)
- Cerebral tumour
- Craniosynostosis.

Acquired
- Post-haemorrhagic (e.g. intraventricular, subdural, subarachnoid)
- Post-infectious (e.g. meningitis, encephalitis).

Management

- Serial head circumference and ventricular index measurements (weekly at first)
- **Assess for signs of raised intracranial pressure (ICP):** bulging fontanelle, separated sutures, open posterior fontanelle at term, vomiting, drowsiness, apnoeas, stiffness, seizures, pupil changes
- Congenital infection (TORCH) screen
- CUSS with ventricular index measurement
- CT/MRI if aetiology unclear
- Consider intervention when ventricular index exceeds 4 mm above the 97th centile for gestational age, or there are clinical signs of raised ICP, or ICP >10 cmH$_2$O (Fig. 11.8)
- Medical management with acetazolamide does not prevent the need for surgery nor improve neurodisability
- Ventricular tap or LP can be used to control raised ICP or rapidly progressive hydrocephalus but does not prevent neurosurgery. Repeated taps should be avoided due to resulting damage to brain tissue. Aim to reduce ICP to 8 cmH$_2$O
- **Neurosurgery:** ventriculoperitoneal (VP) shunt insertion is the definitive treatment. A subcutaneous reservoir device that can be regularly accessed is sometimes implanted in small babies to allow growth to an optimal weight (Fig. 11.9). Other strategies, such as ventricular drainage and endoscopic third ventriculostomy, have been used to delay shunt insertion.

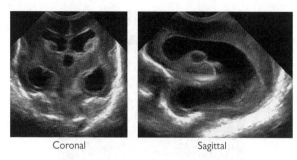

Coronal   Sagittal

Fig. 11.7 Cranial ultrasound showing post-haemorrhagic ventricular dilatation

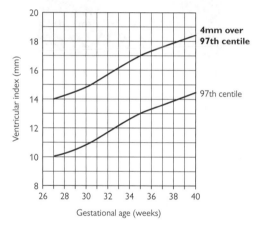

Fig. 11.8 Normal range for ventricular index.
From Levene *Arch Dis Child* 1981;56: 900–904.

Outcome

- Prognosis depends upon the underlying aetiology
- Children with aqueduct stenosis have a generally good outcome
- Premature babies with PHVD have a high incidence of neurodisability
- VP shunts have a high complication rate from infection and blockage with up to 40% requiring revision within 2 years.

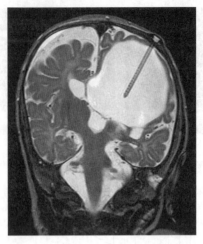

Fig. 11.9 MR scan showing reservoir device inserted into dilated left lateral ventricle.

Neuro-investigations: cranial ultrasound scans

Role: to identify major structural brain abnormalities or haemorrhagic/ischaemic injuries.

- CUSS is a useful modality that is rapid, non-invasive, and widely available
- It utilizes the anterior (or posterior) fontanelle as a window to image structures within the cranium
- Interpretation of images requires experience and expertise.

How to perform a CUSS

- Monitor vital signs carefully for deterioration during scanning
- Use 7.5 or 10 mHz probe
- Clean the probes with an appropriate solution or alcohol wipes
- Liberally apply ultrasound jelly to cover the transducer of the probe
- Apply the probe to the anterior (or posterior) fontanelle
- Adjust the gain (brightness)—if too low, lesions are missed, but if too high, lesions are difficult to differentiate from normal tissue
- Adjust the focal depth (to the level of the lateral ventricles or region of interest)
- Identify abnormalities in both coronal and sagittal planes
- **Coronal views**: align the transducer so that the end marked with a ridge/point is closest the right ear, and label the images 'right' and 'left'. Keeping the transducer applied to the fontanelle, angle the probe backwards (posteriorly) then forwards (anteriorly) to give anterior then posterior views (Fig. 11.10a)
- **Sagittal and parasagittal views**: rotate the transducer 90° with the marked end closest to the nose. Angle the probe laterally to the right then the left (Fig. 11.10b)
- Ensure the entire brain is visualized
- Take still images in the standardized planes shown in Fig. 11.10
- Clean the probe and baby's head when finished
- Record the study by saving or printing still images or on video as part of the patient's medical records
- Write a report in the case notes.

Basic description of findings

- Describe precisely what you see, in addition to using a grading system
- Comment on midline structures (e.g. corpus callosum)
- Describe location of any haemorrhage (e.g. subependymal, intraventricular, or parenchymal), and position of blood within ventricle
- Parenchymal haemorrhages are more echodense than the choroid plexuses
- Comment if there is any ventricular distension. If present, measure ventricular width ('ventricular index') of the right and left lateral ventricles. Ventricular size can be plotted on a percentile chart
- Comment on the periventricular areas (e.g. echogenicity, calcification) and describe location and size of any cysts
- **Ventricular 'index'** (width) = maximum horizontal width of the lateral ventricle, measured in the coronal plane with the third ventricle in view just posterior to the foramen of Munro.

NB **Ventriculomegaly** = large ventricles; **hydrocephalus** = large head circumference due to high pressure in the ventricular system.

(a)

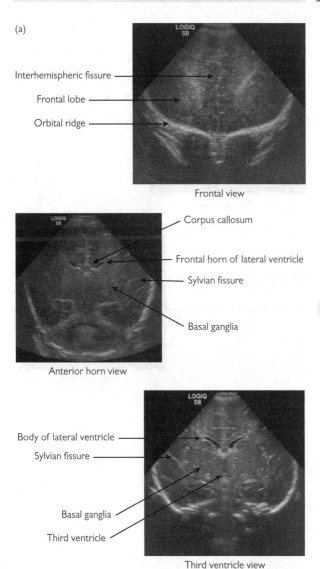

Frontal view

Anterior horn view

Third ventricle view

Fig. 11.10 (a) CUSS planes: coronal views.

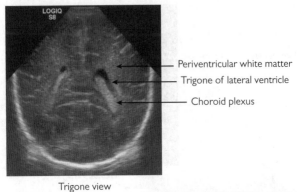

Periventricular white matter
Trigone of lateral ventricle
Choroid plexus

Trigone view

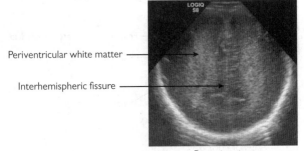

Periventricular white matter

Interhemispheric fissure

Posterior view

Fig. 11.10 (a) CUSS planes: coronal views. (*Contd.*)

(b)

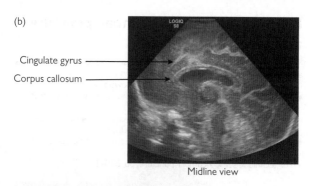

Cingulate gyrus

Corpus callosum

Midline view

Caudothalamic notch

Lateral ventricle

Thalamus

Choroid plexus

Cerebellum

Intermediate parasagittal view

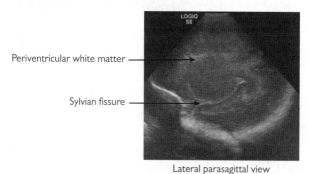

Periventricular white matter

Sylvian fissure

Lateral parasagittal view

Fig. 11.10 (b) CUSS planes: sagittal views.

Neuro-investigations: lumbar puncture and cerebrospinal fluid

Role: diagnostic in cases of suspected sepsis, seizures, or metabolic disease and therapeutic in decreasing intracranial pressure.

There are a few unique considerations in newborns:

- Xanthochromia may be present due to jaundice or old intraventricular haemorrhage
- White cell count may be higher than older children. Normal range for preterms: <30 cells/mm^3 and term: <10 cells/mm^3
- Red cell counts >1000/mm^3 make interpretation impossible and numerical corrections are not validated
- For technique see ➡ Lumbar puncture, pp. 520–1.

Neuro-investigations: electroencephalography

Role: non-invasive assessment of electrical brain activity.

- **Electroencephalography (EEG)** in NICU is challenging (difficulty applying electrodes, electrical noise levels, short recording time, changes with gestational age)
- **Amplitude integrated EEG (aEEG)**: allows continuous monitoring and is relatively easy to interpret, but limited to one or two channels of EEG (Fig 11.11)
- **Normal term EEG**: continuous, moderate voltage, mixed frequency, reactive to stimuli when awake. Continuous, high-voltage, slow (delta) wave pattern in quiet sleep, progressing to rapidly alternating high-voltage bursts and low amplitude intervals. Low-voltage, mixed frequency pattern in active sleep
- **Normal preterm EEG**: tracé discontinu = high-voltage, slow activity with intervals of suppressed activity, intervals become shorter in length with increasing gestational age and EEG is continuous by term. Delta brush = fast waves overlying the delta waves that should not be mistaken for seizure activity, these disappear by term
- **Background activity** reflects cortical function and normal background activity strongly suggests intact cortical function. Non-specific, paroxysmal abnormalities are common and should not be over-emphasized
- **Seizures on EEG**: monophasic, repetitive discharges, or a spike and wave pattern, there is not always a clinical correlate
- **Burst suppression pattern** on EEG predicts poor neurological outcome
- **Electrodes**: even number = right side, odd number = left side, F = frontal, Fp = fronto-polar, P = parietal, C = central, T = temporal, O = occipital, Z = midline, A = auricular.

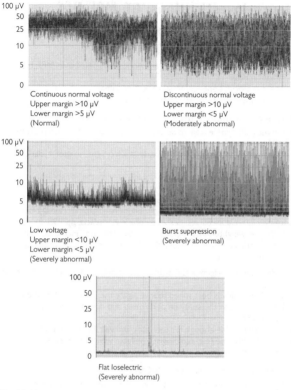

Continuous normal voltage
Upper margin >10 µV
Lower margin >5 µV
(Normal)

Discontinuous normal voltage
Upper margin >10 µV
Lower margin <5 µV
(Moderately abnormal)

Low voltage
Upper margin <10 µV
Lower margin <5 µV
(Severely abnormal)

Burst suppression
(Severely abnormal)

Flat Ioselectric
(Severely abnormal)

Fig. 11.11 Amplitude integrated EEG (aEEG).

Neuro-investigations: CT, MRI, NCS, EMG, and VEP

Computed tomography: head
- Rapid (~5 min), good for bleeds and bones, less detail than MRI, high radiation dose
- Bright = blood, bone, contrast; dark = oedema
- IV contrast enhances vascular areas and abscesses.

Magnetic resonance imaging: brain and spine
- Slower (~30 min), excellent detail, no ionizing radiation, baby must be still for good quality images
- **T1**: 'anatomical' images, white matter = white; grey matter = dark; CSF = black
- **T2**: shows 'water', white matter = dark; grey matter = lighter; CSF = white; oedema = bright
- **Fluid-attenuated inversion recovery (FLAIR)**: dampens CSF signal to detect changes in periventricular areas and subdural haematomas (see ➋ Brain injury in premature babies: periventricular leucomalacia, pp. 298–9)
- **Diffusion-weighted imaging**: shows water 'diffusion', increased signal corresponds to areas of oedema with restricted diffusion soon after ischaemia/infarction.

The decision to perform a CT or MRI can be difficult. Consider these basic questions:
- Which modality is best suited to investigate the (suspected) pathology?
- How quickly can the study be performed and does this make a difference?
- Is the baby stable enough for the study and will the baby lie still?
- Is there someone (e.g. radiologist) available who has experience to interpret the images?

Nerve conduction studies (NCS)
Role: assessment of neuropathies. Skin electrodes along a specific nerve pathway record amplitude, latency, and conduction velocities of nerves.

Electromyography (EMG)
Role: assessment of myopathies. A needle electrode is inserted into muscle groups to record action potentials.

Muscle biopsy

Role: invasive, final-tier investigation for neuromuscular disease. Ideally, should be delayed until a few months of age for better results, but should be carried out in the newborn period if the results may alter management or if the baby is unlikely to survive.

Open surgical biopsy of muscle fibres, usually from the inguinal region, needs to be frozen in liquid nitrogen at the bedside for histology and another sample put on ice for biochemistry.

Visual-evoked potentials (VEP)

Role: assess integrity of the visual pathway. Records EEG response to visual stimulus. Considered following severe hypoxic ischaemic injury.

Neuromuscular disease

Congenital myotonic dystrophy

Autosomal dominant. Reduced fetal movements and polyhydramnios during pregnancy, premature birth.

Clinical features
- *Facial diplegia, hypotonia*, respiratory muscle weakness often requiring support, bilateral talipes equinovarus, flexion contractures of the hips and knees, feeding difficulties
- Weakness is variable from total paralysis to sparse anti-gravity limb movements
- Examine the mother for facial weakness and delayed relaxation after making a fist. Severity of disease in the mother does not predict the baby's course
- Diagnosis: genetic testing of *DMPK* gene on chromosome 19
- Outcome: depends upon the degree of respiratory muscle weakness. Mortality approaches 40% in babies that require prolonged ventilation and withdrawal of care is sometimes appropriate
- Survivors will develop myotonic symptoms from their teens and will have learning difficulties.

Congenital muscular dystrophy

Describes a group of conditions characterized by muscle weakness and dystrophic changes in muscle architecture. Duchenne and Becker muscular dystrophies are inherited, X-linked, and typically present in childhood.

Walker–Warburg syndrome
Severe hypotonia, visual inattention, ocular abnormalities, raised creatinine kinase (CK), MRI shows type II lissencephaly, cerebellar hypoplasia, dystrophic muscle biopsy, *POMT1* gene mutation in some cases.

Muscle–eye–brain disease
Hypotonia, ocular abnormalities not always present at birth, severe learning difficulties, epilepsy; MRI shows pachygyria, polymicrogyria, cerebellar hypoplasia; *POMGTn1* mutation.

Merosin-negative congenital muscular dystrophy
Merosin is an extracellular matrix protein. Signs include hypotonia—upper worse than lower limbs—contractures, massively elevated CK; MRI shows diffuse white matter changes; never achieve walking; *LAMA2* gene mutation.

Merosin-positive congenital muscular dystrophy
Heterogenous group with hypotonia and contractures due to a range of mutations.

Spinal muscular atrophy

Type 1 (Werdnig–Hoffmann disease): the most severe form that affects newborns, leading to death within a year.

Clinical features: alert baby, tongue fasciculations, severe hypotonia, 'jug handle' posture of upper limbs, little or no spontaneous limb movement, respiratory muscle weakness, paradoxical breathing, facial muscles spared, EMG shows fibrillation potentials, *SMN1* gene mutation.

Congenital myopathy

Nemaline myopathy is the most common neonatal form. The severe form presents with polyhydramnios, arthrogryposis, severe weakness, respiratory impairment. The less severe, classical form presents with facial and truncal weakness, and feeding difficulties. Normal CK, EMG is myopathic, muscle biopsy reveals nemaline rods within muscle fibres. *ACTA1* gene mutation in severe form and *NEB* gene mutation in the classical form.

Myasthenia gravis

Transient form

Affects 15% of babies born to mothers with myasthenia gravis, caused by maternal antibodies against AChR crossing the placenta during pregnancy.

Clinical features: appear within hours, generalized weakness, facial weakness, feeding difficulties, fatigability, ptosis, respiratory difficulties. Symptoms resolve by 2 months in most cases. Severity of disease in the mother does not predict severity of the baby's condition.

Management: Babies born to myasthenic mothers should be observed for symptoms for at least 3 days. If symptomatic, give a test dose of neostigmine (150 μg/kg IM slowly), which should markedly improve symptoms within 15 minutes and lasts for around 2 hours. Send blood for AChR antibodies. Nerve stimulation shows a decremental response. Regular oral neostigmine is continued until a few months of age.

Myasthenic syndromes

Some forms of non-transient, inherited defects in the neuromuscular junction may present in the neonatal period. There is weakness of limbs, and respiratory and bulbar muscles but AChR antibodies are negative with no response to neostigmine.

Malformations of the central nervous system

Incidence: 5 per 10,000 births. Most are diagnosed antenatally (see ➲ Routine antenatal screening and diagnosis of fetal anomalies, pp. 2–4).

Neural tube defects (NTD)

- Failure of the neural tube to close during fetal life results in a defect in the vertebral column and possible herniation of its contents. The spectrum includes anencephaly, encephalocele/meningocele, myelomeningocele, spina bifida occulta. See Fig 11.12
- Defects have become less common since routine pre-conceptual folate supplementation and with general improvements in nutrition
- Large defects are identified during antenatal screening and some pregnancies are terminated.

Management
- Make a detailed neurological assessment including muscle tone, joint deformities, sensation, micturition, and bowel opening
- Search for other congenital anomalies (e.g. perform renal USS)
- Neuroimaging: CUSS and MRI of the brain and spinal cord to look for frequent underlying malformations of the central nervous system (CNS)
- Liaise with a neurosurgeon to decide follow-up and timing of neuroimaging.

Encephalocele

The defect is in the skull bone in the midline, occipital in most cases, but sometimes anterior. Brain tissue herniates through this defect, but is covered by skin. Often large, >6 cm diameter. Surgical repair is possible within the first few weeks of life. Outcome depends upon the amount of brain tissue that has herniated through the defect and presence of associated anomalies, but usually poor.

Myelomeningocele

The defect is in the lumbar or thoracic spine. Spinal cord tissue herniates through the defect with a meningeal covering, but may lack skin and leak CSF. There are usually profound neurological abnormalities. Urgent neurosurgical review required for closure of the defect on the first day of age.

There are long-term neurological problems, including hydrocephalus, often requiring a ventriculoperitoneal shunt, learning difficulties, and urinary and bowel incontinence.

Meningocele

There is a defect in the vertebral bodies of the lumbar or sacral spine. The meninges herniate through the defect, but without brain tissue and with a skin covering. The outcome is generally good.

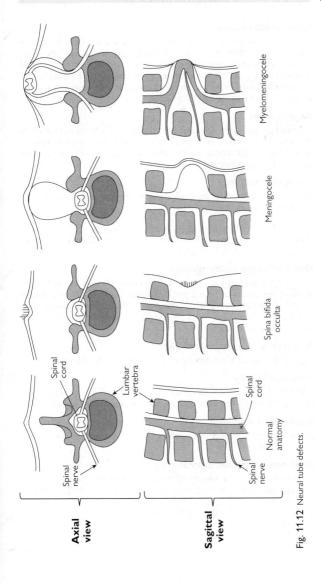

Fig. 11.12 Neural tube defects.

Spina bifida occulta

The defect is in the vertebral bodies of the spine commonly in the lumbosacral region. Both the spinal cord and skin remain intact. Clinical features include a sacral dimple +/− deep pit, sentinel hairy patch, naevus, or overlying fat pad (lipoma). Neuroimaging is needed within 6 weeks to look for underlying cord malformation or tethering. Early neurosurgical repair is advocated for any associated lesions.

Anencephaly

Failure of development of the posterior skull and brain structures above the midbrain. This lethal condition often prompts termination of the pregnancy. Resuscitation is not appropriate and sensitive discussion with parents about palliative care is important.

Holoprosencephaly

Defect in development of the forebrain with poor prognosis. Single ventricle +/− single nostril and eye.

Hydranencephaly

Profound fetal cerebrovascular accident resulting in only small areas of brain tissue at the time of birth. Prognosis is very poor.

Dandy–Walker malformation

A posterior fossa cyst that communicates with the 4th ventricle, with hypoplasia of the cerebellar vermis and hydrocephalus. Often associated with other CNS malformations. It is associated with chromosomal abnormalities (e.g. trisomies 13 and 18). Outcome is variable. Management includes treatment of hydrocephalus.

Agenesis of the corpus callosum

Seen in association with a number of syndromes with CNS involvement.

Megalencephaly

Large head with a variety of causes, including familial, neuronal migration disorders, neurofibromatosis, Soto's syndrome, and metabolic disorders.

Septo-optic dysplasia

Absent septum pellucidum, optic nerve hypoplasia, +/− absent pituitary gland.

Neuronal migration disorders

- *Lissencephaly type I*: (including Miller–Dieker syndrome)—smooth brain lacking gyri/sulci, seizures, learning difficulties, *LIS1* or *DCX* gene mutations
- *Lissencephaly type II*: smooth brain, subcortical heterotopias, hydrocephalus.

Vein of Galen malformations

Rare condition, aneurysms of the vein, identified antenatally or presenting with cardiac failure and intracranial bruit. Poor outcome, transcatheter embolization of feeder vessels in the neonatal period is performed in a few centres.

Further information

Bodensteiner J. The evaluation of the hypotonic infant. *Semin Pediatr Neurol* 2008; **15**: 10–20.

Brouwer A. Neurodevelopmental outcome of preterm infants with severe intraventricular hemorrhage and therapy for post-hemorrhagic ventricular dilatation. *J Pediatr* 2008; **152**: 648–654.

Hellstrom-Westas L. Predictive value of early continuous amplitude integrated EEG recordings on outcome after severe birth asphyxia in full term infants. *Arch Dis Childh* 1995; **72**: F34–38.

Jacobs SE, Berg M, Hunt R, Tarnow-Mordi WO, Inder TE, Davis PG. Cooling for newborns with hypoxic ischaemic encephalopathy. *Cochrane Database Syst Rev* 2013; CD003311.

National Institute for Health and Clinical Excellence 2010 NICE interventional procedure guidance (IPG347). *Therapeutic hypothermia with intracorporeal temperature monitoring for hypoxic perinatal brain injury.* ℘ www.nice.org.uk/guidance/ipg347

Resuscitation Council, UK *Newborn Life Support: Resuscitation at birth*, 4th ed. Resuscitation Council, London, 2016.

Resuscitation Council, UK. Guidelines: Resuscitation and support of transition of babies at birth. 2015. ℘ www.resus.org.uk/resuscitation-guidelines/resuscitation-and-support-of-transition-of-babies-at-birth/

Rutherford MA. MRI of the Neonatal Brain. 2001. ℘ www.mrineonatalbrain.com

Samat HB, Sarnat M. Neonatal encephalopathy following fetal distress: a clinical and electroencephalographic study. *Archives of Neurol* 1976; **33**: 696–705.

Thoresen M. Supportive care during neuroprotective hypothermia in the term newborn: adverse effects and their prevention. *Clin Perinatol* 2008; **35**: 749–763.

Volpe JJ. Hypoxic-ischemic encephalopathy: clinical aspects. In: *Neurology of the newborn*, 5th ed. WB Saunders, Philadelphia, 2002.

Infection

Background

- Newborn infection is common. The risk of infection is higher at lower gestations
- Can be acquired antenatally, during delivery, or postnatally
- Caused by a wide range of organisms.

Factors influencing development of infection

Ability to resist infection
- Undeveloped immune mechanisms:
  - low total numbers of neutrophils and neutrophil progenitors, and reduced neutrophil function
  - low complement levels
  - naïve T and B cell-mediated immunity
  - protective maternal immunoglobulin crosses placenta to fetus only after 28–32 weeks gestation
- Reduced barriers to infection: particularly important with preterm babies
  - fragile +/− immature skin
  - immature gut; may have overgrowth of pathogenic bacteria if delayed feeds or no breast milk
  - impaired mucus membrane +/− ciliary function if needing respiratory support
  - relatively porous blood–brain barrier predisposes to meningitis.

Environment
- Antenatally-acquired infection blood-borne from mother via the placenta
- Perinatally acquired infection from female genital tract:
  - presence of pathogenic organisms (e.g. group B streptococci (GBS), herpes simplex (HSV))
  - rupture of membranes, particularly if prolonged (>18 hours) exposes baby to micro-organisms
- Nosocomial infection from neonatal unit (NNU):
  - warm humid environment (e.g. incubators, ventilator circuits) encourages bacterial growth
  - difficult infection control (crowded, high intensity).

Medical management
- Invasive procedures:
  - intravascular access allows micro-organisms into bloodstream
  - skin easily abraded by routine care and breached by procedures (e.g. phlebotomy)
  - endotracheal tube (ETT) allows access of micro-organisms to respiratory tract
- Antibiotic therapy: frequent use drives antibiotic resistance.

Investigation of suspected sepsis

Basic screen

Once a decision to investigate infection is made, institution of tests and antibiotic therapy should be urgent—aim for <1 hour.

- FBC, blood film
- C-reactive protein (CRP)
- Blood culture: technique is important to avoid contamination; take adequate volume (at least 0.5 ml).

PLUS when clinically indicated

- Placental swabs +/− placental pathology in early onset sepsis
- Chest X-ray (CXR) if respiratory signs (common)
- Lumbar puncture (LP) if neurological signs/symptoms or proven sepsis (raised septic markers or blood cultures positive for organisms other than coagulase negative staphylococci)
- Skin swabs of broken areas, rash, or pustules; swabs of purulent discharge if present
- Individual orifice swabs in virus transport medium for viral detection (e.g. for HSV if generalized sepsis, particularly if deranged liver function or coagulation)
- Urine—preferably clean catch or suprapubic aspiration. Request microscopic exam for yeasts if fungal sepsis is suspected
- AXR if abdomen distended
- ETT secretions
- Nasopharyngeal aspirate for viruses if bronchiolitis is suspected
- Tip of umbilical/central lines and ETT when removed.

Bacterial infection

Incidence
1–8 per 1000 live births. Higher in preterm babies.

Presentation
- Early onset sepsis presents within 48–72 hours of birth:
  - vertically acquired from mother's genital tract
  - often presents with respiratory distress (pneumonia) after aspiration of infected liquor
  - risk factors often present (see ➲ Early onset bacterial infection, pp. 328–9)
  - common organisms are GBS (see ➲ Group B streptococcal infection, pp. 330–1), *Escherichia coli, Listeria*
- Late onset sepsis presents after 48–72 hours:
  - horizontally acquired from the environment or contacts
  - meningitis (and other focal infection) is common
  - common organisms are GBS, *E. coli, Staphylococcus aureus*, other Gram −ve organisms (e.g. *Pseudomonas*).

Outcome
- Mortality 5–15%
- Mortality for early onset > late onset
- Babies who present very soon after birth may have mortality up to 50%.

General antibiotic treatment

General principles
- Choose narrowest appropriate spectrum for clinical circumstances
- Take into account known bacteria for the NNU in question (particularly important for nosocomial infection) and local antibiotic protocols.

Empiric treatment of suspected sepsis

Early onset sepsis—perinatally acquired sepsis (onset <72 hours after birth):
- Benzylpenicillin plus aminoglycoside (e.g. gentamicin)
- Consider amoxicillin/ampicillin instead of benzylpenicillin if risk of listeriosis (e.g. meconium in amniotic fluid <32 weeks gestation)
- Consider aciclovir if HSV suspected.

Late onset sepsis—nosocomial sepsis (onset >72 hours after birth)
- Flucloxacillin or amoxicillin *plus* aminoglycoside (e.g. gentamicin): first-line should cover Gram +ve and Gram –ve organisms known to colonize your NNU
- Progressing to a second-line antibiotic combination should depend on clinical circumstances:
  - positive blood cultures, according to sensitivities
  - failure to respond clinically to first-line antibiotics
- If infection likely, but cultures negative, assess baby's clinical state:
  - baby stable and/or central lines are in place—consider vancomycin for coagulase negative staphylococci (CONS) cover
  - severe illness +/– abdominal sepsis, broaden Gram –ve cover (e.g. meropenem, ceftazidime)
  - concern about NEC—add metronidazole
  - site of infection may require antibiotic with better tissue penetration (e.g. cefotaxime for meningitis)
- If blood cultures grow CONS:
  - take further blood cultures, as isolates may be skin contaminants, some guidelines suggest taking two blood cultures at the onset of late onset sepsis
  - true CONS bacteraemia is unlikely unless there is >1 positive culture with same CONS
  - if there is proven CONS sepsis and a long line (or other central venous line) in situ, can use continuous vancomycin infusion down the long line
- Remove central lines if no clinical improvement or cultures remain positive despite treatment
- Consider fungal sepsis in culture negative sepsis: may add antifungal.

Duration of antibiotics
- Stop all antibiotics after 36–48 hours if cultures and septic markers negative (depends on laboratory timeframe for declaring negative blood cultures)
- Antibiotic course varies depending on type of infection, condition of the baby, change in inflammatory markers, but usually 5–10 days:
  - pneumonia, 10 days; meningitis, 14–21 days depending on the organism. Liaise closely with microbiology.

Early onset bacterial infection

Aetiology
- Vertical acquisition from mother
- Organisms can invade baby via placenta and membranes or by aspiration of infected liquor
- Important organisms include GBS, *E coli* and *Listeria*.

Risk factors
Risk factors to consider when deciding whether to investigate/treat for early onset sepsis:
- Maternal GBS colonization or on mid-stream urine (MSU) in this pregnancy
- Previous baby with GBS disease
- Premature delivery (<37 weeks) following spontaneous labour
- Prolonged pre-labour rupture of membranes (PROM). PROM is considered >18–24 hours (varies with local policies)
- Maternal pyrexia (e.g. >38°C for >1 hour) or other evidence of maternal sepsis (positive blood culture, raised WBC or CRP).

Symptoms and signs (onset <72 hours after birth)
- Respiratory distress (congenital pneumonia), apnoea
- Lethargy, poor feeding, hypotonia
- Irritability, seizures (meningitis)
- Hypoglycaemia, jaundice (particularly <24 hours), metabolic acidosis
- Septic shock, with rapid deterioration and death.

Management
Thresholds to treat vary with local guidelines. National Institute for Health and Care Excellence (NICE) (UK) and American Academy of Pediatrics (US) also provide guidance (see ⊃ Further information, p. 370). The following is general guidance:
- 1 risk factor (early onset bacterial infection) without clinical symptoms/ signs → observe (e.g. hourly for 2 hours, 2 hourly until 12 hours of age)
- 2 risk factors without clinical symptoms/signs → investigate and treat
- Symptoms/signs → review history for risk factors and clinical assessment, with low threshold for investigation and treatment
- If a twin has proven infection, the co-twin should also be treated
- Maternal chorioamnionitis as a single risk factor may be considered an indication for investigation and treatment.

Investigations
- Blood cultures, FBC, and CRP
- CRP may be low at initial septic screen—consider repeating at 18–24 hours
- LP: perform with definite or high suspicion of sepsis or meningitis. Refer to local guidelines—some suggest LP in asymptomatic babies with negative cultures and elevated CRP.

Antibiotics
- Antibiotics should be given as soon as possible, no more than 1 hour after decision to treat
- Benzylpenicillin and gentamicin should be first-line in NNU. Take care using gentamicin on postnatal wards—errors and clinical incidents are common
- Antibiotics should be stopped at 36–48 hours if infection is excluded
- With proven or high suspicion of sepsis, treat for 7 days. If baby is well, particularly if treating for isolated raised CRP, 5 days may be adequate. Longer courses may be indicated with certain organisms, or with slow clinical response. Discuss with microbiologist.

Parent advice
- If there are concerns about potential risk of early onset infection prior to discharge from postnatal ward (either not requiring treatment, or following observation and/or treatment), advise parents to watch for signs/symptoms:
  - abnormal behaviour (e.g. abnormal cry, reduced activity)
  - hypotonia
  - poor feeding
  - abnormal temperature
  - rapid breathing
  - colour change.

Group B streptococcal infection

Background
- Maternal carriage varies in different populations: UK ~25%
- Incidence of neonatal GBS disease 0.7 per 1000 live births (UK); up to 1.8 per 1000 in US
- Mortality of identified invasive GBS disease 5–15% (higher in preterm)
- 90% of babies with GBS sepsis present at birth or in first 12 hours.

Intrapartum antibiotic prophylaxis
Risk factor based approach
- Recommended by Royal College of Obstetricians and Gynaecologists (RCOG); prevents 50–70% of neonatal GBS sepsis
- Treat with IV benzylpenicillin 4 hourly; if mother penicillin sensitive, RCOG recommends vancomycin
- The following should be considered strong risk factors and indications for intrapartum prophylaxis:
  - previous baby with GBS disease
  - treated this pregnancy for GBS infection
  - vaginal swab positive for GBS this pregnancy
  - maternal pyrexia >38°C for more than 1 hour (mother should get broad spectrum cover for this as treatment is for chorioamnionitis, which may be due to organisms other than GBS)
- More controversial risk factors and indications for prophylaxis include:
  - preterm labour
  - prolonged ROM (>18–24 hours—definition varies between local policies)
- Not indicated if elective Caesarean section with no labour and intact membranes.

Screening-based approach
- Not routinely followed in UK; recommended in populations with high colonization rates (e.g. US; prevents 65–85% of GBS sepsis)
- Low vaginal or rectovaginal swab into enriched medium at ~35 weeks
- Intrapartum prophylaxis given for:
  - swab positive for GBS
  - labour before swab result available.

Management of babies in whom intrapartum treatment was indicated
Some aspects of management can be controversial. Remember to consult local guidelines.

Term
- Mother has a single risk factor (see ➲ Intrapartum antibiotic prophylaxis, this chapter, p. 330)
  - observations for 12–24 hours postnatally
  - if baby symptomatic, screen (blood culture, FBC, and CRP) and treat
  - if baby remains well, give advice to parents regarding signs of sepsis after discharge

- Mother has at least two risk factors (see ➋ Intrapartum antibiotic prophylaxis, p. 330), and has had no treatment or antibiotics <4 hours before delivery. Screen and treat
- If mother has had at least 1 dose IV penicillin or ampicillin >4 hours before delivery, GBS should be assumed to have been adequately treated and GBS is removed as a risk factor. Therefore, treat as already described taking the GBS treatment into account. NB This does not pertain to maternal IV antibiotic treatment for suspected chorioamnionitis
- Symptomatic babies should also have LP if no contraindications.

Preterm (<37 weeks)
Follow protocol for term babies taking prematurity as a risk factor (e.g. baby needs only one further risk factor to be screened and treated if intrapartum treatment was inadequate).

Treatment

- GBS cover only: IV benzylpenicillin; otherwise benzypenicillin and gentamicin
- If culture positive for GBS continue with penicillin alone
- If cerebrospinal fluid (CSF) culture positive for GBS and no improvement in clinical condition and/or markers of sepsis within 48 hours, consider repeating LP (see ➋ Specific infections: meningitis, pp. 332–3).

Duration of treatment

- Septicaemia: 5–10 days (discuss with consultant and microbiologist)
- Meningitis: 14 days minimum
- Arthritis: 2–3 weeks
- Osteomyelitis: 3–4 weeks.

Specific infections: meningitis

Organisms
- GBS and *E. coli* are responsible for over 60% of cases
- Other causes: *Listeria*, other Gram –ve organisms, *Candida*; CONS if a ventriculoperitoneal shunt in situ
- Enterovirus, HSV.

Clinical features
- Non-specific signs of sepsis (e.g. temperature instability, apnoea, hyperglycaemia)
- Bulging fontanelle, seizures, altered level of consciousness, etc., are late signs and associated with long-term neurological sequelae.

Investigations
CSF analysis
In general, there should be a low threshold for performing lumbar punctures.

Contraindications to performing LP
- Baby too sick: treat with appropriate antibiotics and defer LP until condition improved
- Severe coagulopathy or thrombocytopenia: consider platelet transfusion prior to LP
- Local sepsis over LP site
- Known non-communicating hydrocephalus: ventricular tap is then necessary.

Interpretation of CSF results
- Normal values:
  - CSF WBC count in term babies <20 × 10⁶/l; in preterm babies (<37 weeks gestation) <27 × 10⁶/l. If CSF blood-stained, compare ratio of RBC:WBC counts in blood and CSF
  - CSF protein in term babies 0.6 g/l; in preterm babies 1.0 g/l.

Viral polymerase chain reaction (PCR)
Detection of virus in CSF is diagnostic. A negative result does not necessarily exclude these viruses. Discuss with virology.

Blood culture
Neonatal meningitis is usually secondary to septicaemia.

Treatment
- Supportive care paramount: ABC, ventilation, inotropic support, anticonvulsants
- Choice of antibiotics: empirical therapy (organism unknown)— amoxicillin *and* cefotaxime → once the organism is known, treatment can be changed as necessary. Consider adding aciclovir if herpes simplex is suspected

- For bacterial pathogens, consider repeating LP:
  - after 48 hours of treatment to document adequacy of treatment, particularly if clinical signs and/or markers of infection have not improved
  - if deterioration occurs during antibiotic course

Persistent infection may indicate a focus (e.g. obstructive ventriculitis, sub-dural empyema, multiple small vessel thrombi).

- Consider cranial CT/MRI scan to exclude abscesses or subdural collections if there is a delay in treatment response (e.g. failure to sterilize the CSF within 48 hours)
- Cranial ultrasound 1–5 days into treatment and prior to discharge. Consider MRI scan if concerns about neurological status or cranial ultrasound scan
- Length of treatment:
  - *GBS*: 2 weeks
  - *Gram –ve organisms*: 3 weeks
  - more prolonged treatment may be indicated if there has been delayed sterilization of CSF (i.e. >48 hours)
  - *viral aetiology*: herpes encephalitis needs 14–21 days aciclovir; discuss with virology (see Perinatal herpes simplex virus, pp. 360–1)
- Electrolytes need to be monitored to assess for syndrome of inappropriate antidiuretic hormone secretion (SIADH)
- Hearing screening prior to discharge
- Long-term monitoring for neurodevelopmental impairment, hydrocephalus, etc.

Specific infections: urinary tract infection

Suspected urinary tract infection (UTI)

- A diagnosis of UTI can only be confidently made from a suprapubic aspiration, clean catch, or catheter specimen of urine. Microscopy, culture, and sensitivity (MC&S) results from a bag specimen of urine are only of use if the results are negative
- Check urinanalysis using Multistix® *and* send specimen to microbiology for urgent MC&S. The sample should be kept in the fridge while awaiting transport to the laboratory.
- Start IV antibiotics (e.g. amoxicillin and gentamicin) while awaiting sensitivities
- Check U&E's, FBC, and CRP, repeating daily if any concerns.

Confirmed UTI

As for suspected UTI, plus:
- Arrange renal tract US scan
- Change the antibiotics according to sensitivities from MC&S
- Continue antibiotics for 7 days
- Once treatment course of antibiotics is discontinued, start prophylactic trimethoprim 2 mg/kg at night. This should be continued until results of the follow-up scans are known. May require long-term prophylaxis
- Arrange micturating cystourethrogram (MCUG) and dimercaptosuccinic acid scan (DMSA) for 8 weeks, and arrange review after these investigations
- Consider paediatric nephrology referral if abnormalities found on MCUG and/or DMSA.

Specific infections: sticky eyes and conjunctivitis

Mucoid discharge or 'sticky eye' in the first week of life is common and is not usually due to infection.

- If mild discharge persists it is likely to be due to a non-canalized lacrimal duct, 96% of which spontaneously resolve by 1 year of age
- If discharge is heavy, purulent, or obviously involves the conjunctiva, or if the eye is red or swollen:
  - send a swab for MC&S
  - prescribe topical chloramphenicol or sodium fusidate drops or ointment every 4 hours for 5 days. Check swab result after 24–48 hours and change antibiotics according to sensitivities if necessary.

Gonococcal ophthalmitis (ophthalmia neonatorum)

Presents with early, profuse discharge usually within first week of life.

- Send urgent swab and Gram stain (Gram –ve diplococci)
- Hourly eye irrigation with sterile normal saline
- IV benzylpenicillin for 7 days or single dose of ceftriaxone. Check sensitivities and discuss antibiotic regimen with microbiologist as necessary
- Consider empirical treatment for concomitant *Chlamydia*
- May need ophthalmology review
- Refer mother and partner to genito-urinary (GU) clinic.

Chlamydial conjunctivitis

Usually occurs at 5–10 days. Suspect if eye discharge is not improving on chloramphenicol or if there are concomitant respiratory symptoms:

- Swab each eye with specific chlamydial swabs
- Oral erythromycin for 14 days
- Refer mother and partner to GU clinic.

Specific infections: umbilical sepsis

- Umbilicus is an important portal of infection in early newborn period; preventable with good cord care
- Commonest pathogen is *S. aureus*
- If the umbilicus is unduly 'sticky', clean with an alcohol swab or other antiseptic solution. Further treatment is unnecessary. Swabs for MC&S are not useful
- If there is a purulent discharge or the surrounding skin is erythematous (umbilical flare), arrange the following:
  - bacterial swab
  - blood culture
  - start IV flucloxacillin and gentamicin until culture results are known, and review antibiotic combination according to culture and sensitivity results. Continue IV antibiotics for 5–7 days
  - if umbilical lines are in situ, consider removal.

Specific infections: osteomyelitis and septic arthritis

Aetiology
- Most commonly S. aureus or GBS
- May also be due to Gram –ve bacilli or Candida
- Osteomyelitis may coexist with a septic arthritis
- Commonest mechanism of infection is the haematogenous route
- It is important to exclude septic arthritis in a baby with sepsis, particularly in S. aureus sepsis and/or when osteomyelitis is suspected.

Clinical features
- Non-specific signs of sepsis
- Pseudoparalysis of the affected limb
- Incidental finding on X-ray of a baby with multisystem disease. Multiple sites may be affected
- Consider if a baby has persistently positive blood cultures despite adequate antibiotic treatment.

Investigations
- Blood culture and inflammatory markers (although CRP is normal in about 50% of cases)
- X-ray: abnormalities often appear within 7 days (unlike older children)
- Ultrasound should be used to look for subperiosteal abscesses and to assess adjacent joints for septic arthritis. MRI scan may also be useful
- Bone scan: is often not helpful in neonates
- Consider skeletal survey, as neonatal osteomyelitis may be multifocal
- Bone biopsy or joint aspiration
- MSU and CSF culture: likelihood of metastatic spread is high.

Management
- An orthopaedic opinion should be sought as soon as possible. Septic arthritis is an orthopaedic emergency
- **Antibiotics:** be guided by Gram stain of pus, etc.—first-line or if no organism found, then start IV flucloxacillin and gentamicin empirically
- Treatment should last for 4–6 weeks.

Prognosis
Worse than for older children: 30–50% develop limb shortening.

MRSA and other resistant organisms

Incidence

- In UK paediatric population, meticillin-resistant *S. aureus* (MRSA) increased from 0.9% to 13% of *S. aureus* septicaemias between 1990 and 2000
- Biggest problem on NNUs; 42% of cases in British Paediatric Surveillance Unit survey 2005–2006 in babies <1 month old
- Predominantly hospital acquired, but increasing incidence of community-acquired.

Surveillance

- Some NNUs will screen all new admissions
- For *ex utero* transfer, ask referring hospital for baby's MRSA status prior to transfer and screen baby on admission
- Liaise closely with Infection Control on any positive results or concerns.

Prevention

- Avoid introduction of MRSA positive patients where possible—is admission absolutely necessary?
- Hand hygiene (hand washing and the use of alcohol gel) is the mainstay of prevention (see Box 12.1)
- Every baby should have alcohol gel/handwash beside their cot, which must be used before and after each time the baby is handled.

Avoiding spread once MRSA isolated

- Isolate colonized/infected baby, in side/separate room if possible
- Discharge baby as soon as possible
- Where possible, staff should not work between colonized and non-colonized babies
- Colonized babies should not be handled without gloves and plastic apron
- Hands should be decontaminated and/or disinfected on entering the isolation room, before and after contact, and prior to leaving isolation room
- Care should be taken not to touch surfaces unless necessary
- Use baby's own cotside pens—not your own
- Colonized babies should remain isolated until discharge from the unit.

Treatment of MRSA sepsis

- Unlike adults, babies do not tend to be decontaminated due to lack of data on safety, although some units have nonetheless introduced decontamination protocols
- IV vancomycin usually effective
- May require adjunctive therapy for better tissue penetration (particularly if baby presents with multiple abscesses, bone, or joint involvement). Consider rifampicin.

Box 12.1 Hand washing, hand decontamination, and disinfection

- Hands and forearms should be washed each time the NNU is entered
- After hand washing, always apply alcohol gel and allow to dry before handling babies
- Use alcohol gel on entering and leaving all clinical areas, and before and after each patient contact
- No rings (wedding rings are often excepted) or watches to be worn, sleeves above elbows, no ties
- If hands become contaminated (body fluids, etc.) wash with soap and water
- If you have trouble with the condition of your skin, the procedure should be as follows:
  - wet hands
  - wash hands with liquid soap, and rinse
  - while hands still wet, apply moisturizer
  - dry hands with paper towel
  - rub in alcohol gel.

Fungal sepsis

Incidence

- *Candida* colonization very common (20–60%) in newborns on NNU
- Fungal sepsis affects 1–5% of very low birth weight (VLBW) babies (<1500 g), higher incidence in US than UK.

Commonest pathogens

- *Candida albicans* (~75% cases)
- *Candida parapsilosis*
- Aspergillosis, *Trichophyton*, *Malassezia furfur*.

Risk factors

- Extreme prematurity
- Fungal colonization (may occur at birth)
- Central lines
- Postnatal steroids
- Total parenteral nutrition (*Malassezia furfur* especially associated with prolonged use of IV lipid)
- Antibiotic use (broad spectrum antibiotics/prolonged use)
- NEC.

Prevention

- Hand washing
- Minimize invasive procedures
- Early enteral feeding
- Minimal and rational use of antibiotics
- Antifungal prophylaxis (see ➔ Prophylaxis, this chapter, p. 341).

Presentation

Congenital fungal sepsis

- Associated with intrauterine contraceptive devices and cervical suture
- Spreads over mucocutaneous surfaces (not blood-borne), and presents with skin involvement and pneumonia.

Nosocomial fungal sepsis

As with bacterial sepsis, may present with:

- Temperature instability
- Erythematous maculopapular rash
- Jaundice
- Abdominal distension/aspirates/vomiting
- Respiratory deterioration
- Cardiovascular instability
- Carbohydrate +/− lipid intolerance.

Diagnosis

Remember to consider fungal infection, especially in at-risk babies who present with signs of sepsis and fail to respond to antibiotics. Early diagnosis and treatment are more likely to lead to a favourable outcome. Look for signs of mucocutaneous infection during daily examination and treat promptly.

Investigations

To confirm diagnosis and location(s) of fungal infection:
- FBC and film: WBC changes and thrombocytopenia may not be present at the onset of infection
- Skin swabs of all suggestive skin lesions in babies at risk of invasive fungal sepsis
- Chase placental swabs and placental pathology
- Blood cultures (peripheral and from indwelling lines)
- Suprapubic aspirate of urine (or catheter specimen)
- Lumbar puncture
- Endotracheal aspirates
- Cranial US scan (poor outcome with parenchymal lesions)
- Abdominal US scan (looking at renal tract and for abscesses)
- Ophthalmology review (looking for retinal involvement)
- Echocardiogram (looking for endocarditis).

Prophylaxis

The Cochrane review from 2015 suggests that fungal (particularly *Candida*) sepsis can be prevented with prophylactic antifungal therapy, but mortality is unchanged. Both IV fluconazole and oral/topical nystatin have been used, although neither has become widespread. Concerns exist about fungal resistance from fluconazole prophylaxis.

Treatment

Oropharyngeal and/or topical candidiasis
- Treat topical perineal *Candida* with oral therapy, as well as topical therapy to prevent re-infection
- Nystatin is commonly used
- Continue topical treatment for 7 days after lesions have healed.

Suspected or proven fungal septicaemia
- Remove invasive lines
- Therapy should be refined once sensitivities are known
- Continue treatment for 21 days or until cultures negative
- Three main treatment options: amphotericin, liposomal amphotericin, and fluconazole.

Disseminated candidiasis—isolation of fungi from sterile body sites (e.g. CSF or retina/renal involvement)
- **Combined therapy:** amphotericin and flucytosine
- Continue both drugs for minimum 4 weeks
- Take blood cultures at least 5 days before planned discontinuation date
- Fungal meningitis can result in hydrocephalus.

Medications used in systemic fungal infection

Amphotericin

- Broad antifungal cover
- Poor central nervous system (CNS) penetration
- Side effects include fever/rigors, renal impairment, hypokalaemia, hypomagnesaemia, bone marrow suppression
- Requires a test dose and increasing doses over 3–5 days
- Continue treatment for 21 days or until blood culture is negative (whichever is longer).

Liposomal amphotericin

- Same spectrum with fewer (especially nephrotoxic) side effects than amphotericin (although more expensive)
- May have less renal tract penetration than amphotericin
- Also requires a test dose and increasing doses over 3–5 days.

Fluconazole

- More resistance, especially in non-albicans spp.
- Good urinary penetration (excreted via kidneys)
- Bone marrow depression with high serum levels
- Dose interval changes with postnatal age
- Treat for 21 days or until blood culture negative (whichever is longer).

Flucytosine

- Synergistic effect with amphotericin
- Good CSF penetration and excreted by kidneys—improves fungal clearance
- Can depress liver and bone marrow function.

Congenital infection: general principles

- Traditionally described as the 'TORCH' infections—toxoplasmosis, rubella, cytomegalovirus (CMV), HSV. TORCH infections are not all truly congenital, but often perinatal (e.g. HSV)
- Non-bacterial pathogens associated with neonatology also include syphilis, human immunodeficiency virus (HIV), varicella zoster virus (VZV), human T-cell leukaemia virus (HTLV), hepatitis B (HBV) and hepatitis C (HCV), parvovirus B19, Zika virus, and enteroviruses
- Think before ordering congenital infection investigations on babies:
  - some infections can be ruled out on clinical evidence alone (e.g. perinatal HBV and HCV are almost always asymptomatic and don't cause neonatal jaundice)
  - serological diagnosis may be made on mother's blood; and some viral infections excluded by testing mother (e.g. HBV and HCV, HIV, HTLV)
  - baby's serology may reflect mother's long-term past infections
  - baby's IgM not always reliable as a marker of congenital infections (e.g. CMV)
- Diagnosis may be best done by direct detection:
  - molecular techniques such as PCR to detect viral genomes
  - rapid culture
  - immunofluorescence for viral proteins (e.g. CMV in urine)
- Some infections need follow-up for up to 18 months before maternal antibody has decayed to exclude congenital infection (e.g. toxoplasmosis, syphilis, HCV, HIV)
- In late-booking mothers ensure screening serology (e.g. HBV, HIV, syphilis) is available as soon as possible after birth
- A history of travel during the pregnancy may be relevant (e.g. Zika virus)
- Important to seek advice on diagnosis with virology.

Congenital infection: clinical features

See Table 12.1.

Other things to note
- IUGR is suspicious particularly if symmetrical
- Purpura or petechiae usually due to thrombocytopenia. 'Blueberry muffin' appearance may be caused by extramedullary haemopoiesis in the skin
- Hepatosplenomegaly usually indicates extramedullary haemopoiesis
- Parvovirus can cause both aplastic and haemolytic anaemia, and may lead to hydrops
- Pneumonitis may present in preterm infants with unexpectedly severe chronic lung disease
- Cerebral calcification widespread in toxoplasmosis; periventricular in CMV.

Investigations
- Do not request a 'TORCH screen'
- Try to make a presumptive diagnosis and send appropriate laboratory investigation requests
- Discuss tests in advance with virology.

Table 12.1 Congenital infections: clinical features

	Toxo	Rubella	CMV	Parvo	Entero	Syph	Others
IUGR	√	√	√			√	Zika
Cardiac							
– structural	√	√	√				
– inflammation			√	√	√		
Ocular							
– cataract		√					
– chorioretinitis	√	√	√				
– conjunctivitis							Chlamydia
Hepatic (jaundice, hepatitis)	√	√	√		√		HSV
Haematological							
– purpura/ petechiae	√	√	√			√	HSV
						√	
– anaemia				√			
Hepato-splenomegaly		√	√			√	
Respiratory (pneumonitis)			√		√		
Neurological							
– microcephaly	√	√	√				Zika
– calcification	√		√				
– hydrocephalus	√			√			
– encephalitis		√			√		
– deafness		√	√				

CMV: cytomegalovirus; Entero: enterovirus; HSV: herpes simplex virus; IUGR: intrauterine growth restriction; Parvo: parvovirus B19; Syph: syphilis; Toxo: toxoplasmosis.

Congenital infection: hepatitis B

- Babies can acquire HBV perinatally or postnatally
- Neonatal HBV is usually asymptomatic and has a high incidence of chronic infection (90%)
- There is universal antenatal screening of mothers for HBV in the UK
- Maternal serology (and in some units maternal viral load) is used to interpret the risk of perinatal transmission:
  - HB surface antigen (HBsAg) indicates maternal carrier status
  - HB e antigen (HBeAg) correlates with viral replication and high levels of virus (i.e. high infectivity)
  - HB e antibody (anti-HBe) correlates with the loss of replicating virus and with lower levels of virus (i.e. low infectivity)
  - viral load may be useful where there is unknown 'e' status or baby is negative for HBeAg and anti-HBe. Viral load >10^6 indicates high infectivity
- Transmission risk from HBeAg positive mother is 70–90% without immunization and <10% after immunization. If a mother is HBsAg positive and anti-HBe positive the transmission without immunization is about 10%
- There is no contraindication to breastfeeding.

Hepatitis B immunization

- In the UK, HB immunization is given only to babies considered at risk of HBV. In many other countries universal immunization is recommended
- Where there is high risk of transmission (see Table 12.2) the baby should receive both HB immunoglobulin (HBIG) and commence the HBV vaccination schedule. Otherwise HB vaccination alone is sufficient.
- If required, HBIG should be given within 24 hours of birth
- Initial dose of vaccine should be given within 24 hours of birth
- Subsequent doses are generally given at 1, 2, and 12 months of age (accelerated schedule)
- Serology should be checked subsequently (at 4–6 weeks after 4th dose) and further vaccination arranged as necessary.

Table 12.2 Risk factors for acquisition of neonatal hepatitis B and recommended treatment of baby

Risk factors	Baby should receive	
	HBV vaccine	HBIG
Mother HBsAg +ve and HBeAg +ve	Yes	Yes
Mother HBsAg +ve, e-markers not present or not determined*	Yes	Yes
Mother has acute HBV during pregnancy (HBc IgM +ve)*	Yes	Yes
Very low birth weight baby <1500 g and mother HBsAg +ve (regardless of e antigen status)	Yes	Yes
Mother HBsAg +ve, HBeAg -ve, anti-HBe +ve*	Yes	No
Mother HBsAg -ve, but has blood-borne virus risk factors, e.g. IVDU, HCV +ve, HIV +ve (depends on local protocols)	Yes	No
Father HB carrier	Yes	No

*Advice may vary in units where HB viral load is used to assess infectivity.

HB: hepatitis B; HBc: HB core; HBeAg: HB e antigen; HBIG: HB immunoglobulin; HBsAg: HB surface antigen; HBV: hepatitis B virus; HCV: hepatitis C virus; HIV: human immunodeficiency virus; IVDU: intravenous drug user.

Congenital infection: HIV

- Perinatal acquisition of HIV is a particular problem in the developing world, where treatment of pregnant women during pregnancy and perinatally is still often unavailable
- Despite enormous improvements in antenatal retroviral treatment (ART) in developed countries (including the UK), new diagnoses of HIV in infancy remain static because of the steady increase in the number of HIV infected women giving birth
- In the UK, transmission rates have fallen over the last 10–15 years from 25% to <1%.

Antenatal management

- There is universal antenatal screening offered to mothers for HIV in the UK
- HIV-positive women should be managed in a multi-disciplinary team
- Although the first reductions in perinatal HIV transmission were achieved by perinatal ART (predominantly zidovudine) and elective Caesarean section, increasingly women are having highly active anti-retroviral treatment (HAART) to completely suppress their viral load with a view to enable them to have vaginal delivery.

Neonatal investigations

- Blood should be taken from the baby (**NB** Cord blood is not suitable due to potential contamination with maternal blood)
- **Virology:** HIV antibody and HIV DNA PCR
- FBC and liver function tests (LFTs).

Neonatal management

- Mainly involves prevention of mother to child transmission by 'post-exposure prophylaxis' (PEP)
- Breastfeeding is contraindicated in developed countries as risk of transmission outweighs risks associated with formula milks. In developing countries it may be safer for HIV-positive mothers to exclusively breastfeed than to formula feed
- Bacillus Calmette-Guérin (BCG) should not be given until negative HIV DNA PCR at 3 months
- Treatment may vary according to local guidelines, maternal viral load, CD4 count, maternal ART, and compliance. Plan for neonatal treatment should be made antenatally
- Ask advice from GU medicine team, infection, or virology specialists
- Risk of transmission is increased if:
    - maternal viral load high (>50 copies/ml) or unknown due to late presentation or failure to attend clinic
    - there has been inadequate maternal treatment in pregnancy
    - prematurity (<36 weeks), ruptured membranes >4 hours prior to delivery (unless planned vaginal delivery), chorioamnionitis, placental abruption
- Presumed low risk of transmission:
    - low maternal viral load (<50 copies/ml) will usually be due to treatment with combination therapy or zidovudine (AZT) alone to reduce vertical transmission

- commence AZT as soon as possible after birth (within 4 hours)
- dose of AZT varies with gestation
- AZT is the only ART with an IV preparation and can be given to babies not on oral feeds
- Concern about high risk of transmission:
  - consideration for combination PEP for the baby postnatally should be given if the risk of transmission is increased
  - combination PEP will generally consist of triple ART, such as AZT, lamivudine and nevirapine, although this will depend on maternal ART.

Follow-up

- Neonatal ART will normally continue for 4 weeks after birth
- Only babies considered at high risk of transmission will need to start co-trimoxazole after completing their ART
- Follow-up bloods will include HIV DNA PCR at 6 weeks and 3 months, and HIV antibody test at 18 months to confirm disappearance of maternal antibody
- Be aware that mothers may not disclose their HIV status to partners, GP, or other family members, so take care with confidentiality.

Congenital infection: hepatitis C

- There is no universal antenatal screening offered to mothers for HCV in the UK. Only women considered high risk will be screened (e.g. women known to be HBV or HIV positive, or women with a history of intravenous drug use)
- Mothers found to be HCV antibody positive antenatally should be tested for HC RNA PCR
- Babies of mothers who are HC RNA positive have a 2.5–12% risk of acquiring HCV perinatally. Babies of mothers who are HCV antibody positive, but RNA negative have a 0.3% risk
- HCV is unlikely to present in the neonatal period and usually causes a low-grade chronic hepatitis in childhood. The natural history of the progression of vertically transmitted HC is currently not known.

Postnatal management

- Check mother's HBV and HIV status from antenatal testing
- Babies are often recommended to receive HB vaccine course regardless of mother's HBV status due to the similar risk profiles
- Breastfeeding should not be discouraged as the risks are likely to be negligible
- Recommended investigations are as follows:
  - 6–8 weeks and 6 months HC RNA PCR
  - 12 months HC RNA PCR and HC antibody
  - if HC antibodies are positive at 12 months they should be repeated at 18 months to confirm loss of maternal antibody
- Refer to paediatric hepatology or gastroenterology clinic if RNA PCR is positive at any time or if antibodies are still detectable at 18 months.

Congenital infection: Zika virus

Background
- Congenital Zika Syndrome recognized in 2015 in central/South America
- Arbovirus. Transmitted predominantly by the *Aedes aegypti* mosquito.
- Usually asymptomatic or mild illness in adults
- The risk of birth defects appears low; sequelae more severe if infection occurs in early gestation.

Presentation
- Commonest presentation is microcephaly. Other clinical findings: IUGR, hypertonia, seizures, microphthalmia, cataracts, ocular calcification, hearing abnormalities
- Imaging findings: cerebral calcification, ventriculomegaly, cerebral and cerebellar atrophy, cortical migrational abnormalities.

Investigation
Maternal
- Consider in women with symptoms of infection within 2 weeks of travel to areas with active Zika transmission
- Blood and urine for Zika RNA PCR and Zika serology
- Amniocentesis if fetal abnormality with a positive travel history.

Baby
Where mother travelled to high risk area during pregnancy or within 4 weeks of conception:
- Perform clinical assessment for signs of congenital infection (See ➔ Congenital infection: clinical features, p. 346)
- Baby has abnormalities and mother has been not been tested → Zika virus tests on mother and baby
- Investigations should include:
  - placenta for histopathology and Zika virus PCR
  - FBC and film, clotting, U&E, LFT, CRP
  - paired maternal and neonatal serum for Zika virus IgG and IgM
  - EDTA blood, saliva, stool for Zika virus PCR ; CSF for Zika PCR if neurological concerns
  - consider investigations for other congenital infections
  - neuroimaging: cranial ultrasound in all babies; MRI scan if concerns
  - ophthalmology assessment and hearing screening

Follow up
- All babies should be followed up until 1 year
- Neurology/neurodevelopmental follow-up in babies with abnormalities
- Repeat ophthalmology and audiology assessment at 3–6 months.

Congenital infection: syphilis

- Syphilis is caused by the spirochete, *Treponema pallidum*. Prevalence is rising in the UK
- All mothers are screened for syphilis at booking. If positive, the woman should be referred to GU clinic:
  - some women will be known to have had effective treatment in the past and will not be treated again during the pregnancy
  - some women will not be known to have had treatment or considered likely to have latent disease. These women should receive treatment with penicillin during pregnancy
  - a minority of women will be found to have active disease (primary or secondary syphilis) and will be treated with penicillin
- Parenteral (IM) penicillin treatment for syphilis completed at least 4 weeks before delivery prevents most congenital syphilis.

There are a few difficulties for neonatal practice:
- Congenital syphilis can be asymptomatic but cause significant (preventable) problems for the child later
- None of the available tests are perfect:
  - there is no test to define at birth if an infant has been infected
  - there is no test to ensure that a mother has not been reinfected since treatment.

Infants not needing investigation or serological screening from birth

- Where it is known that the mother has been cured prior to pregnancy, and the GU specialist is confident there has been no reinfection, the mother will not have been treated again in pregnancy. This infant required no testing. This requires close liaison with GU team.

Infants needing only clinical and serological screening over first year

- Maternal syphilis serology confirmed positive and treated during this pregnancy with penicillin *and* completed treatment at least 4 weeks before delivery.

Infants needing investigation and treatment in newborn period

Infant asymptomatic, but 'inadequate' maternal treatment

- Criteria have been published for diagnosing congenital syphilis. See ➔ Further information, p. 370
- Never treated
- Treated during this pregnancy, but not adequately—not with parenteral penicillin (e.g. erythromycin), or parenteral penicillin treatment incomplete or completed less than 4 weeks before delivery.

Infant unwell with symptoms consistent with congenital syphilis

Signs and symptoms suggestive of congenital syphilis include: IUGR, hydrops, rhinitis, rashes (especially soles and palms, perioral, and perianal), condylomata lata (especially perineal), osteochondritis and periostitis, hepatosplenomegaly, thrombocytopenia and anaemia, meningitis, renal impairment.

Investigation

- Serology (see ➲ Serological and clinical screening, this chapter, p. 355)
- FBC, LFTs
- X-rays: request long bone films
- Lumbar puncture.

Treatment and follow-up

- Benzylpenicillin IV for 10 days, procaine benzylpenicillin IM for 10 days, and a single dose of benzathine benzylpenicillin IM have all been recommended. Discuss with infection specialist
- Regular repeat serology screening
- Symptomatic infants with negative IgM should have repeat IgM at 4 and 8 weeks, as there can be a delayed IgM response in infants
- Observe for signs of late syphilis: developmental delay, 8th nerve deafness, interstitial keratitis, abnormal bones and joints, abnormal teeth
- Outlook for congenital syphilis treated at birth is good, but treponemes may remain in the eye (interstitial keratitis). Refer to paediatric ophthalmologist.

Serological and clinical screening

See Box 12.2.
- Screening is done at birth, and repeated at 3 and 6 months, and 1 year
- IgM is most useful at birth, then *Treponema pallidum* particle agglutination (TPPA)/IgG/rapid plasma reagin (RPR) during follow-up
- If baby is IgM positive at birth, recall for full investigation and treatment
- Maternal antibodies will disappear over the first year. Once a baby is negative (TPPA/IgG and RPR) no further testing is necessary
- Infants should be investigated, and treated or re-treated if titres are rising. Treated infected infants may have persistent low levels of IgG/TPPA, but RPR tests should be negative.

Box 12.2 Quick guide to available serological tests for syphilis

- **IgM enzyme immunoassay (EIA):** for treponemal IgM; presence highly suggestive of active infection; absence does not exclude active infection
- **IgG EIA:** for treponemal IgG; presence suggestive of infection, does not distinguish previous or latent infection, and is likely to be due to maternal antibody transfer in the infant unless levels are increasing
- **RPR:** non-treponemal test that has replaced the VDRL (venereal disease reference laboratory test). Both are raised in acute infection, and titres fall in response to effective treatment
- **TPPA:** does not distinguish between active and previously treated infection.

Congenital infection: cytomegalovirus

Background
- CMV is a herpes virus, seropositivity in adults varies from 50 to >90%
- CMV infection in the newborn baby can be congenitally or perinatally/ postnatally acquired
- For presentation of an infant with congenital CMV, see ➲ Congenital infections: clinical features, p. 346 and Table 12.1
- Perinatal acquisition of CMV usually has no long-term implications for the baby.

Investigations
- Virology tests:
    - urine for CMV viral PCR (this test is definitive for congenital CMV in the first 2 weeks of life)
    - saliva and bronchial washings if available
    - other investigations may include blood for CMV PCR, or IgM
    - also check maternal CMV serology (IgG and IgM)
- LFTs, clotting, and FBC (anaemia, thrombocytopenia)
- For the diagnosis of congenital CMV, it is essential to collect urine within the first 2 weeks of life, otherwise perinatal infection (as opposed to congenital infection) cannot be ruled out
- Cranial US scan (and consider need for MRI scan)
- Ophthalmology assessment
- Hearing screening: a negative hearing screen at birth does not rule out the possibility that hearing loss may occur later.

Management
- Antiviral treatment should be discussed with infection or virology specialists
- Most babies congenitally infected with CMV shed virus in urine and body secretions, so barrier nursing is indicated
- Ganciclovir has been used for life threatening infection
- Evidence has emerged recently that long-term hearing loss in babies born with congenital CMV central nervous system disease can be prevented with a regimen of IV ganciclovir or oral valganciclovir
- The dose and length of treatment is debatable. Neutropenia and thrombocytopenia are possible side effects
- Long-term follow-up to assess hearing and neurodevelopment will be necessary.

Congenital infection: rubella

- Congenital rubella may be expected to increase with reduced uptake of mumps, measles, and rubella (MMR)
- Classical congenital rubella exhibits a triad of cataract, congenital heart disease and nerve deafness (for other presentations, see ➔ Congenital infection: clinical features, p. 346 and p. 347)
- Confirmation of maternal rubella immune status and immunization history, and whether there has been a rubella-like illness in pregnancy is important
- Rubella serology is no longer part of pregnancy screening in the UK.

Investigations

- Virology tests:
  - viral serology on baby for rubella IgM
  - check maternal booking viral serology (if done) and order current maternal IgG and IgM
  - further specialist tests such as rubella PCR or culture may be advised by virologist
- LFTs, clotting, and FBC
- Cranial ultrasound scan (and consider need for MRI scan)
- Cardiology opinion and echocardiogram
- Ophthalmology assessment
- Hearing screening.

Treatment

- There is no safe, proven, effective treatment for congenital rubella
- Most babies congenitally infected with rubella shed virus in urine and body secretions, so barrier nursing is indicated.

Congenital infection: toxoplasmosis

Background

- Highly variable. Relatively high rate in France has led to an antenatal screening programme. No screening in UK
- Risk of congenital infection rises as pregnancy progresses, but sequelae more severe with infection early in pregnancy. Overall risk of congenital infection following maternal infection in pregnancy 20–50%
- Evidence for effectiveness of antenatal treatment after maternal infection is weak.

Presentation

- Majority of babies are asymptomatic at birth
- Classical congenital toxoplasmosis exhibits a triad of chorioretinitis, hydrocephalus, and intracranial calcification (for other presentations, see ➲ Congenital infection: clinical features, p. 346 and p. 347).

Investigation

Discuss with infection and virology specialists.

Maternal

- Take a thorough maternal history during pregnancy including possible exposure (travel, handling, or ingestion of previously uncooked meat, kittens/cat litter) and illness (lymphadenopathy, fatigue, viral-like illness). Note that such illness prior to conception is unlikely to be relevant to a diagnosis of congenital toxoplasmosis
- Review results of antenatal US scans and maternal serology results if available
- Send maternal serology after discussion with virologist.

Baby

- Diagnosis is by a combination of serology, looking for IgM and/or IgA initially, then following IgG through the first year of life. IgG avidity and PCR are also used. Liaise with virology.
- FBC and film, U&Es, LFTs
- Urinalysis
- Ophthalmology assessment
- Cranial ultrasound scan (and consider need for MRI scan)
- Hearing screening.

Management

- Breastfeeding by an infected mother provides no risk to her infant
- Infected babies are not contagious
- Even in moderately affected babies, considerable improvement can occur with aggressive treatment
- Symptomatic babies:
  - pyrimethamine, sulfadiazine and folinic acid
  - continue all three for 1 year, monitor LFTs and FBC every 4–6 weeks (risk of myelosuppression and hepatitis)
- Asymptomatic infants with positive serology. Treatment of these babies is not straightforward. Discuss individual cases with infection and virology specialists.

Follow-up

- Infants born to women with a definite toxoplasma infection in pregnancy will need to be followed for up to 18 months. Frequency of testing will be determined by rate of maternal IgG decay or appearance of infant's intrinsic immune response to toxoplasma
- Monitor liver and marrow function
- Ophthalmology review as suggested by paediatric ophthalmologists
- Audiology assessment according to hearing screening result or clinical indication
- Neurosurgical referral if hydrocephalus occurs.

Perinatal herpes simplex virus

Incidence varies between populations, higher in US than UK, but is approximately 1 per 3000 to 20,000 live births.

Pathogenesis

- Infant usually acquires HSV at the time of delivery, through direct contact with infectious secretions or lesions
- HSV-2 in 70–85%
- Transmission far more likely in primary than secondary infection as there is no maternal antibody to afford protection
- Risk to individual baby is difficult to quantify due to the high incidence of asymptomatic maternal infection and the unknown extent of viral shedding between episodes (50–70% of babies are born to asymptomatic mothers).

Presentation

- Typically at 7–14 days
- Often initially non-specific, with irritability, lethargy, fever, or failure to feed
- Consider in any babies with sepsis-like illness, particularly if deranged LFTs and/or coagulation.

The three classical presentations are:

Skin-eye-mouth (SEM) disease

- Disease localized to mucous membranes
- May progress to encephalitis or disseminated disease.

CNS disease/encephalitis

- Can be isolated or occur in association with SEM or disseminated disease
- Encephalitis is present in 70% of neonatal herpes
- 10% mortality with treatment, high rate of neurological impairment at follow-up.

Disseminated disease

- Multi-organ involvement: encephalitis, pneumonitis, hepatitis, disseminated intravascular coagulation, keratoconjunctivitis
- Frequently no skin lesions present
- Mortality 60% with treatment.

By the time diagnosis is made, many infants have severe disease and have developed complications.

Management

Prevention

- Babies born to mothers with active lesions thought to be primary should be advised to have elective Caesarean section. Otherwise vaginal delivery is reasonable
- Breastfeeding is not contraindicated, as long as there are no breast lesions.

Asymptomatic baby and mother with active lesions

- Send swabs for viral HSV detection from vesicular lesions, conjunctiva, throat, nasopharynx +/− anal and vulval
- Observe for skin or scalp rashes (especially vesicular lesions), respiratory distress (neonatal HSV infection may cause pneumonitis), seizures, signs of sepsis
- Babies born to mothers without genital lesions or those born by Caesarean section may be discharged early, but parents should be instructed to look out for any rashes or signs of viraemia. Babies born vaginally to mothers with active lesions should be observed for at least 4 days.

Babies with suspected herpes simplex infection

- Investigations:
  - EDTA blood and CSF for HSV PCR
  - urine and blood for HSV culture
  - FBC, LFTs, clotting (look for evidence of viral hepatitis)
- Treatment is often delayed as babies assumed to have bacterial sepsis; early treatment has better outcome
- If signs of viraemia are present or the diagnosis is strongly suspected start IV aciclovir
- Treatment in proven cases should be for at least 14–21 days
- Barrier nurse, preferably in an isolation room.

Outcome

- Mortality from virtually nil (isolated SEM disease) to 60% (disseminated disease) in treated babies
- High rate of neurological impairment at follow-up in babies with encephalitis (up to 80%)
- Recurrent disease can occur and may require repeated or long-term treatment.

Perinatal chickenpox

Maternal chickenpox

- Herpes zoster (shingles) infection in mother is not an indication for concern in the newborn
- If mother develops chickenpox ≥7 days before birth, the baby is likely to have received maternal antibodies transplacentally, therefore varicella zoster immunoglobulin (VZIG) or other treatment is not indicated
- If mother develops chickenpox from <7 days before birth until 7 days after birth, VZIG should be given
- There is no contraindication to breastfeeding
- The mother and baby should be isolated from other mothers and babies
- The appearance of any vesicular lesions in a newborn should be treated with IV aciclovir whether VZIG has been given or not
- Shingles in infancy or childhood may occur following perinatal chickenpox
- Maternal chickenpox during early pregnancy is associated with embryopathy (microcephaly, microphthalmia, limb atrophy, etc.), risk: 2–12 weeks ~0.5%, 12–28 weeks ~1.4%, >28 weeks 0%.

Chickenpox contact (baby within 1 month of birth)

- Contact is defined as being in the same room for 15 minutes or more, or face-to-face conversation for 5 minutes or more or living in the same house. Chickenpox is infectious from 48 hours before the rash and until ~5–7 days after (traditionally taken as when all lesions have become scabs)
- If a baby is ≤28 weeks gestation and/or ≤1000 g at birth, regardless of mother's previous chickenpox exposure, they are unlikely to have received adequate antibody transplacentally and should be given VZIG
- If baby is >28 weeks gestation, the mother should have her chickenpox serology performed, regardless of history of chickenpox (this may be done on booking blood samples)
  - if mother is seropositive for VZV, the baby is likely to be immune, and will not need prophylaxis or treatment
  - if maternal serology is negative, the baby requires VZIG
- Anyone with chickenpox infection must not visit NNU until no longer infectious
- Any chickenpox contacts must not visit the NNU from days 7 to 21 after the contact
- Babies who are contacts should be isolated (and cohorted if there are more than one) from days 7 to 21 after contact (or from days 7 to 28 after contact if they received VZIG).
- Breastfeeding of babies exposed to maternal chickenpox should be encouraged. If the mother has chickenpox lesions close to the nipple, milk should be expressed until the lesions have crusted. The baby should be protected from chickenpox by VZIG, and so can receive expressed breast milk

- Babies who are contacts should be nursed by staff who are immune to chickenpox
- When indicated, VZIG should be given as soon as possible, certainly within 72 hours of contact, but is recommended up to 10 days following contact
- If other family members have chickenpox at home and the mother is seronegative, discharge should be delayed until the baby is at least 7 days old.

Treatment of chickenpox in neonates

- Request that a virologist performs lesion scrape for electron microscopy and viral culture
- Treat with IV aciclovir if within first 1 month of life, regardless of previous provision of VZIG, or maternal chickenpox status.

Tuberculosis and BCG vaccination

Tuberculosis (TB) is due to infection with *Mycobacterium tuberculosis*.

Management of baby with TB contact

- Mother diagnosed with 'open' TB and on treatment ≤2 weeks
  - breastfeeding contraindicated
  - CXR for baby to exclude disease
  - start baby on isoniazid prophylaxis 10 mg/kg daily, and pyridoxine if breastfed
  - refer to specialist
  - follow-up diagnostic testing at 6 weeks: tuberculin skin test, +/− interferon gamma release assay (IGRA)
  - withhold BCG until 6 months
  - household should be screened
- Immediate family member with recently diagnosed 'open' TB; or 'closed' TB prior to screening other family members
  - start baby on isoniazid prophylaxis 10 mg/kg daily, and pyridoxine if breastfed
  - household should be screened
  - consider tuberculin skin test/BCG based on maternal screening
- Mother with TB disease on adequate treatment >2 weeks before birth
  - BCG for baby at birth
  - household should be screened.

Neonatal tuberculosis

- Neonates are very susceptible to *Mycobacterium tuberculosis*
- Virtually all infections are acquired postnatally from maternal TB; less commonly close household contacts; rarely from staff with open TB
- Can be acquired antenatally (congenital TB).

Congenital tuberculosis

- Occurs with maternal miliary TB or a recent primary infection
- 50% of mothers are previously undiagnosed.

Mode of transmission

- Infection from genital tract rare, usually results in abortion or stillbirth
- Transplacental:
  - haematogenous leads to primary focus in liver
  - via amniotic fluid by ingestion or aspiration.

Presentation

- Asymptomatic at birth, but most have an abnormal CXR and are symptomatic by 2–3 weeks
- Symptomatic at birth, very sick, and may be infectious:
  - hepatosplenomagaly, lymphadenopathy, fever
  - respiratory distress, pleural effusions
  - meningitis (present in 1/3 of cases)
  - papules and petechiae, discharging ear.

Diagnosis
- Microscopy for acid-fast bacilli: only 10% +ve
- PCR: 25–83% +ve
- Culture (takes 6 weeks)
- Tuberculin skin test may be –ve for 3 months
- Diagnosis often has to rely on making the diagnosis in the mother.

Treatment
- Isoniazid, rifampicin, and pyrazinamide + ethambutol or streptomycin, until sensitivities known
- Continue appropriate antituberculous medication for 9–12 months.

Bacillus Calmette-Guérin vaccination

- BCG vaccine is a live attenuated strain of *Mycobacterium bovis*
- Neonatal BCG vaccination provides 50–70% protection against all forms of TB and 70–80% protection against miliary TB and TB meningitis
- High-risk group if:
    - any member of household has TB or has had it in the past
    - any member of household born in Africa, Asia (excluding Japan but including Cyprus and Turkey), South or Central America (including Caribbean)
    - any member of household likely to visit these areas for >1 month
    - refugees
    - in homeless accommodation
    - travellers
- Provision of BCG in the community depends on prevalence and local practice
- Contraindications to BCG vaccination:
    - immunosuppressive medication or condition
    - generalized skin sepsis
    - sepsis
- No need for prior tuberculin test <6 years unless resident in area of high TB prevalence
- Intradermal injection
- Parents should be informed that pinhead, dry, red pimples commonly appear after 2–6 weeks and may last several months.

Immunizations relevant to the neonatal unit

This follows the guidance from the Department of Health Joint Committee on Vaccination and Immunization (the UK 'Green Book'):

- Immunizations are offered to preterm babies just as for the newborn in general, and at ages not corrected for gestation
- Live vaccines (BCG, oral polio, and MMR) are contraindicated for 3 months following dexamethasone, because of its immunosuppression
- Parents must give consent for any course of immunizations. Record the administration of any immunization including site of administration and batch numbers
- The anterolateral aspect (too lateral injects the fascia lata) of the thigh is most commonly used for IM injections. The deltoid may also be used in bigger babies.

Diphtheria, tetanus, pertussis, meningococcus C, polio, *Haemophilus influenzae* B, Pneumococcus, meningococcus B

- These are administered in different combinations (see Table 12.3) at 2, 3, and 4 months, but generally delayed if baby is very unwell or deteriorating
- Diphtheria, tetanus, pertussis (acellular) (DTaP), *Haemophilus influenzae* type B (HiB), and polio come in the '5 in 1' preparation. Meningococcus C (MenC), meningococcus B (MenB), and pneumococcal vaccines are currently given separately
- There is probably an increased risk of apnoea in preterm infants for 24–48 hours following routine immunization. This may be due to the pertussis component. Ensure adequate monitoring during this period.

Hepatitis B

See also → Congenital infection: hepatitis B, p. 348.
- VLBW babies (<1500 g) are recommended to have HBIG in addition to immunization
- It is not clear how immunogenic the vaccine is in preterm infants, so serology should be checked 6–8 weeks after the third dose, to guide the need for an extra booster.

BCG

See → Tuberculosis and BCG vaccination, pp. 364–5.

Influenza

- Indicated in infants with chronic lung disease (needing oxygen/ventilatory support by 36 weeks corrected) >6 months of age
- It is administered in two half-adult doses (i.e. 0.25 ml) 1 month apart.

Table 12.3 Summary scheme of current UK infant immunizations

Chronological age (months unless indicated)	Hepatitis B*	DTaP-polio-HiB	MenC	Pneumo	Influenza*	RSV*	MMR	Rotavirus	MenB
0	√								
1	√								
2	√	√		√				√	√
3	√	√	√					√	
6–8 weeks after 3rd HB	Serology (preterm)								
4		√		√					√
First autumn					√ ×2	√ ×5			
12–13	√ and serology		√ (+ HiB)	√			√		√

*Where indicated—see ⟳ Hepatitis B. p. 366; ⟳ Influenza, p. 366; ⟳ Respiratory syncytial virus, p. 368 in this chapter.

DTaP: diptheria-tetanus-acellular pertussis vaccine; HiB: *Haemophilus influenzae* type B vaccine; MenB: meningitis B vaccine; MenC: meningitis C vaccine; MMR: measles, mumps, and rubella vaccine; pneumo: Pneumococcus vaccine; RSV: respiratory syncytial virus vaccine.

Respiratory syncytial virus

- Humanized monoclonal antibody (IgG) against respiratory syncytial virus (RSV)—palivizumab—is available for passive immunization. The effect lasts a month, so it must be given monthly during the RSV season (about October to February)
- Indicated in babies with chronic lung disease, although the definition in this context varies between units. Consult local guidelines. Usually given in babies at home in oxygen. See ⊃ Bronchiolitis on the neonatal unit pp. 146–7.

Rotavirus

Live attenuated oral vaccine, given at 2 and 3 months of age.

- Caution is needed if the vaccine is delayed, as this increases incidence of associated intussusception
- Advice is to give to parents of preterm babies regardless of gestation or whether the baby is an inpatient on NNU. There is no evidence for transmission of infection from live attenuated virus between babies in the NNU environment, but strict hand hygiene should be observed.

Further information

Further information

Cleminson J, Austin N, McGuire W. Prophylactic systemic antifungal agents to prevent mortality and morbidity in very low birth weight infants (review). Update *Cochrane Database Syst Rev* 2015; 24(10):CD003850.

Department of Health. *Immunization against infectious disease*, The Green Book. DoH, London, 2013.

Hughes RG, Brocklehurst P, Heath P, Stenson B. *Prevention of early onset neonatal Group B streptococcal disease*, Royal College of Obstetricians and Gynaecologists, Guideline No. 36, Second edition, July 2012.

Johnson AP, Sharland M, Goodall CM, et al. Enhanced surveillance of MRSA bacteraemia in children in the UK and Ireland. *Arch Dis Child* 2010; **95**: 781–785.

Klein JO, Remington JS, Marcy SM. *Infectious diseases of the fetus and newborn infant*. WB Saunders, Philadelphia, USA, 2010.

National Institute for Health and Clinical Excellence (2012) NICE clinical guideline CG149. *Antibiotics for the prevention and treatment of early-onset neonatal infection.* ℘ www.nice.org.uk/CG149

National Institute for Health and Clinical Excellence (2011) NICE clinical guideline CG117. *Clinical diagnosis and management of tuberculosis, and measures for its prevention and control.* ℘ www.nice.org.uk/CG117

Polin RA, Committee on Fetus and Newborn. Management of neonates with suspected or proven early-onset bacterial sepsis. *Pediatrics* 2012; **129**: 1006–1015.

Taylor GP, Clayden P, Dhar J, et al. British HIV Association guidelines for the management of HIV infection in pregnant women 2012. *HIV Medicine* 2012; **13**: 87–157.

Kingston M, French P, Higgins S, et al. UK national guidelines on the management of syphilis 2015. *Int J STD AIDS* 2016; **27**(6): 421–46.

Chapter 13

Metabolic problems and jaundice

Hypoglycaemia: overview

Definition

Blood glucose <2.6 mmol/l.

- Low point-of-care testing (POCT) blood glucose results should be confirmed with a laboratory sample (but treatment should not be delayed if <1.5 mmol/l)
- Normal term babies commonly have blood glucose levels <2.6 mmol/l, particularly in the 1st 24 hours (more common in breastfed babies), but are not at risk of any long-term sequelae because they can utilize alternative fuels (e.g. ketone bodies, lactate). Therefore, blood glucose analysis should not be routinely performed on healthy, term babies.

Babies at risk of clinically relevant hypoglycaemia/causes of neonatal hypoglycaemia

- Increased demand/decreased supply:
  - preterm
  - intrauterine growth retardation (IUGR)
  - hypothermia
  - infection
  - hypoxia ischaemia
  - polycythaemia
- Hyperinsulinism:
  - infant of a diabetic mother
  - haemolytic disease of the newborn
  - hyperinsulinism hyperammonaemia syndrome (HIHA)
  - transient neonatal hyperinsulinism
  - Beckwith–Wiedemann syndrome
  - persistent hyperinsulinaemic hypoglycaemia of infancy (previously called nesidioblastosis)
  - islet cell adenoma
- Endocrinopathies:
  - pituitary (e.g. growth hormone deficiency, septo-optic dysplasia)
  - adrenal (e.g. congenital adrenal hyperplasia)
- Carbohydrate metabolism disorders:
  - glycogen storage disease
  - galactosaemia
- Organic acidaemias
- Liver failure
- Fat oxidation defects: MCAD (medium-chain acyl CoA dehydrogenase), LCHAD (long-chain 3-hydroxyacyl CoA dehydrogenase), and VLCAD (very long-chain acyl CoA dehydrogenase) deficiency.

Investigation of persistent or severe hypoglycaemia

These should be carried out if hypoglycaemia is severe and/or persistent.

Box 13.1 shows the key points in the investigation of neonatal hypoglycaemia.

Box 13.1 Key points in the investigation of neonatal hypoglycaemia

- Laboratory samples should be collected at the same time hypoglycaemia is confirmed by POCT
- The key investigation is the presence or absence of ketones—this should be assessed at the time of the hypoglycaemic episode by blood POCT or urine dipstick testing (or sending a blood/urine sample to the laboratory)
- Low or absent urine ketones = hypoketotic hypoglycaemia (caused by hyperinsulinism, fat oxidation defects, or liver failure)
- Ketotic hypoglycaemia—all other causes.

Blood tests
- Glucose
- Electrolytes
- Liver enzymes
- Insulin + c-peptide
- Acylcarnitines
- Cortisol
- Free fatty acids
- Growth hormone
- Lactate
- B-hydroxybutyrate
- Ammonia (if hyperinsulinism confirmed)
- Galactose-1-phosphate uridyl transferase.

Urine tests
- Ketones
- Organic acids.

Hypoglycaemia: management

Suggested guidelines are as follows, but local guidelines should also be referred to.

Determine whether the baby is at risk from hypoglycaemia

If at risk, minimize risks

- Feed early (i.e. as soon as possible after birth and within 30 minutes) or if enteral feeding is contraindicated, start IVI 10% glucose
- Check blood sugar before 2nd, 3rd, and 4th feeds, and until there have been at least two satisfactory measurements (i.e. ≥2.6 mmol/l)
- If the baby is already on IV fluids.

Calculate glucose intake

Glucose intake (mg/kg/min) = (ml/h × % glucose)/[6 × weight (kg)]

Ensure that the glucose intake is adequate:
- Term: 3–5 mg/kg/min
- Preterm: 4–6 mg/kg/min
- Small for gestational age: 6–8 mg/kg/min
- Consider hyperinsulinism if: >10 mg/kg/min.

Treatment of babies at risk from hypoglycaemia

- If sugar <1.5mmol/l:
  - admit to neonatal unit (NNU)
  - confirm hypoglycaemia with laboratory blood glucose assay
  - give IVI 10% glucose 2 ml/kg bolus followed by an infusion. Initial infusion rate: 6 mg/kg/min (= 3.6 ml/kg/h 10% glucose). If IV glucose already running, increase infusion rate or glucose concentration to 8 mg/kg/min
  - recheck glucose after 15 minutes initially and then frequently until stable, aiming for blood glucose 3–4 mmol/l
- If sugar 1.5–2.5mmol/l:
  - feed immediately and recheck blood sugar after 30 minutes
  - if blood sugar still low, consider admission and IVI glucose
- Investigate if hypoglycaemia recurrent/persistent (see ➔ Hypoglycaemia: overview, pp. 372–3)
- If the baby requires a glucose concentration of 15% or greater, it should be given via a central venous line
- If the hypoglycaemia is persistent, or IV access is unobtainable, or the underlying diagnosis is hyperinsulinism, give glucagon 100 µg/kg IV or IM. Refer to local endocrine/metabolic team for further management if hyperinsulinism is suspected
- If the hypoglycaemia is secondary to hyperinsulinism, further treatment with a glucagon infusion, or diazoxide (+ chlorthiazide), or a somatostatin analogue may be required. Check ammonia levels to exclude hyperinsulinism hyperammonaemia (HIHA).

Infants of diabetic mothers

The risk of complications in fetus/baby is related to the degree of maternal glycaemic control. The risks therefore differ depending when glycaemic control is poor—poor glycaemic control in very early pregnancy is related to ↑ risk of congenital malformations; whereas in later pregnancy it is associated with neonatal hypoglycaemia.

Management of infants of diabetic mothers

- Obstetric/midwifery team should inform neonatal unit staff of maternal history
- Check antenatal ultrasound scan results and examine carefully for signs of macrosomia, congenital abnormalities (congenital heart disease, sacral agenesis, microcolon, neural tube defects), signs of respiratory distress, and heart murmurs
- Routine NNU admission is not recommended and babies of women with diabetes should not be separated from their mothers unless there is a clinical complication or there are abnormal clinical signs that warrant admission
- Monitor baby for hypoglycaemia (starting within 2–4 hours of birth):
    - encourage breastfeeding and start feeds as soon as possible after birth (within 30 minutes)
    - continue feeds at frequent intervals (2–3 hourly) until blood glucose monitoring can be discontinued
    - check blood sugar before 2nd, 3rd, and 4th feeds, and until there have been at least two satisfactory measurements (i.e. ≥2.6 mmol/l)
    - See ➲ Treatment of babies at risk from hypoglycaemia, p. 374, if blood sugar <2.6 mmol/l
- Observe baby for signs of polycythaemia and jaundice. Blood tests (serum bilirubin, full blood count, calcium, and magnesium) should be carried out if any clinical signs are present
- Echocardiogram if heart murmurs or other signs of cardiac disease present (congenital heart disease or transient hypertrophic (septal) cardiomyopathy)
- Discharge to community care is not recommended before 24 hours of age and should only occur after medical/midwifery staff are satisfied that blood glucose levels are maintained and the baby is feeding well.

Hyperglycaemia

Definition
- There is no agreed definition for hyperglycaemia in neonates
- Two consecutive levels >7–10 mmol/l may be considered significant.

Pathophysiology
- Usually transient and secondary to other disorders
- Glycosuria leading to osmotic diuresis may result from hyperglycaemia, but renal threshold low (particularly in preterm) and may even occur in the presence of normoglycaemia
- Hyperglycaemia in neonates does *not* cause ketosis or acidosis
- Glucose levels >20 mmol/l may be associated with adverse neurological outcome (although evidence for a causal link is weak).

Aetiology
- Excess glucose intake
- Pain/stress (increased catecholamines → anti-insulin effect)
- Infection
- Drugs (e.g. steroids, adrenaline)
- Relative insulin resistance/decreased insulin secretion—transient phenomenon seen in extremely low birth weight (ELBW) infants
- Neonatal diabetes mellitus (very rare, often transient in babies that are small for gestational age).

Management
The algorithm in Fig. 13.1 shows the suggested management of neonatal hyperglycaemia. General principles:
- Confirm POCT blood glucose analysis results with laboratory assay (although POCT methods are more reliable than when used for monitoring hypoglycaemia)
- Investigate as appropriate for any of the causes listed under aetiology (e.g. sepsis)
- Avoid over-treating and causing hypoglycaemia: **hypoglycaemia is more dangerous than hyperglycaemia**
- Avoid glucose levels >20 mmol/l
- Insulin infusion at 0.05–1.0 U/kg/h may be needed. A sliding scale with 4–5 steps should be used. Suggested starting regime (may need adjustment depending on response):
  - <10mmol/l: no insulin
  - 10–12mmol/l: 0.05 U/kg/h
  - 12–16mmol/l: 0.1 U/kg/h
  - 16–20mmol/l: 0.15 U/kg/h
  - >20mmol/l: 0.2 U/kg/h
- Check blood glucose within 1 hour of starting insulin infusion and 1 hour after any change in rate
- Introduction of enteral feeding as soon as it is tolerated may hasten sugar control by inducing gut hormone secretion.

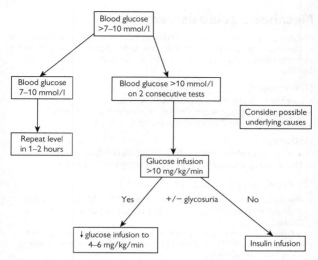

Fig. 13.1 Suggested management of neonatal hyperglycaemia.

Metabolic acidosis: overview

Metabolic acidosis is a common finding in sick (often preterm babies) and is often associated with sepsis and poor tissue perfusion. Inborn errors of metabolism (IEM) may be considered if metabolic acidosis is severe or persistent.

Definition
- Low pH associated with decreased base excess
- Further investigation and treatment of metabolic acidosis may be considered if pH <7.25 with base excess <−7 to −10.

Aetiology
Anion gap may help to distinguish causes of metabolic acidosis.
The following equation shows how the anion gap is calculated:

$$\text{Anion gap} = \left(Na^+ + K^+\right) - \left(HCO3^- + Cl^-\right)$$

- Metabolic acidosis with increased anion gap (>16–20 mmol/l) is due to an accumulation of acids, often lactate, but also other organic acids. Causes:
  - *tissue hypoperfusion*: baby may be haemodynamically unstable with low blood pressure and poor perfusion, and/or may have suffered hypoxic ischaemic insult
  - *inborn errors of metabolism* (see Table 13.1): ↑ lactate and/or ketosis usually present
- Metabolic acidosis with normal anion gap (<16–20 mmol/l) represents a loss of buffer (usually bicarbonate) or may occur with hyperchloraemia. Causes:
  - renal tubular acidosis/low renal bicarbonate threshold (common in preterm)
  - iatrogenic from excess chloride intake (usually from NaCl given for hypovolaemia or from total parenteral nutrition (TPN))
  - from gastrointestinal losses (loose, watery stool).

Investigation (see Table 13.1)
- Consider further investigation for IEM (and referral to specialist metabolic team) in severe or persistent metabolic acidosis with raised anion gap
- Key investigations are:
  - blood gas
  - anion gap
  - ketones (urine dipstick or laboratory urinalysis)
  - glucose
  - lactate
  - acylcarnitines
  - urine organic acids.

Table 13.1 Inborn errors of metabolism—key investigations

	Ketones	Glucose	Lactate	Other investigations
Organic acidaemias	+	Normal or ↑	Normal or ↑	Urine organic acids Ammonia
Ketolysis defects	+	Normal or ↑	Normal	Fibroblasts
Respiratory chain defects	+	Normal or ↓	↑	CSF lactate MRI brain
Gluconeogenesis defects	+	↓	↑	Urate Examine for hepatomegaly
Adrenal insufficiency	+	↓	Normal	Electrolytes Cortisol
Pyruvate disorders	+/−	Normal or ↑	↑	Lactate/pyruvate ratio
Fat oxidation defects	−	↓	↑	Acylcarnitines
Renal tubular acidosis	−	Normal	Normal	Blood gas/ bicarbonate Urine pH Urinary amino acids
Villous atropy	−	Normal	Normal	Gut biopsy

CSF: cerebrospinal fluid; MRI: magnetic resonance imaging.

Metabolic acidosis: management

Fig. 13.2 shows suggested management of metabolic acidosis in neonates.

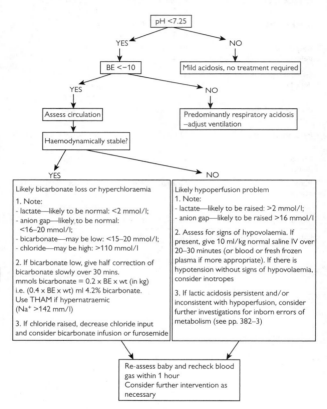

Fig. 13.2 Suggested algorithm for management of metabolic acidosis in neonates.
BE: base excess; THAM: tris-hydroxymethyl aminomethane.

Inborn errors of metabolism presenting in neonates

Incidence
Rare individually, but total approximately 1 in 3000–4000 live births.

Clinical presentation
- Presentation is usually non-specific, but may appear as dysmorphism, sepsis, or severe persistent metabolic acidosis. Check history for:
  - parental consanguinity
  - previous multiple miscarriages, stillbirths, or sudden unexpected death in infants (SUDI) or sudden infant death syndrome (SIDS)
  - maternal illness in pregnancy (e.g. acute fatty liver of pregnancy, HELLP syndrome); may occur in pregnancies with fetus with long chain fat oxidation defects
  - increased fetal movements (*in utero* seizures)
- Inborn errors typically present at times of metabolic stress—the neonatal period being a classic time
- Neonatal presentation is classified into three groups:
  - *Failure to make or break complex molecules*: usually dysmorphic at birth, but may be normal and become progressively more obvious as storage accumulates (e.g. Smith–Lemli–Opitz, Zellweger)
  - *Intoxication*: symptom-free period prior to decompensation, whilst toxic metabolites build up after enteral feeding established. Classically present on day 3 (e.g. aminoacidopathies, urea cycle defects, organic acidaemias, sugar intolerance (galactosaemia)). Presentation is similar to sepsis
  - *Energy insufficiency*: may present immediately (e.g. lactic acidosis) or later (sometimes after neonatal period). Includes conditions that only present if delay in fuel provision (e.g. respiratory chain defects, pyruvate metabolism defects, fat oxidation defects, glycogen storage disease, defects in gluconeogenesis)
- Examine carefully for dysmorphism, organomegaly, and ocular signs.

Investigations (see Table 13.1)
These should be taken at the time of decompensation—this will avoid the need for 'stress tests' later. Results should be discussed with the local paediatric metabolic team.

Blood
- FBC and film
- Clotting profile
- U&Es
- Liver enzymes
- Glucose
- Blood gas
- Lactate
- Ammonia (free flowing sample)
- Acylcarnitines
- Amino acids
- Blood for DNA storage.

Urine
- Ketones (blood POCT, urine dipstick, or laboratory urinalysis)
- Reducing substances
- Organic acids
- Amino acids.

Secondary investigations
Depending on results of blood and urine investigations:
- Neuro-imaging (MRI) (e.g. basal ganglia changes in mitochondrial disorders)
- Echocardiography (e.g. cardiomyopathy in respiratory chain disorders, fat oxidation disorders, Pompe's disease)
- ECG
- EEG
- Tandem mass spectrometry for specific diagnosis
- Skin biopsy, muscle biopsy, liver biopsy.

Post-mortem specimens
Occasionally, a baby may present with severe unexplained illness leading to death within a short time of presentation, which could possibly indicate an IEM. Following discussion with parents and the local paediatric metabolic team it may be appropriate to take the following samples (as well as recommending a post-mortem examination):
- **Blood:** two lithium heparin samples stored in fridge (4°C) and freezer (−20°C) + four blood spots on a blood spot screening card + EDTA sample
- **Urine:** stored in freezer (−20°C)
- **Skin biopsy:** stored in culture medium or saline in fridge (4°C)
- **Muscle biopsy:** snap frozen in liquid nitrogen
- **Liver biopsy:** snap frozen in liquid nitrogen.

Management of suspected inborn errors of metabolism
- Discuss all results with local paediatric metabolic team
- Stop feeds
- **Promote anabolism:** start 10% glucose and add insulin if becomes hyperglycaemic, rather than cut glucose concentration. **NB** High concentration glucose can exacerbate the lactic acidosis of pyruvate and respiratory chain defects, therefore use 5% glucose in suspected primary lactic acidosis
- Correct any associated biochemical disturbances
- Specific treatments that may be recommended include clearing toxic metabolites with either dialysis or drugs, use of enzyme cofactors, and other specific treatments:
  - *dialysis*: lactate, organic acids, ammonia, leucine
  - *drugs*: e.g. phenylbutyrate or sodium benzoate for urea cycle defects; carnitine, glycine for organic acidaemias
  - *enzyme cofactors*: e.g. biotin, thiamine, riboflavin
  - *other specific treatment*: e.g. enzyme replacement, liver or bone marrow transplantation
- Genetic counselling and screening of siblings recommended if indicated.

Metabolic bone disease

Definition
Inadequate bone mineralization in preterm babies. Also known as osteopenia or rickets of prematurity.

Pathogenesis
- Inadequate phosphate and calcium uptake *in utero* followed by poor postnatal intake in the presence of high growth velocity
- Not usually due to vitamin D deficiency (although it is important to prevent this by prescribing multivitamins) or parathyroid hormone deficiency
- Phosphate is critical as unlike calcium may be preferentially used for other metabolic processes
- Two-thirds of fetal accretion of phosphate and calcium normally occurs in the 3rd trimester
- Normal requirements postnatally in preterm babies:
  - *phosphate*: 2.1–2.6 mmol/kg/day
  - *calcium*: 2.5–3.0 mmol/kg/day
- 180 ml of:
  - breast milk provides approximately 0.9 mmol phosphate + 1.6 mmol calcium
  - breast milk + breast milk fortifier (BMF) or preterm formula provides approximately 2.0 mmol phosphate + 3.6 mmol calcium.

Clinical picture
- Osteopenia occurs in approximately 50% preterm babies <1000 g and 30% preterm babies <1500 g, particularly if exclusively breastfed
- Biochemical changes of abnormal mineral metabolism occur initially
- Radiological changes of reduced bone mineralization (osteopenia) follow biochemical abnormalities
- Abnormal bone remodelling with generalized osteopenia, cupping, splaying, and fraying of the metaphyses of long bones, with fractures and craniotabes occurring later if treatment is delayed or insufficient
- Slower linear growth occurs and may result in reduced height in later childhood.

Investigations
- Raised alkaline phosphatase (ALP). Normally a preterm baby's ALP rises to ×2–3 maximum adult value (i.e. 250–375 IU/l) by 2–3 weeks of age and then falls. An ALP >1200 IU/l in the neonatal period is associated with a long-term linear growth deficit
- Hypophosphataemia (i.e. <1.8–2.2mmol/l)
- Calcium normal or raised, but may be low in advanced disease
- Urinary Ca/P ratio >1 (due to P depletion).

Additional investigation by imaging is rarely necessary.

Management (prevention and treatment)

- **Prevent vitamin D deficiency:** 400 IU/day in multivitamins (usually prescribed shortly after reaching full enteral feeds/around 2 weeks) +/– colecalciferol 400 IU/day
- **Prescribe phosphate (starting dose usually 1 mmol/kg/day) if either:**
  - VLBW (i.e. birth weight <1500 g) and on unfortified breast milk (or non-preterm formula)
  - ALP >500 IU/l
  - plasma phosphate <1.8 mmol/l
- Add calcium (starting dose usually 1 mmol/kg/day) if:
  - P >1.8 mmol/l
  - ALP high or rising
  - radiological changes suggestive of metabolic bone disease of prematurity.

NB Plasma Ca may be normal.

- Ca and P can each be added to the milk, but avoid adding together to prevent precipitation
- Gentle physiotherapy and avoidance of immobility are also likely to have a role in improving bone mineral accretion
- Consider additional vitamin D (colecalciferol or alfacalcidol) if ALP remains >1000 IU/l despite adequate P and Ca
- If still unresponsive, investigate renal tubular function (P loss)
- **VLBW babies on TPN:** aim to supply at least 1.5 mmol/kg/day P and 1.5 mmol/kg/day Ca, increasing as necessary
- After discharge from hospital: if on breast milk only, consider continuing added phosphate until 6 months corrected age. Alternatively, stop phosphate supplements at around the time of discharge and check bone biochemistry 2 weeks later and subsequently as necessary.

Neonatal jaundice

Physiological jaundice

Jaundice becomes apparent when serum bilirubin (sBR) >80–100 μmol/l. Although approximately 60% of term babies become visibly jaundiced during the first week of life, only about 1% require treatment.

Jaundice is more common in preterm babies with approximately 80% incidence in the first week.

Causes of physiological jaundice
- Haemolysis due to:
  - bruising
  - antibody induced
  - relative polycythaemia
  - ↓ lifespan of RBCs (term 70 days, preterm 40 days)
- Immature hepatic enzyme systems
- 'Shunt' bilirubin from breakdown of non-RBC haem pigments
- ↑ Enterohepatic circulation (likely explanation for risk of prolonged jaundice in breastfed babies).

Non-physiological jaundice

Jaundice requiring investigation and treatment is more likely to be non-physiological. Therefore, investigate jaundice and consider treatment if:
- Onset <24 hours after birth
- sBR >250 μmol/l by 48 hours or >300 μmol/l by 96 hours of age
- Rapidly rising sBR (>100 μmol/l/24 h)
- Lasting >14 days (term) or >21 days (preterm)
- Conjugated hyperbilirubinaemia.

Non-physiological jaundice is associated with conditions known to cause or increase risk of jaundice
- Haemolysis:
  - haemolytic disease of the newborn (Rh, etc.)
  - ABO incompatibility
  - hereditary spherocytosis
  - glucose-6-phosphate dehydrogenase (G6PD) deficiency
  - pyruvate kinase (PK) deficiency
  - α-thalassaemia
- Polycythaemia
- Extravasated blood
- Increased enterohepatic circulation (may be caused by breast milk)
- Congenital hypothyroidism
- IEM (e.g. galactosaemia)
- Rare liver enzyme deficiencies (e.g. Crigler–Najjar syndrome).

Haemolytic disease of the newborn

See **➐** Haemolytic disease of the newborn, pp. 402–3.

Routine assessment of jaundice in all newborn babies

Identify babies as being more likely to develop significant jaundice if they have any of the following factors:

- <38 weeks gestation
- Previous sibling with neonatal jaundice requiring phototherapy
- Exclusively breastfed
- Onset of visible jaundice <24 hours.

In all babies:

- Check whether there are factors associated with an increased likelihood of developing significant jaundice soon after birth
- Examine the baby for jaundice at every opportunity especially in the first 72 hours.

When looking for jaundice (visual inspection):

- Check naked baby in bright (preferably natural) light
- Examine sclerae, gums, and blanched skin
- Ensure babies with factors associated with an increased likelihood of developing significant jaundice receive an additional visual inspection by a healthcare professional during the first 48 hours of life.

Measuring bilirubin in babies with jaundice

- Assessment of babies with jaundice should not rely on visual inspection alone to estimate the bilirubin level
- Transcutaneous bilirubinometers can be used to measure transcutaneous bilirubin level (tBR) if ≥35 weeks gestation and >24 hours old (although newer generation transcutaneous bilirubinometers are also suitable for lower gestations)
- If a transcutaneous bilirubinometer is not available, or if <35 weeks gestation or <24 hours old, measure serum bilirubin (sBR)
- If tBR >250 µmol/l, check sBR.

Investigation of jaundice in the first week of life

Maternal

- ABO group
- Rh D group
- Serum screen for unusual iso-immune antibodies.

Infant

- ABO group
- Rh D group
- Direct Coombs test
- Serum bilirubin.

If severe jaundice

- FBC and film
- Reticulocyte count
- G6PD level
- U&Es
- Investigation of sepsis as appropriate.

Treatment of jaundice

The aim of treating jaundice is to reduce the risk of bilirubin encephalopathy, which causes acute and chronic neurological dysfunction. Damage (also known as kernicterus) is caused to predisposed areas of the brain (brainstem and basal ganglia in particular). This results when the plasma albumin-bilirubin binding capacity is exceeded and lipid-soluble free unconjugated bilirubin is then able to cross the blood–brain barrier.

- Treatment thresholds are controversial, but most centres follow guidelines from the UK National Institute for Health and Care Excellence (NICE) or the American Academy of Pediatrics (AAP) for well, term babies. Also refer to local guidelines
- For preterm babies guidelines have been developed so that treatment is started at lower bilirubin levels due to limited post-mortem findings that kernicterus can occur at these lower levels compared to term babies
- Treatment thresholds should also be lower for babies who are sick (e.g. septic, acidotic, or with hypercarbia) with evidence of haemolysis or with rapidly rising serum bilirubin (>8.5 μmol/l/h)
- Ensure that any baby presenting with jaundice is well-hydrated, but routine additional feeds and fluids are not necessary
- **Phototherapy:**
  - used to treat moderately severe unconjugated hyperbilirubinaemia in order to reduce the need for exchange transfusion
  - phototherapy photo-oxidizes and isomerizes bilirubin →↑ excretion via urine and bile
  - continuous multiple phototherapy (also called intensive phototherapy) should be considered if sBR rapidly rising (>8.5 μmol/l/h), within 50 μmol/l below the exchange transfusion threshold after 72 hours age, or if it fails to respond to single phototherapy (i.e. continues to rise or does not fall within 6 hours of starting)
  - complications of phototherapy are mainly minor, and include loose stool, increased transcutaneous fluid loss, and rashes
  - parents should be reassured that side-effects and complications of phototherapy are minor and that short breaks for feeding, changing, etc. should be encouraged (unless continuous multiple phototherapy required)
  - eye protection should be used routinely
- Exchange transfusion:
  - used to treat severe unconjugated hyperbilirubinaemia, often with concomitant anaemia, most commonly due to haemolysis
  - should be considered when sBR is at recommended treatment threshold, or lower if there are clinical signs suggestive of acute bilirubin encephalopathy
  - effective by diluting bilirubin, removing sensitized red blood cells and correcting anaemia
  - double-volume exchange transfusion is performed via arterial and central venous lines over several hours, replacing the baby's blood volume twice with donor blood (see ➲ Exchange transfusion, p. 518)

- complications of exchange transfusion include infection and other line-related complications, fluid and electrolyte disturbance, thrombocytopenia, coagulopathy, and transfusion reaction
- Intravenous immunoglobulin (IVIG)
  - IVI 500 mg/kg over 4 hours
  - used in haemolytic disease of the newborn (HDN) due to Rhesus or ABO incompatibility (see ➜ Haemolytic disease of the newborn, pp. 402–3) as an adjunct to continuous multiple phototherapy and/or exchange transfusion if sBR continues to rise >8.5 µmol/l/h
  - IVIG has been shown to reduce the need for exchange transfusion in HDN, but increases the incidence of late anaemia.

Suggested thresholds for the treatment of jaundice

- Table 13.2 shows sBR thresholds for management of babies ≥38 weeks gestation with jaundice, as recommended by NICE
- Guidelines for babies of <38 weeks gestation can be found at: ✍ www.nice.org.uk/guidance/cg98.

Table 13.2 Serum bilirubin (sBR) thresholds for management of babies ≥38 weeks gestation with jaundice, as recommended by NICE

Age (h)	sBR (µmol/l)			
0	–	–	>100	>100
6	>100	>112	>125	>150
12	>100	>125	>150	>200
18	>100	>137	>175	>250
24	>100	>150	>200	>300
30	>112	>162	>212	>350
36	>125	>175	>225	>400
42	>137	>187	>237	>450
48	>150	>200	>250	>450
54	>162	>212	>262	>450
60	>175	>225	>275	>450
66	>187	>237	>287	>450
72	>200	>250	>300	>450
78	–	>262	>312	>450
84	–	>275	>325	>450
90	–	>287	>337	>450
96+	–	>300	>350	>450
Action	Repeat sBR in 6–12 h	Consider phototherapy and repeat sBR in 6 h	Start phototherapy	Perform exchange transfusion unless sBR falls <treatment threshold while treatment being prepared

Prolonged jaundice

Definition
- Visible jaundice lasting >2 weeks in a term baby or >3 weeks in preterm
- More common in breastfed babies
- Prolonged jaundice is usually harmless but may be an indicator of serious liver disease and therefore requires investigation.

Investigation
- If well with normal colour of stools and urine, investigation should be initiated at 3 weeks in all gestations:
  - total bilirubin
  - conjugated bilirubin (>25 µmol/l is significant)
  - liver enzymes
  - urine culture
- If total bilirubin >250 µmol/l and conjugated bilirubin <25 µmol/l
  - mother's and baby's blood group (if not already known)
  - direct antiglobulin test (DAT)
  - FBC + film
  - coagulation profile
  - G6PD
  - thyroid stimulating hormone (TSH)
- If conjugated hyperbilirubinaemia and/or pale stools/dark urine, do tests listed under the first two bullet points and:
  - urinary reducing substances
  - coagulation profile
  - liver ultrasound
  - α_1-antitrypsin level/*PiZZ* genotype
  - galactose-1-phosphate uridyl transferase (GAL-1-PUT)
  - hepatitis viral serology
  - investigations for IEM (lactate, plasma amino acids, urine organic acids)
  - genetic studies for cystic fibrosis +/− immune reactive trypsin
  - cortisol
  - ferritin
  - immunoglobulins
  - autoantibodies
  - urate.

Conjugated hyperbilirubinaemia

Causes of conjugated hyperbilirubinaemia

- TPN cholestasis
- Viral hepatitis (hepatitis B, CMV, herpes virus, rubella, HIV, coxsackievirus, adenovirus)
- Other infections (toxoplasmosis, syphilis, bacterial)
- Haemolytic disease (due to excessive bilirubin)
- Metabolic (α_1-antitrypsin deficiency, cystic fibrosis, galactosaemia, tyrosinaemia, Gaucher's and other storage diseases, Rotor syndrome, Dubin–Johnson syndrome)
- Biliary atresia
- Choledochal cyst
- Bile-duct obstruction from tumours, haemangiomas, etc.

Further information

American Academy of Pediatrics Subcommittee on Hyperbilirubinemia. Management of hyperbilirubinemia in the newborn infant 35 or more weeks of gestation. *Pediatrics* 2004; **114**: 297–316.

Champion M, Fox G. *Inherited metabolic disease: a guide for neonatologists.* Orphan Europe Ltd, Henley-on-Thames, UK, 2007.

National Institute for Health Care and Excellence (2015) NICE guidelines (NG3). *Diabetes in pregnancy: management from preconception to the postnatal period.* ℛ www.nice.org.uk/guidance/ng3

National Institute for Health Care and Excellence (2010, updated 2016) NICE clinical guidance (CG98). *Jaundice in newborn babies under 28 days.* ℛ www.nice.org.uk/guidance/cg98

Haematological problems

Neonatal haematology: general information

Background

Haematological problems in the newborn period are common. These problems may arise in a variety of ways unique to the newborn period:

The baby's haemopoietic and other systems are still developing

This in itself can cause problems, or lead to problems when babies are stressed by prematurity or illness, for example:

- Anaemia of prematurity—extremely common; results from immature erythropoiesis, reduced erythropoietin response, and phlebotomy
- High incidence of sepsis—immature granulopoiesis, with relatively low neutrophil progenitor numbers and immature neutrophil function predispose to sepsis—often associated with neutropenia
- Placental insufficiency leads to impairment of haemopoiesis and a triad of polycythaemia, neutropenia, and thrombocytopenia
- The risk of haemorrhage is increased by low levels of clotting factors.

Interaction between mother and the fetus or newborn

- Transplacental passage of antibodies may result in haemolysis in Rhesus incompatibility, or platelet destruction in alloimmune thrombocytopenia
- Fetal or perinatal acquisition of infection such as parvovirus infection leading to aplastic anaemia.

Genetic abnormalities

- Haemolytic anaemia due to red cell disorders (e.g. G6PD deficiency, hereditary spherocytosis)
- Babies with Down syndrome may have a variety of haematological problems, including thrombocytopenia, polycythaemia, and transient abnormal myelopoiesis (TAM).

The basics

Haemopoiesis

- A basic knowledge of the process of haemopoiesis is useful in understanding fetal and neonatal haematological problems (see Fig. 14.1)
- All blood cells are derived from multipotent stem cells capable of dividing or differentiating. Once a stem cell's fate is decided towards the production of blood cells, it further differentiates to become a lineage-specific progenitor cell, such as an erythroid, megakaryocyte, or myeloid progenitor
- Proliferation and differentiation is regulated by cytokines ('colony-stimulating factors'). Each blood cell lineage has a particular cytokine (e.g. erythropoietin, Epo) that is its prime regulator and which can stimulate massive increases in production of these cells if required

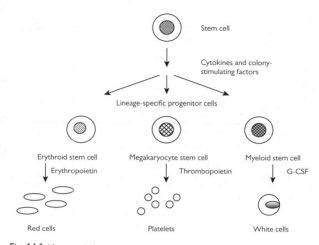

Fig. 14.1 Haemopoiesis.
G-CSF: granulocyte colony-stimulating factor.

- Haemopoiesis occurs in different places in the embryo and fetus dependent on gestation. In the second trimester, the liver is the main haemopoietic organ. The bone marrow only takes over this function during the third trimester. There is a lull in erythropoiesis in the first weeks following birth accompanied by a fall in Epo levels
- These dynamic changes in haemopoiesis during fetal and neonatal life make the newborn, particularly preterm, baby vulnerable to haematological problems.

Haemoglobin (Hb) synthesis

- Hb consists of the protein 'globin' bound to the red 'haem' pigment. The globin is made up of four polypeptide chains, which determine the type of haemoglobin. Hb synthesis occurs in the mitochondria of red cells.
- HbF has two alpha (α) and two gamma (γ) chains and predominates in fetal life. It has a higher oxygen affinity to compensate for the relatively hypoxic *in utero* environment. Adult HbA is made up of two α-chains and two β-chains (see Fig. 14.2).

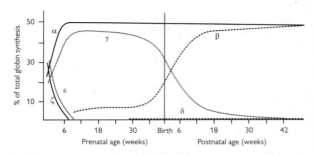

Fig. 14.2 Fetal and neonatal production of globin chains for haemoglobin.

Adapted from Olivieri N. 1997. Fetal erythropoiesis and the diagnosis and treatment of hemoglobin disorders in the fetus and the child. *Seminars in Perinatology* 21(1): 64. Reprinted with permission from Elsevier.

Anaemia

Background

Incidence will vary according to the definition. Many babies will have Hb levels below the normal range (e.g. 140–200 g/l in term newborns, see Table 14.1), although not all of these require investigation or treatment. Anaemia is almost universal in the premature population.

Aetiology

- **Blood loss:**
  - antepartum haemorrhage (especially vasa praevia, which although uncommon may be catastrophic)
  - feto-maternal haemorrhage (may be acute or chronic)
  - feto-fetal haemorrhage (twin-to-twin transfusion syndrome, ➔ see Multiple births, p. 12, acute or chronic)
  - umbilical cord accidents
  - intraventricular haemorrhage (IVH)
  - pulmonary haemorrhage
- **Haemolysis** (see ➔ Haemolytic disease of the newborn, pp. 402–3)
- **Iatrogenic** (blood sampling): this is the commonest cause of anaemia in the preterm baby
- **Anaemia of prematurity:** this is a multifactorial condition due to:
  - immature erythropoiesis
  - reduced erythropoietin production in response to hypoxia
  - illness
  - recurrent phlebotomy
- **Bone marrow disorders**—uncommon (e.g. Fanconi anaemia, Diamond Blackfan anaemia).

Presentation

Anaemia may produce multi-organ dysfunction due to inadequate tissue oxygen delivery:

- **Respiratory:** increased respiratory distress, raised oxygen requirement, apnoea
- **Cardiovascular:** hypotension, tachycardia, prolonged capillary refill, lactic acidosis
- **Other:** lethargy, feed intolerance, poor weight gain (debatable).

Acute anaemia is likely to produce symptoms and signs. Babies with chronic anaemia may be asymptomatic down to very low Hb levels.

Table 14.1 Normal Hb values

	Preterm		Term	Postnatal term babies		
	28 weeks	34 weeks	40 weeks	1 day	1 week	2 weeks
Hb (g/l) mean (range)	145	150	168 (140–200)	184 (150–230)	170 (130–220)	168 (130–200)

Management

The mainstays of treatment are:
- **Prevention:** reduce phlebotomy losses by only performing necessary blood tests; utilize near patient testing and micro-samples; use technology such as transcutaneous monitoring. Iron, vitamins, and folic acid supplementation are also important
- **Resuscitation and supportive care:** ABC
- **Transfusion.**

Blood transfusion

Indications for red cell transfusions
- Over the last 20 years there has been an increasing attempt to limit transfusion, due to its potential complications and the lack of a good evidence base for the previously rather liberal approach
- Recent studies by Bell et al. and Kirplani et al. have informed current practice (see ➲ Further information, this chapter, p. 422). Restrictive guidelines reduce donor exposure and associated problems, but may be associated with adverse neurodevelopmental outcomes
- Decision to transfuse will depend on the acuteness of presentation, and the presence of symptoms and signs.

Transfusion should be considered in the following:
- Significant blood loss
- Signs of shock (hypotension, tachycardia, lactic acidosis, poor perfusion) in the presence of low or falling Hb
- Hb <100–110 g/l in a baby requiring ventilation or nCPAP. Hb threshold will be lower in older babies if stable on respiratory support
- Hb <80 g/l in a stable growing preterm if requiring nasal cannula oxygen, or has tachycardia of >180, or tachypnoea >80 or increasing apnoeas
- Hb <70 g/l in any stable, growing preterm baby.

Thresholds are likely to be higher in any unstable baby (e.g. sepsis, cardio-vascular instability, perioperatively, etc.). Low reticulocyte count (<100 × 10^9/l) may give an indication of likelihood of needing subsequent transfusion in an anaemic preterm baby; however, will not usually be useful in deciding to transfuse or not.
- Acute symptomatic anaemia is an emergency and urgent transfusion of uncrossmatched O RhD negative red cells may be required. Some hospitals will have these available on the labour ward.
- Multiple paediatric packs from a single adult donor should be allocated to minimize donor exposure in babies who are likely to require more than one transfusion. An adult pack will produce up to six paediatric packs. This is particularly relevant in sick and/or preterm babies.
- Transfuse 15–20 ml/kg (depending on the increment required) or use the formula of desired rise in Hb (g/l) × weight × 4 ÷ 10, slowly over 4 hours. Consider >15 ml/kg if the desired increment >30 g/l.
- More than 20 ml/kg is not usually required except in circumstances such as ongoing blood loss.

- Evidence suggests that furosemide need not be used routinely with blood transfusion in the newborn. Consider if there is:
  - pre-existing fluid overload (tachycardia, tachypnoea, hepatomegaly, oedema, rise in O_2 requirement)
  - patent ductus arteriosus (PDA) with evidence of cardiac failure or other cause of congestive cardiac failure
  - chronic lung disease
  - renal failure.

Haemolytic disease of the newborn

Aetiology

Immune

Transplacental passage of antibody directed at fetal blood cells. Direct anti-globulin test (DAT) is almost always positive:
- Rhesus incompatibility
- ABO incompatibility
- Others: other Rhesus groups (c, C, e, E), Kell, Kidd, Duffy.

Non-immune
- Red cell membrane disorders—hereditary spherocytosis (most common), hereditary elliptocytosis
- Red cell enzyme disorders—G6PD deficiency (most common), pyruvate kinase deficiency
- Haemoglobinopathies (rarely in the newborn period).

Rhesus incompatibility
- Mother Rh negative, raised maternal anti-D titre, baby Rh positive
- Massive fall in incidence since introduction of anti-D prophylaxis in 1970s
- Anti-D prophylaxis is now given routinely in all Rh negative pregnancies and to all Rh negative women who deliver Rh positive babies
- Significant Rhesus iso-immunization occurs due to failure of anti-D prophylaxis (e.g. missed abortion, silent antepartum haemorrhage, healthcare error)
- Risk of neonatal disease predicted by maternal anti-D titre:
  - unlikely if titre <4 U/ml
  - 10% when titre 10–100 U/ml
  - 70% when titre >100 U/ml
- Usually associated with a degree of anaemia, which can be severe.

ABO incompatibility
- Mother O positive, baby almost always A positive. Most ABO incompatible mother–infant pairs do not have immune haemolysis. Only 1% of O positive women have sufficient IgG antibodies
- No previous pregnancy history required
- Associated anaemia uncommon.

Presentation
- Severe jaundice in the first week of life; babies may present from the community after early discharge
- Early jaundice, particularly <24 hours
- Antenatally with high or rising maternal antibody titres +/– fetal anaemia or hydrops. Some babies will have had intrauterine transfusion
- Prolonged jaundice.

Investigation
See **➔** Neonatal jaundice, pp. 386–7.

Management

Refer to jaundice in Metabolic chapter (see ➲ Neonatal jaundice, pp. 386–7; ➲ Treatment of jaundice, pp. 388–9; ➲ Prolonged jaundice, p. 390) and exchange transfusion in Practical Procedures chapter (see ➲ Exchange transfusion, p. 518).

- Rapid and adequate assessment:
  - do not delay commencing phototherapy if baby is thought (clinically) to have significant jaundice. Transcutaneous bilirubin measurement can be helpful for initial assessment
  - baby with Rhesus incompatibility may have significant anaemia
  - baby may present with significant neurological symptoms and signs due to kernicterus
- Resuscitation and supportive care:
  - ABC, particularly if preterm, anaemic, or hydropic
  - attention to fluid balance; dehydration may exacerbate jaundice
- Phototherapy
- Exchange transfusion indicated if:
  - bilirubin rapidly rising (e.g. >8–10 µmol/l per hour) despite adequate phototherapy
  - severe hyperbilirubinaemia insufficiently responsive to phototherapy and supportive care
  - significant anaemia (Hb <100 g/l)
- **Intravenous immunoglobulin:** only for immune haemolysis—this has been shown to reduce the need for exchange transfusion, but increase the incidence of late anaemia.

Follow-up

- Parents should be counselled about recurrence in subsequent pregnancies
- Outpatient clinic follow-up to check for late anaemia at 4–6 weeks
- Folate supplementation may protect against late anaemia (500 µg/kg/day until 3 months)
- Ensure hearing screen is performed if baby has had exchange transfusion or significant jaundice (serum bilirubin >350 µmol/l).

Polycythaemia

Background

- Defined as a central venous or arterial packed cell volume (PCV) >65%
- Occurs in up to 5% of newborns
- Clinical significance lies in the increase in blood viscosity that occurs as PCV rises, leading to reduced blood flow and oxygen delivery to tissues.

Aetiology

Increased incidence with:

- **Intrauterine hypoxic states**: intrauterine growth retardation (IUGR), maternal diabetes, maternal smoking
- **Increased blood volume**: recipient of twin-to-twin transfusion (see twin-to-twin transfusion ◑ in Multiple births, p. 12)
- **Fetal abnormalities** (e.g. Down syndrome).

Presentation

Babies are often asymptomatic. Multi-organ involvement can occur secondary to reduced tissue perfusion:

- Plethoric facies
- Lethargy, hypotonia, poor sucking
- Irritability, convulsions
- Tachypnoea
- Cyanosis
- Hypoglycaemia
- Jaundice.

Complications

- Cerebrovascular occlusion
- Renal vein thrombosis
- Necrotizing enterocolitis
- Myocardial ischaemia
- Thrombocytopenia.

Investigations

- Haemoglobin
- Arterial or free-flowing venous PCV. PCV that is obtained from laboratory on FBC is calculated. A more accurate PCV is obtained by centrifuging a capillary sample
- If twin, check twin's PCV, as they may be anaemic (due to twin-to-twin transfusion syndrome).

Management

- In all babies at risk, ensure adequate hydration
- Actively treat if:
    - central venous or arterial PCV >70, even if asymptomatic
    - central venous or arterial PCV >65, if significant symptoms
- Hydrate with IV fluids and stop oral feeds
- If inadequate response to hydration, perform a dilutional exchange transfusion (see ➊ Dilutional exchange transfusion, p. 519):
    - use 0.9% saline as dilutional fluid
    - avoid umbilical catheterization if possible (risk of NEC)
    - volume needed for exchange (ml) =
      total blood volume × [(observed PCV − desired PCV)]/observed PCV
    - neonatal blood volume = 85 ml/kg (approx.)
    - desired PCV = 55%
    - aliquots used: 5–20 ml/kg (lower part of range for preterm babies).

Neutropenia

Background
- Definition: mild 1.0–1.5 × 10⁹/l; moderate 0.5–1.0 × 10⁹/l; severe 0.2–0.5 × 10⁹/l; very severe <0.2 × 10⁹/l.
- A degree of neutropenia is a common finding in the newborn period. Unlikely to cause problems unless neutrophils fall <0.5 × 10⁹/l.

Aetiology
- **Infection:** usually bacterial, don't forget fungal and viral
- **Placental insufficiency:** IUGR, maternal hypertensive disorders (secondary to reduced granulocytopoiesis)
- **NEC**
- **Hypoxia ischaemia**
- **Spurious:** beware machine differentials as FBC analysers do not always count neutrophils accurately in the newborn period. Always confirm with a manual differential on a blood film
- **Other:**
  - *reduced production:* Kostmann syndrome (bone marrow shows maturation arrest), Fanconi syndrome, Shwachmann–Diamond syndrome (associated abnormalities may be present)
  - *immune destruction:* alloimmune, autoimmune (e.g. systemic lupus erythematosus (SLE); see ⦿ Thrombocytopenia, pp. 408–9).

Investigation
- Request blood film to confirm
- If baby <5 days old, moderate neutropenia (0.5–1.5 × 10⁹/l) and significant placental insufficiency no investigations necessary
- Severe neutropenia (<0.5 × 10⁹/l), no previous history of placental insufficiency or >5 days old:
  - careful clinical assessment
  - septic screen
  - look for associated abnormalities.

Treatment
- Supportive care
- There is not a good evidence base for using granulocyte colony-stimulating factor (G-CSF). Cochrane review (2003) suggests that there may be an improved outcome in babies with neutropenic sepsis, however, a large randomized controlled trial is required.

Thrombocytopenia

Background

- *Definition:* mild 100–150 × 10^9/l; moderate 50–100 × 10^9/l; severe <50 × 10^9/l
- Occurs in 1–4% of newborns, but in up to 70% of preterm babies requiring intensive care.

Aetiology

Preterm

Early

Apparent in the first 72 hours of life—usually resolves spontaneously if uncomplicated. 75% of neonatal thrombocytopenic episodes.

- Extreme prematurity
- Placental insufficiency: IUGR, maternal pre-eclampsia → reduced megakaryocytopoiesis
- See also aetiology for Term babies.

Late

Occurs after 72 hours, although may develop prior to recovery of platelet count from early thrombocytopenia:

- Infection: usually bacterial—don't forget fungal and viral (especially CMV, but other congenital infection too)
- NEC.

Term

Neonatal alloimmune (NAITP)

- Fetal and newborn platelet destruction from transplacental passage of maternal antibodies against paternally inherited platelet antigens similar to haemolytic disease of the newborn. Most common antibodies are against HPA1a antigen
- Thrombocytopenia is often severe
- May present with petechiae at first newborn examination. There is a high risk of bleeding (e.g. intracranial, which may occur antenatally) probably due to concomitant reduced platelet function.

Neonatal autoimmune thrombocytopenia

- Also due to maternally derived anti-platelet antibodies. Mother is usually also thrombocytopenic (e.g. immune thrombocytopenia (ITP), SLE)
- Although thrombocytopenia may be severe, bleeding is uncommon
- Platelet count may fall after birth, so babies of mothers with ITP should have at least two platelet counts after birth to ensure they are stable
- All babies of mothers with unexplained thrombocytopenia should have a platelet count performed after birth.

Infection
Congenital infections: viral (e.g. CMV, toxoplasmosis), bacterial, fungal.

Hypoxia ischaemia
Often accompanied by coagulopathy (DIC).

Other rarer causes
- Reduced production (e.g. Fanconi syndrome, thrombocytopenia-absent radius syndrome, congenital amegakaryocytic thrombocytopenia)
- Sequestration (e.g. splenic, Kasabach–Merritt).

Treatment
- Assess bleeding, i.e. IVH, pulmonary, gastrointestinal tract, petechiae, urine
- There is currently a poor evidence base and little agreement about what threshold to use for platelet transfusion. Suggested thresholds are:
  - platelet count: <50 × 10^9/l and bleeding and/or sick
  - *preterm*: platelet count <30 × 10^9/l
  - *term*: platelet count <20 × 10^9/l
- If NAITP, treat urgently with HPA1a-negative platelets
- If maternal ITP (or NAITP with consumption of HPA1a-negative platelets), give IV immunoglobulin, 0.4 g/kg/day over 4 hours for 5 days. If unresponsive, consider platelet transfusion +/− steroids after consultation
- Platelet transfusion (unmatched) for other indications
- Remember to check whether platelet count has responded to treatment
- Some unit policies suggest prophylactic platelet transfusion at platelet count <50 × 10^9/l for invasive procedures (e.g. lumbar puncture) and non-steroidal treatment for PDA. For surgery, discuss prophylactic transfusion with anaesthetist +/− surgeon if the platelet count is <100 × 10^9/l. It may be appropriate to ensure platelets are available in theatre.

Investigation
See Fig. 14.3.

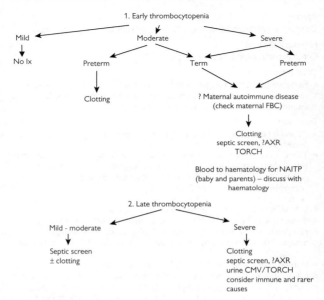

Fig. 14.3 Investigation of neonatal thrombocytopenia.

AXR: abdominal X-ray; CMV: cytomegalovirus; FBC: full blood count; Ix: intervention; NAITP: neonatal alloimmune thrombocytopenia; TORCH: Toxoplasmosis, Other (syphilis, varicella-zoster, parvovirus B19), Rubella, Cytomegalovirus (CMV), and Herpes infections.

Neonatal clotting abnormalities

Background

- Newborn babies have relatively low concentrations of many of the coagulation factors compared with adults—these may not reach adult levels for months after birth
- The procoagulant and anticoagulant systems in newborn haemostasis are usually balanced
- A variety of disease processes and disorders can exacerbate this haemostatic immaturity and lead to significant haemorrhage
- Some rare disorders of coagulation can present with major haemorrhage in the newborn period.

Box 14.1 lists the tests that may be performed when a coagulation profile is requested, and Box 14.2 lists the causes of neonatal clotting abnormalities.

Box 14.1 Tests that may be performed when requesting coagulation profiles

Prothrombin time (PT) or PT ratio

- Assesses fibrinogen (I), prothrombin (II), V (common pathway), VII, and X (extrinsic pathway)
- Prolonged in multiple deficiencies, such as those occurring with prematurity, liver failure, vitamin K deficiency, and DIC (single deficiencies of these are rare).

Activated partial thromboplastin time (APTT) or APTT ratio

- Assesses I, II, V (common pathway), VIII, IX, XI, and XII (intrinsic pathway)
- Prolonged in multiple deficiencies (as with list under PT), haemophilia, and with heparin contamination.

Fibrinogen concentration

Reduced in DIC or liver dysfunction.

Thrombin time (TT)

- Assesses fibrinogen (function and concentration) and is very sensitive to heparin contamination
- Prolonged in DIC and heparin contamination.

Reptilase time (RT)

Similar to TT (assesses fibrinogen), but unaffected by heparin.

Fibrin degradation products (FDPs)/d-dimers

Raised in DIC.

Box 14.2 Aetiology of neonatal clotting abnormalities

Prematurity
- Many coagulation factor concentrations are lower at lower gestations
- ↑ PT, ↑ APTT, fibrinogen <1.5 g/l (but probably abnormal if <1.2).

DIC
- Most commonly seen following hypoxia ischaemia and sepsis
- Thrombocytopenia, ↑ PT, ↑ APTT, ↓ fibrinogen, ↑ TT, ↑ RT, ↑ FDP/ d-dimers.

Vitamin K deficient bleeding
Haemorrhagic disease of the newborn (see ➲ Vitamin K deficiency bleeding and the administration of vitamin K, pp. 418–19).
- Vitamin K dependent factors are II (prothrombin), VII, IX, and X
- ↑ PT, ↑ APTT, normal fibrinogen, normal platelets, low factor assays II, VII, IX, X, raised PIVKA-II (undercarboxylated or abnormal factor II) levels.

Liver disease
- Impaired production of clotting factors
- Perform a coagulation screen in assessment of conjugated hyperbilirubinaemia
- ↑ PT, ↑ APTT, may have lowish fibrinogen and platelets, all factor assays low.

Inherited disorders
- Commonest are haemophilia A (factor VIII) and haemophilia B (factor IX) deficiencies
- Normal PT, ↑ APTT, normal fibrinogen and platelets, ↓ specific factor assay.

Heparin contamination
- Normal PT, ↑ APTT, normal fibrinogen, ↑ TT, normal RT.

Investigations
See Fig. 14.4.
- FBC and coagulation screen will usually be adequate—usually includes PT, APTT, fibrinogen
- It is reasonable to take a clotting screen from a heparinized line in small, difficult babies if you take 2 ml of dead space first and interpret the result accordingly. You can ask the laboratory to correct for heparinization (e.g. reptilase time)
- In the absence of an obvious cause of significantly deranged coagulation (e.g. perinatal hypoxia ischaemia, NEC), discuss with haematology and consider performing specific factor levels
- Ratios are calculated from adult norms. Coagulation results are rarely given with gestation or age-matched normal ranges. Therefore, interpret results with caution—neonates commonly have ratios 1.0–1.5 and these are likely to be normal.

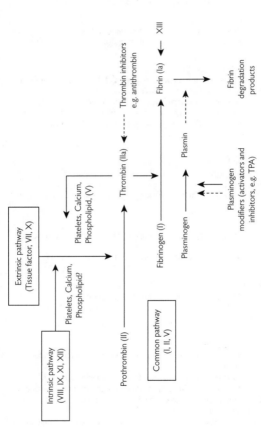

Key: TPA – tissue plasminogen activator; ⟶ procoagulant pathway; ----▸ anticoagulant pathway;

Fig. 14.4 Coagulation regulation.

Treatment

Always take coagulation screen results in tandem with platelet count. Evidence for treating deranged coagulation in the absence of bleeding is poor. Thresholds for treatment are outlined in Box 14.3.

Management

- Treat underlying problem (sepsis, HIE, acidosis, etc.)
- **Phytomenadione (Vitamin K):** ensure it has been given; may require repeated doses, particularly for raised PT/international normalized ratio (INR)
- **Fresh frozen plasma (FFP):** first line treatment for all babies who are bleeding, start with 15 ml/kg
- **Cryoprecipitate:** if fibrinogen remains low (<0.8 g/l) despite FFP; D/W haematology
- **Platelet transfusion**
- **Fibrinogen concentrate:** consider in refractory low fibrinogen (especially in DIC); discuss with haematology
- **Specific factor concentrate:** if specific deficiency found.

Box 14.3 Threshold for treatment

Normal ranges are gestation and laboratory-specific.

Mildly deranged (PT and APTT ratios <1.5; fibrinogen >1.2 g/l)
- Very common, especially in preterm
- No treatment.

Moderately deranged (PT and/or APTT ratios 1.5–2.0 and/or fibrinogen 0.8–1.2 g/l)
Usually requires treatment only if baby has significant bleeding.

Markedly deranged (PT and/or APTT ratios >2.0 and/or fibrinogen <0.8 g/l)
Requires treatment if:
- Bleeding is present
- Baby is unwell
- At high risk of bleeding, especially preterm babies in the first week of life
- Associated with severe thrombocytopenia (platelet count <50 × 10⁹/l)
- Specific disorder suspected or diagnosed.

Haemophilia

- Haemophilia A is an X-linked deficiency of factor VIII; haemophilia B is an autosomal recessive deficiency of factor IX
- Presentation may be with:
  - family screening (FHx negative in 30% as new mutation)
  - minor haemorrhage (oozing from umbilicus, heel prick, or circumcision site)
  - major haemorrhage (intracranial haemorrhage in 2–4%)
- Haemophilia A can be diagnosed at birth as factor VIII levels should be within adult range at birth
- Haemophilia B—factor IX levels are normally low at birth, so diagnosis in newborn period is difficult unless deficiency is severe (levels <15%).

Vitamin K deficiency bleeding and the administration of vitamin K

Refer also to ➲ Neonatal clotting abnormalities, pp. 412–15.

Background
- All babies should receive vitamin K at birth
- Incidence:
  - *classical*: 1–2 in 1000 in untreated, newborn babies
  - *late*: 5 in 10,000 untreated babies

An increased risk of malignancy was reported in the early 1990s to be associated with the administration of IM vitamin K to the newborn. Subsequent studies demonstrated that solid tumours are certainly no more common in children given IM vitamin K. However, it has not been possible to definitely prove that there is no increased risk of leukaemia. If there is a leukaemia risk, it is extremely small and insignificant compared with the dangers of vitamin K deficiency bleeding.

Pathogenesis
- Newborn babies are relatively deficient in vitamin K
- Breast milk is low in vitamin K (formula milks are all fortified)
- Liver disease (e.g. neonatal hepatitis, biliary atresia) reduces production of vitamin K dependent factors.

Presentation
- **Early (<24 hours):** may be due to abnormal maternal vitamin K metabolism (e.g. maternal anticonvulsants)
- **Classical (1–7 days):** almost always in babies who have not had vitamin K prophylaxis who are breastfed
- **Late (1–8 weeks):** either have same risk factors as for classical presentation (plus may have missed later oral doses) or have hepatic disease.

Management

Prophylaxis
- Current NICE (National Institute for Health and Care Excellence) guidance is that all babies should receive IM vitamin K
- If parents refuse IM dose, they should be offered oral dosage. This option is felt to be not as good as there may be problems with supply of, and compliance with, 2nd and 3rd doses—although taken properly there is probably not a difference in vitamin K deficiency bleeding risk between IM and oral dosing

- Doses:
  - **IM phytomenadione MM:** once only at birth: BW ≥2.5 kg: 1 mg; BW <2.5 kg: 0.4 mg/kg

  or

  - **Oral phytomenadione MM:** all babies should have a dose at birth and at 1 week; breastfed babies only (<2 bottles formula/day) need a third dose at 4–6 weeks; all doses 2 mg
- It is not recommended to give vitamin K IV routinely as the depot effect of the IM injection is lost. However, if an IV dose only is given at birth further doses will be needed (IM or oral)
- If parents refuse administration of vitamin K, they should have the risks explained by a senior member of the neonatal team.

Thrombosis and thrombophilia

See also ➔ Arterial thrombosis, in Iatrogenic problems, pp. 460–1.

Background

- Neonates are at relatively high risk of thrombosis
- Commonest presentation is secondary to vascular access devices (e.g. peripheral arterial lines, umbilical lines, cardiac catheterization)
- Spontaneous thrombosis may present with renal vein thrombosis, neonatal stroke (most commonly middle cerebral artery)
- Rarely associated with hereditary thrombophilia.

Risk factors

- Arterial or venous access
- Polycythaemia
- IUGR
- Perinatal hypoxia ischaemia
- Maternal diabetes
- Prematurity.

Investigation of hereditary thrombophilia
See Box 14.4.

Management

- Imaging with Doppler ultrasound in large vessel thrombus is useful to assess size of clot
- Remove offending line.

Venous thrombosis
- Clinically important thrombosis requiring anticoagulation may include:
  - pulmonary embolus
  - thrombosis proximal to and including femoral or axillary veins
  - totally occlusive thrombus (ultrasound will delineate degree of residual blood flow)
  - limb- or organ-threatening thrombus
- Discuss anticoagulation with senior.

Box 14.4 Investigation for hereditary thrombophilia

- Thrombophilia is due to the presence of genetically determined procoagulant, or the deficiency of natural anticoagulant activity
- Consider investigation for inherited thrombophilia in spontaneous or significant thrombus
- Discuss with haematology. Tests look for abnormalities in activity, levels, or expression of:
  - Protein C
  - Protein S
  - Antithrombin III
  - Factor V Leiden
  - Prothrombin
- Testing for thrombophilia in the immediate newborn period at presentation may give spurious results: wait until 3 months of age.

Arterial thrombosis
- Loss of peripheral pulses after arterial cannulation may be due to vessel spasm, thrombus or, rarely, dissection
- Remove arterial catheter
- GTN patch: half a 5 mg patch (beware: some patches lose efficacy when cut) may relieve spasm; can be replaced daily if ongoing ischaemia
- Limb or organ threatening ischaemia should be considered for anticoagulation and/or thrombolysis
- Discuss anticoagulation and/or thrombolysis with senior.

Further information

Bell EF, Strauss RG, Widness JA, et al. Randomized trial of liberal versus restrictive guidelines for red blood cell transfusion in preterm infants. *Pediatrics* 2005; **115**:1685–1691.

British Committee for Standards in Haematology. Transfusion guideline for neonates and older children. *Br J Haematol* 2004; **124**: 433–453.

Kirplani H, Whyte RK, Anderson C, et al. The Premature Infants in Need of Transfusion (PINT) study: a randomized, controlled trial of restrictive (low) versus liberal (high) transfusion threshold for extremely low birth weight infants. *J Pediat* 2006; **149**: 301–307.

McNinch A, Busfield A, Tripp J, et al. Vitamin K deficiency bleeding in Great Britain and Ireland: British Paediatric Surveillance Unit surveys, 1993–94 and 2001–2. *Arch Dis Child* 2007; **92**: 759–766.

Monagle P, Chan AK, Goldenburg NA, et al. Antithrombotic therapy in neonates and children. *Chest* 2012; **141**: e737S–801S.

National Institute for Health and Care Excellence (2006, updated 2015) NICE Clinical Guideline (CG37). *Postnatal care up to 8 weeks after birth.* ℘ www.nice.org.uk/guidance/cg37

Olivieri N. Fetal erythropoeisis and the diagnosis and treatment of hemoglobin disorders in the fetus and child. *Sem Perinatol* 1997; **21**: 64.

Roberts J, Murray NA. Neonatal thrombocytopenia: causes and management. *Arch Dis Child* 2003; **88**: F359–364.

Whyte RK, Kirplani H, Asztalos EV, et al. Neurodevelopmental outcome of extremely low birth weight infants randomly assigned to restrictive or liberal hemoglobin thresholds for blood transfusion. *Pediatrics* 2009; **123**:207–213.

Nephrological and urological problems

Fetal and neonatal renal function

- Nephrogenesis starts in the 1st trimester and is completed by 36 weeks gestation
- Fetal urine production is the primary determinant of amniotic fluid volume, and amniotic fluid volume is essential for fetal lung growth. Fetal renal disease due to bilateral obstructive uropathy (e.g. posterior urethral valves) or severe renal parenchymal disease (e.g. bilateral multicystic dysplastic kidneys) has a poor prognosis due to the risk of pulmonary hypoplasia
- Glomerular filtration rate (GFR) is lower in the fetus and preterm babies compared with term babies, and increases approximately 8× between 28 weeks and term
- GFR continues to increase postnatally (GFR at term <5% adult values) initially due to a fall in renal vascular resistance
- Renal tubular function is immature in preterm neonates (<32 weeks), this leads to:
  - high fractional excretion of sodium (FENa) → hyponatraemia
  - low urine concentrating capacity → ↑ risk of dehydration
  - low capacity to excrete acid (H^+ ions) + low bicarbonate threshold → metabolic acidosis.

Antenatally diagnosed renal pelvis dilatation/hydronephrosis

The purpose of investigating and treating antenatally diagnosed renal pelvis dilatation (RPD) is to minimize the risk of missing clinically significant hydronephrosis (e.g. due to vesico-ureteric reflux or pelvi-ureteric junction (PUJ) obstruction), which may predispose the patient to recurrent urinary tract infection during childhood, and in turn contributes to the risk of chronic renal failure in older children and adults.

The guideline algorithm (Fig. 15.1) has been developed with the paediatric nephrology/urology team in our hospital in order to minimize the risk of missing clinically significant hydronephrosis. Opinion on investigation and management of this condition varies widely and local guidelines should be referred to if available.

- In all cases, check the antenatal details carefully
- RPD or hydronephrosis = dilatation of the renal pelvis >10 mm and/or dilatation of the calyces and/or ureters
- High risk: males with bilateral RPD who may have posterior urethral valves (PUV). Need investigation immediately after birth and referral/discussion with the local paediatric nephrology/urology team
- Low risk babies: the initial renal tract US scan should be delayed until around 1 week of age so that hydronephrosis is not missed due to the relative oliguria occurring during the first 24–48 hours
- Antibiotic prophylaxis (usually trimethoprim or cefotaxime once daily) is recommended for RPD. The need for ongoing antibiotics should be considered when initial investigations are complete.

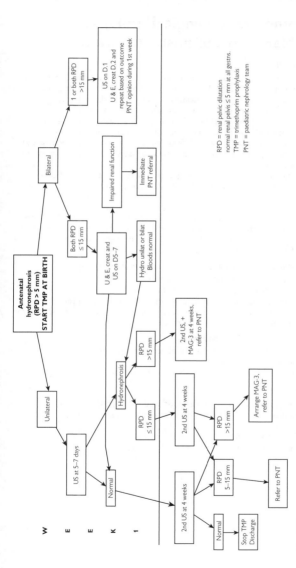

Fig. 15.1 Postnatal management of antenatally detected hydronephrosis.

Common nephrological/urological problems on the postnatal ward

Delayed passage of urine

It is normal for babies to pass urine within 24 hours of birth. If >24 hours:

- Check antenatal history for oligohydramnios or other abnormalities on antenatal scans (e.g. abnormalities of kidneys or urinary tract)
- Examine baby checking for signs of sepsis, dehydration, urinary retention, and abnormalities of the external genitalia and lower spine
- If history and examination normal, consider confirming subsequent passage of urine by using a urine collection bag. If urine still not passed over next 4–8 hours, check blood biochemistry and request a renal tract ultrasound scan
- If renal tract ultrasound scan suggests urinary retention or other abnormality, discuss with paediatric nephrology/urology team.

Hypospadias

Meatus abnormally placed on ventral side of penis. May be glandular (mild), coronal (moderate), or on base of penis or perineal (severe). Sometimes associated with chordee (ventral curvature of penis) or meatal stenosis (therefore, essential to check urine stream).

Mild hypospadias (glandular hypospadias and no chordee)

- Usually needs no treatment as a neonate
- Check stream (may be poor if meatus stenotic)
- Warn not to circumcise as foreskin may be needed for surgery
- Arrange paediatric surgeon/urologist outpatient referral for 3–6 months (or urgent review if urine stream poor).

Moderate or severe hypospadias

- Assess presence of testes and if absent, consider ambiguous genitalia
- Arrange renal US scan
- Request early paediatric surgery/urology opinion.

Micropenis

- True micropenis is rare and is associated with hypopituitarism
- An apparently short penis is more common, usually buried in suprapubic fat
- Normal stretched penile length ~3 cm. If <2.5 cm, consider further investigations and referral to paediatric endocrinologist.

Undescended testes

Testes are usually palpable at term, but may be retractile. Small, under-developed scrotal sac implies maldescent:

- If unilateral inform parents of findings and ask GP to review at 6 weeks
- If there are bilateral impalpable testes then check for associated anomalies such as prune-belly syndrome (bilateral undescended testes, absence of anterior abdominal wall musculature, and urinary tract abnormalities), ambiguous genitalia, and Prader–Willi syndrome. Arrange renal US scan
- If unilateral or bilateral undescended testes have not descended by 6 months then refer to paediatric surgeon/urologist. Orchidopexy usually done at 1–2 years, or sooner if other associated problems (e.g. hernia).

Hydrocele

Occur due to failure of the processus vaginalis to completely close:

- Distinguish from hernia (may require US scan)
- Reassure parents and inform that highly likely to resolve spontaneously by 1 year of age
- Refer to paediatric surgeon if present at 1 year or refer earlier if problems develop (e.g. associated hernia or enlarging tense hydrocele).

Posterior urethral valves

- Membrane causes partial or complete obstruction of posterior urethra
- Almost exclusively occurs in males
- May be diagnosed antenatally with oligohydramnios, or anhydramnios if obstruction complete or nearly complete, and rarely → poor prognosis due to pulmonary hypoplasia
- Ultrasound, either antenatally or postnatally likely to show distended, trabeculated, thick-walled bladder, ureteric and upper renal tract dilatation, and renal dysplasia
- Antenatal fetal urine analysis shows ↑ sodium and amino acid levels
- Antenatal intervention with vesico-amniotic shunt insertion sometimes performed
- May require resuscitation and respiratory support if severe oligohydramnios results in pulmonary hypoplasia
- Examine carefully, noting signs of respiratory distress, abdominal musculature (may have 'prune-belly'), lower back for spinal abnormalities, genitalia, and anus
- Check blood pressure, blood tests for renal function and electrolytes
- Postnatal investigation by renal tract US scan and micturating cystourethrogram (MCUG) via a suprapubic catheter (see Fig. 15.2)
- Treatment is by endoscopic (transurethral) ablation of the valve tissue
- Chronic renal failure and urinary incontinence are common long-term problems.

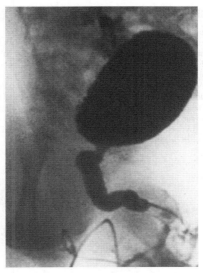

Fig. 15.2 Micturating cystourethrogram (MCUG) showing distended, trabeculated, thick-walled bladder, and ureteric and upper renal tract dilatation due to posterior urethral valves (PUVs).

Polycystic kidney disease

- Autosomal dominant polycystic kidney disease (ADPKD) may be diagnosed in the fetus and neonate by US scan but otherwise does not present until progression to end-stage renal failure after ~30 years of age. The disease is due to a mutation of *PKD1* or *PKD2* genes.
- Autosomal recessive polycystic kidney disease (ARPKD) is rare and of variable severity. A single gene mutation (6p21) with variable expression causes maldevelopment of distal collecting ducts with tubular dilatation ('cysts'). Clinical presentation ranges from antenatal renal failure with oligohydramnios and fatal pulmonary hypoplasia to chronic renal failure with severe hypertension in older children or adults. ARPKD is also associated with hepatic fibrosis.

Multicystic dysplastic kidneys

- Non-functioning, irregular cysts form during fetal life (Fig. 15.3)
- May be unilateral or bilateral and often diagnosed antenatally
- If unilateral, frequently involute
- If bilateral, may → poor prognosis due to oligo- or anhydramnios and pulmonary hypoplasia, +/− postnatal renal insufficiency
- Renal agenesis may be a form of multicystic dysplastic kidney disease where antenatal involution has occurred. Bilateral form of this = Potter's syndrome.

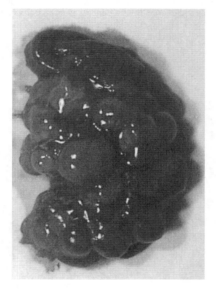

Fig. 15.3 Multicystic dysplastic kidney from post-mortem of a baby who died from bilateral renal disease, anhydramnios, and severe bilateral pulmonary hypoplasia.

Congenital nephrotic syndrome

- May be caused by congenital infection (TORCH, syphilis), or rarely autosomal recessive (Finnish type), or associated with a disorder of sexual differentiation, Denys–Drash syndrome (mutation of *WT-1* gene on chromosome 11)
- Placenta is macrosomic, baby often born preterm with oedema, low serum albumin, and facial dysmorphism
- Initial support is with careful fluid and electrolyte management with albumin replacement. Medical reduction of renal protein losses may be achieved using indometacin or angiotensin converting enzyme (ACE) inhibitors. Long-term definitive treatment requires bilateral nephrectomy and interim dialysis, pending eventual transplantation. Prognosis is poor.

Bladder extrophy

- Rare abnormal development of cloacal membrane
- Commoner in males
- Bladder opens onto anterior abdominal wall, with separation of pubic bones and epispadias
- Requires referral to a specialist centre for bladder reconstruction.

Acute renal failure

Definition
Sudden and severe reduction in GFR resulting in anuria/oliguria (<1 ml/kg/h) and increased creatinine.

Assessment and management
Need to differentiate pre-renal, renal, and post-renal causes
See Table 15.1.
- Assess hydration by clinical examination:
  - capillary refill
  - blood pressure
  - core-peripheral temperature gap
  - weight (compare with birth weight or previously measured weight)
  - skin turgor
  - serum Na
- Renal tract ultrasound scan to exclude obstructive (post-renal) causes, dysplastic kidneys, and to document flow in renal arteries and veins
- Calculation of fractional excretion of sodium (FENa, %) may be useful in term babies. This is not 100% sensitive or specific at determining whether acute renal failure is pre-renal, renal, or post-renal, and has limited value in extremely preterm babies and if furosemide has been given:
  - FENa = (urine Na/serum Na) × (serum creatine/urine creatine) × 100
  - *Pre-renal*: FENa <1–3% (up to ~6% in preterms)
  - *Renal*: FENa >1–3%.

Table 15.1 Aetiology/classification

Pre-renal	Renal	Post-renal
Hypovolaemia	Post-hypoxia ischaemia	Obstructive uropathy (e.g. posterior urethral valves)
Haemorrhage		
Severe dehydration		
3rd space losses (e.g. necrotizing enterocolitis)		
Normovolaemic hypotension	Sepsis	
Sepsis		
Low cardiac output (perinatal hypoxia ischaemia, congenital heart disease, etc.)		
Altered renal blood flow	Drugs (e.g. ACE inhibitors, indometacin, aminoglycosides)	
Renal vessel thrombosis	Acute presentation of chronic renal disease	
	Bilateral cystic dysplastic kidneys	
	Polycystic kidney disease	

Optimize respiratory and circulatory support
- Ventilatory support to maintain normal blood gases
- Inotropic support to maintain normal blood pressure and perfusion
- Consider low dose dopamine (2–3 µg/kg/min) to improve perfusion.

Optimize fluid and electrolyte balance
- If hypovolaemic or dehydrated give 10–20 ml/kg bolus (isotonic saline or colloid depending on cause) over several minutes or 1–2 hours (depending on acuity of fluid loss) and reassess
- Consider furosemide (bolus dose up to 5 mg/kg or infusion 0.1–2 mg/kg/h) once hypovolaemia or dehydration corrected depending on response
- If not dehydrated, fluid restrict (urine output plus insensible and GI losses (i.e. urine output + approx. 30 ml/kg/24 h if in closed, humidified incubator))
- Consider central venous access for hypertonic solutions of glucose (may be needed if severely fluid restricted)
- Monitor fluid input and output accurately (urine and GI losses)
- Monitor electrolytes at least 12-hourly
- Treat hyperkalaemia if potassium >6.5 mmol/l (see ➲ Hyperkalaemia, pp. 78–9)
- Treat hyperphosphataemia with oral calcium carbonate if possible to continue enteral feeds
- Treat metabolic acidosis with sodium bicarbonate (initially half correction followed by continuous infusion) in order to maintain normal plasma pH and bicarbonate levels
- Indications for dialysis in acute renal failure in neonates:
  - gross fluid overload
  - intractable hyperkalaemia
  - severe metabolic acidosis, not correctable within fluid input limits
  - hyperphosphataemia/hypocalcaemia.

Peritoneal dialysis in neonates

Peritoneal dialysis is usually more practical than haemodialysis in neonates. It can be carried out on the neonatal unit, but requires support from a paediatric neonatology team (PNT). The technique uses the peritoneum as a semi-permeable membrane, which allows solutes to diffuse from the circulation into the dialysis fluid, which is placed in the peritoneal cavity.

Technique for peritoneal dialysis
See ➲ Peritoneal dialysis catheter insertion, p. 527.
- **Analgesia:** IV morphine and local 1% lidocaine
- Insert peritoneal dialysis catheter percutaneously via trocar or Seldinger into peritoneal space (can use chest drain) lateral to rectus sheath and just below umbilicus level. A 13–16 FG size Tenckhoff type catheter is preferable in term babies, in order to minimize risk of bowel perforation. Smaller-sized catheters, or even chest drains or large bore IV cannulae may be used in smaller preterm babies
- Connect appropriate warm dialysis fluid (with 1 unit/ml heparin added) as advised by PNT

- An automatic gravity flow system can be used in term babies, but preterm babies requiring smaller cycle volumes must be managed manually
- Set flow rate of gravity flow system, using volumes of 15 ml/kg initially with no dwell time. Increase up to 40 ml/kg as indicated, or tolerated, or suggested by PNT
- Record dwell, and total cycle times, and volumes dialysed
- Use 30-minute cycles initially. Adjust as advised by PNT
- Peritoneal catheter may need to be repositioned and flushed intermittently
- IV calcium is often required. Adjust according to blood levels
- Monitor blood glucose levels 4-hourly
- Monitor for signs of peritonitis. Prophylactic broad-spectrum antibiotics may be added to dialysis fluid or given IV
- Send peritoneal fluid sample daily for MC&S
- Adjust all drug dosages for renal failure (some drugs may be 'dialysed out')
- See Table 15.2 for complications of peritoneal dialysis in neonates.

Haemofiltration

Haemofiltration is the removal of plasma water and solutes across a permeable membrane. It requires a net pressure gradient between hydraulic and hydrostatic pressure, which favours filtration, and oncotic pressure, which opposes it. Haemofiltration may be considered if peritoneal dialysis is contraindicated (e.g. in a baby with severe necrotizing enterocolitis) or if peritoneal dialysis is unsuccessful.

Haemodialysis

Haemodialysis may be necessary if solute removal is inadequate with haemofiltration. In this, dialysis fluid is run through the ultrafiltrate compartment of the filter in the opposite direction to blood flow.

Haemofiltration and haemodialysis are technically difficult in small babies, and if required, prognosis is poor.

Table 15.2 Practical problems and complications of peritoneal dialysis in neonates

Trauma from catheter insertion (bowel perforation, etc.)	↑ Risk in small preterm infants due to relatively large size of catheter
Fluid leakage from catheter site	
Catheter blockage	↓ Risk by regular flushing of catheter
Infection	Catheter site; peritonitis
Hyperglycaemia	↑ Risk in small preterm infants due to relatively large surface area of peritoneum
'Failed' dialysis	↑ Risk in small preterm infants due to relatively large surface area of peritoneum with greater permeability. Need short dwell times, larger volumes, and ↑ glucose in dialysate
Respiratory failure	Due to abdominal distension
Haemodynamic instability	

Endocrinology

Disorders of sexual differentiation

Sexual differentiation is determined by a combination of sex chromosomes and hormones. Disorders of sexual differentiation (DSD) occur as combinations of abnormal chromosomes, gonads, and genital phenotype. Disordered phenotypic sex is also commonly referred to as ambiguous genitalia.

Fetal sexual differentiation

- Bipotential gonads and internal structures
- Müllerian duct: precursor for ♀ internal genitalia
- Wolffian duct: precursor for ♂ internal genitalia
- Testosterone and anti-Müllerian hormone (AMH) cause regression of ♀ structures
- Testosterone and dihydrotestosterone cause development of ♂ internal and external genitalia respectively
- In the absence of AMH, ♀ structures survive and form ♀ internal genitalia
- *SRY* gene on the Y chromosome is an essential gene for male differentiation, there are many other important genes implicated for normal ♂ and ♀ differentiation.

46 XX DSD

Clinical presentation

Cliteromegaly, labial fusion, phenotypic sex reversal.

Causes

- Congenital adrenal hyperplasia—accounts for 90% (see ➲ Adrenal insufficiency, pp. 444–6)
- Gonadal dysgenesis
- Ovotesticular DSD
- Prenatal androgen exposure from maternal source (rare).

46 XY DSD

Clinical presentation

Micropenis, cryptorchism, hypospadias, phenotypic sex reversal.

Causes

- Abnormal androgen production including 5α-reductase deficiency, (converts testosterone to dihydrotestosterone)
- Abnormal androgen sensitivity—partial androgen insensitivity syndrome or complete androgen insensitivity syndrome
- Gonadal dysgenesis.

45 XO/46 XY DSD

Clinical presentation

Variable presentation, ♂ or ♀ phenotype (98% have ♂ phenotype). May have streak gonads that present a gonadal tumour risk.

Other sex chromosome abnormalities

- 45 XO Turner's syndrome (incidence 1:2000 to 1:5000)
  - clinical features: ♀ phenotype, gonadal dysgenesis, streak gonads, webbed neck, low set ears, broad chest, lymphoedema, congenital cardiac disease (coarctation of the aorta), renal abnormalities (horseshoe kidney)
- 47 XXY Kleinfelter syndrome (incidence 1:500 to 1:1000 males)
  - clinical features: ♂ phenotype, hypotonia, micropenis, hypospadias, cryptorchism, possible learning difficulty
- Other rare combinations of sex chromosomes are possible and may have associated DSD.

Isolated abnormalities

- Micropenis: phallus length <2.5 cm. Can be part of DSD or normal variant
- Hypospadias: distal (incidence 1:200); mid (incidence 1:450); proximal (incidence 1:900). Of proximal: 30% genetic cause; 70% idiopathic. Refer to urology.

⚠ Advise parents to avoid circumcision before surgical repair of hypospadias.

- Cryptorchism: unilateral undescended testes—7% at term; 3% at 3 months. Long-term presents a testicular tumour risk.

⚠ Bilateral impalpable undescended testes—need investigation as for DSD.

Diagnosis

Clinical evaluation

- BP, perfusion, hydration, jaundice, midline defects, length, weight
- Look for associated abnormalities: cardiac, skeletal, renal, etc.
- Document anatomy of external genitalia: position of gonads, phallus length, position of urinary meatus, scrotal/labial fusion, anogenital distance
- Prader staging
- External masculinization score (EMS) range 0–12 (Fig. 16.1).

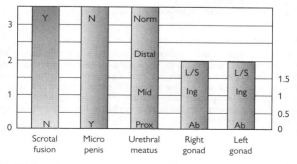

Fig. 16.1 External masculinization score (EMS).

First-line investigations
- Day 1
  - fluorescent in situ hybridization (FISH)/polymerase chain reaction (PCR) for sex chromosomes
  - comparative genomic hybridization (CGH) array/karyotype
  - cortisol, electrolytes, glucose, blood gas
- Day 3
  - cortisol, electrolytes, glucose, blood gas
  - 17-OHP (17-hydroxyprogesterone)
  - pelvis and adrenal ultrasound
  - save serum
- Second-line investigations for 46 XX DSD (CAH most common diagnosis)
  - urinary steroid profile—ideally take >36 hours and before steroid replacement is started
  - urine electrolytes and osmolality
  - monitor electrolytes
  - monitor glucose levels
  - adrenocorticotropic hormone (ACTH)
  - dehydroepiandrosterone sulphate (DHEAS), androstenedione, and testosterone
  - plasma renin activity
  - tetracosactide stimulation test—measure cortisol baseline and peak response. Normal peak 450–600 nmol/l
- Second-line investigations for 46 XY or 45 XO/46 XY DSD
  - testosterone and dihydrotestosterone
  - AMH: normal range newborn female 0–60 pmol/l, newborn male 0–2000 pmol/l
  - inhibin B
  - luteinizing hormone (LH), follicle-stimulating hormone (FSH)
  - HCG stimulation test—if positive confirms presence of testes. Positive test if testosterone > normal limit for prepubertal range, or increase > ×2 baseline value
  - imaging: MRI pelvis
  - examination under anaesthetic, +/− laparoscopy, +/− gonadal biopsy.

Principles of sex assignment

Discuss investigations and any uncertainty with the parents. Sex assignment needs an individual and flexible approach and it is important not to guess the sex if there is uncertainty. There is a legal requirement in the UK to assign a sex by 6 weeks of age. Involve a paediatric endocrinologist and regional specialist centre early. Later considerations include fertility, future tumour risk, surgical and hormonal options, requirement for ongoing specialist support and counselling.

Adrenal insufficiency

Hormones

- Adrenal cortex:
  - zona glomerulosa produces a mineralocorticoid: aldosterone
  - zona fasciculata produces corticosteroids: cortisol, deoxycorticosterone, and corticosterone
  - zona reticularis produces androgens: DHEAS, androstenedione
- Adrenal medulla produces catecholamines: adrenaline and noradrenaline
- The adrenal gland is under the influence of the pituitary hormone ACTH, which is in turn under the control of corticotropin-releasing hormone (CRH) from the thalamus
- Cortisol production is stimulated in response to stress such as birth, hypoglycaemia, illness, and pain.

Fetal and neonatal adrenal function

- The fetal adrenal gland is formed of a zona glomerulosa, zona fasciculata, and a large fetal zone
- In preterm infants the fetal zone predominates until term
- The fetal zone produces androgens and regresses and remodels after birth to form the zona reticularis
- Cortisol peaks after delivery and falls by day 7.

Clinical presentation of adrenal insufficiency

- Neonatal collapse
- Hyponatraemia with salt-losing crisis, dehydration, metabolic acidosis, and hypoglycaemia
- Hyperkalaemia
- Virilization of ♀; penile enlargement in ♂
- Hyperpigmentation.

Causes

- Hypopituitarism
- Congenital adrenal hyperplasia (CAH)
- Adrenal hypoplasia congenita
- Aldosterone resistance
- Bilateral adrenal haemorrhage
- Maternal causes: high dose steroids or Cushing's disease.

Congenital adrenal hyperplasia

- 21-hydroxylase deficiency accounts for 90–95%. Other forms include 11β-hydroxylase deficiency and 17α-hydroxylase deficiency
- ↓ Cortisol production →↑ ACTH release from the pituitary and 2° adrenal hyperplasia
- ↓ Mineralocorticoid production in the majority; however 11β-hydroxylase deficiency is associated with ↑ mineralocorticoid production, salt retention, and hypertension
- ↑ Sex hormone production, 2° virilization—classic: salt wasting (two-thirds) or simple virilizing (one-third)
- Non-classic: ↑ androgens, polycystic ovary syndrome, glucocorticoid stress deficiency (Fig. 16.2).

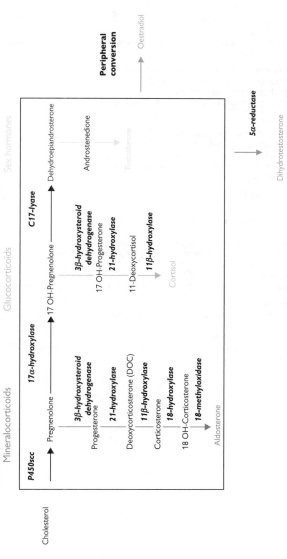

Fig. 16.2 Adrenal hormone pathway.

Adrenal hypoplasia congenita
- Rare X-linked
- Clinical presentation: salt-losing crisis, hyperpigmentation (2° ↑ ACTH), faltering growth.

Aldosterone resistance (pseudohypoaldosteronism)
- Autosomal dominant, Types I and IIB
- High aldosterone and renin levels
- Treat with salt supplements, thiazide diuretics.

Diagnosis
- As for XX DSD investigations (see ➔ Disorders of sexual differentiation, pp. 440–2)
- Tetracosactide test
- For neonatal collapse—investigations for other causes such as sepsis and metabolic disorders.

Management

Acute
- Correct dehydration and shock with oral/IV fluid
- IV hydrocortisone 4–6 hourly
- Fludrocortisone (first check plasma renin activity)
- Replace sodium deficit: IV sodium supplementation until normalized, then oral sodium supplements
- Treat hyperkalaemia (see ➔ Hyperkalaemia, pp. 78–9)
- Treat hypoglycaemia (see ➔ Hypoglycaemia: management, pp. 374–5).

Maintenance
- Oral hydrocortisone tds; titrate to androstenedione, testosterone level, and 17-OHP levels
- Oral sodium supplements qds, up to 1 year
- Emergency care plan for intercurrent illness after discharge from hospital.

Pituitary disorders

- Anterior pituitary hormones: ACTH, thyroid stimulating hormone (TSH), LH, FSH, prolactin, growth hormone (GH)
- Posterior pituitary hormones: ADH (antidiuretic hormone)
- The hypothalamic-pituitary axis is functional by 20 weeks gestation
- Pituitary hormone deficiencies may be congenital or acquired, isolated or multiple hormone deficiencies
- Multiple or combined hypopituitarism ('panhypopituitarism') has an incidence of ~1:8000 and may present with severe hypoglycaemia and seizures (see ➡ Hypoglycaemia: overview, pp. 372–3)
- Clinical presentation depends on which hormones are deficient.

GH deficiency

- Incidence of isolated GH deficiency ~1:3500
- Neonatal presentation suggests severe deficiency.

Clinical presentation

- Clinical features: hypoglycaemia, hypotonia, seizures, nystagmus, conjugated hyperbilirubinaemia, hypothermia
- Physical phenotype: infant immature, prominent forehead, midline defects, low muscle mass, high-pitched cry, micropenis
- Associated midline defects; hypotelorism, hypertelorism, cleft palate, septo-optic dysplasia.

Causes

- Idiopathic
- Partial or complete pituitary stalk agenesis
- Anterior pituitary hypoplasia
- Ectopic pituitary
- Septo-optic dysplasia.

Diagnosis

- Imaging: cranial ultrasound (for midline defects), MRI with pituitary views
- Pituitary function tests: GH, IGF-1, ACTH, cortisol, TSH, free T4, LH, FSH, prolactin, glucose
- Growth hormone deficiency dynamic testing: glucagon stimulation test, growth-hormone releasing hormone (GHRH) test. Seek advice from paediatric endocrinologist.

Management

- GH from 6 months, earlier if growth failure severe.

Diabetes insipidus (DI)

For DI/sodium balance (see ➡ Sodium balance, pp. 76–7).

Clinical presentation

- Hypernatraemic dehydration, weight loss, seizures, vomiting, jaundice.

Causes
- Central DI: posterior hypopituitarism, ADH deficiency—isolated or in combination with other pituitary hormone deficiencies. Often improves with time
- Nephrogenic DI: renal insensitivity to ADH.

Diagnosis
- Fluid input/output monitoring
- Pituitary function tests
- Urinary and serum electrolytes and osmolality (urine inappropriately dilute compared to plasma). Normal urine osmolality 300–900 mOsm/kg. Normal plasma osmolality 275–295 mOsm/kg. With dehydration, urine osmolality should be at 3–4× that of plasma
- Test dose of vasopressin.

Management
- Vasopressin or desmopressin—IV/nasal; monitor electrolytes.

Syndrome of inappropriate ADH (SIADH)
Clinical presentation
- Hyponatraemia with fluid overload, weight gain, seizures.

Causes
Inappropriately high ADH secretion commonly in response to:
- Respiratory disease, neurological disease, sepsis, and pain.

Diagnosis
- Fluid input/output monitoring
- Serum and urinary electrolytes and osmolality (urine inappropriately concentrated compared to plasma).

Management
- Fluid restriction
- Treat underlying disease.

ACTH deficiency
See ➜ Adrenal insufficiency. pp. 444–6.

TSH deficiency
See ➜ Thyroid disorders, pp. 450–1.

LH and FSH deficiency
See ➜ Disorders of sexual differentiation, pp. 440–2.

Thyroid disorders

Hormones

- TSH released from the pituitary under the influence of TRH
- TSH stimulates the thyroid to synthesize and release thyroxine (T4) and triiodothyronine (T3)
- T4 is deiodinated peripherally to the active compound T3.

Fetal and neonatal thyroid function

- During fetal life, TSH, T4, and T3 gradually increase, and inactive reverse T3 (rT3) gradually falls
- Maternal T4 crosses the placenta well in the first trimester, but this decreases with increasing gestational age
- At birth there are sudden surges in TSH, T4, and T3 which return to near normal levels by 3 days of age. This is less in preterms, and T4 may take some weeks to rise to normal levels.

Neonatal hypothyroidism

- Neonatal hypothyroidism occurs in 1:3500 live births
- Compensated or uncompensated hypothyroidism
- Transient hypothyroidism is most pronounced in extreme prematurity
- Risk of neurodevelopmental delay.

Causes

- Aplastic, hypoplastic, or ectopic thyroid
- Rarely hypothalamic or hypopituitary (TSH usually not ↑)
- Rarely caused by maternal hypothyroidism.

Maternal hypothyroidism

- Causes: Hashimoto's thyroiditis, iodine deficiency, congenital aplasia, congenital hypoplasia, treated Grave's disease
- Thyroid receptor antibodies in Hashimoto's are unlikely to cross the placenta so the risk of neonatal hyper- or hypothyroidism is low.

Clinical presentation

- At birth: large for gestational age, post-mature, umbilical hernia, +/– goitre, +/– RDS
- First few weeks: sleepy, poor feeding, constipation, abdominal distension, hypothermia, poor perfusion, oedema, prolonged jaundice
- Late signs: cretinous appearance, growth failure, delayed development, hearing loss.

Diagnosis

- TSH on newborn bloodspot screening taken 4–7 days after birth (**NB** will not pick up the rare cases of hypothalamic/pituitary hypothyroidism)
- Confirm with full thyroid function tests (TFTs)—T3, free T4, and TSH
- Thyrotropin releasing hormone (TRH) stimulation and radioisotope scanning rarely indicated in newborn, but if so must be done before or immediately after starting treatment
- If maternal hypothyroidism is due to treated maternal Graves' disease, there is a risk of neonatal hyperthyroidism.

Management

- Delay in starting treatment beyond the first few weeks of life compromises neurodevelopment, particularly if initial T4 levels are very low
- Immediately start thyroxin 10–15 µg/kg once daily (**NB** treatment of hypothyroidism in preterm babies has unclear benefits, therefore currently not recommended)
- Monitor TFTs weekly, then 2–3 monthly
- At 1–2 years stop treatment temporarily and reassess thyroid function.

Neonatal hyperthyroidism

Causes

- Usually maternal hyperthyroidism
- McCune-Albright syndrome (rare).

Maternal hyperthyroidism

- Usually Graves' disease, caused by TSH receptor-stimulating immunoglobulins (TSI)—IgG that cross the placenta. Can be present even if maternal disease previously treated medically or surgically
- TSI are sometimes balanced by thyroid inhibiting immunoglobulins (TIIs), which also cross the placenta
- Only 1–2% neonates affected if mother has (or has had) Graves' disease. More likely, if TSI levels are high or if mother required treatment during pregnancy. Usually results in neonatal hyperthyroidism
- Maternal antithyroid drugs (particularly propylthiouracil) may cross the placenta and cause fetal hypothyroidism; goitre and bradycardia.

Clinical presentation

- Antenatal: fetal tachycardia, arrythmias, and hydrops, which require treatment by using maternal antithyroid medication
- First 1–2 weeks: symptoms of thyrotoxicosis; irritability, poor feeding, weight loss, diarrhoea, goitre, eye signs, hypertension, hepatosplenomegaly, jaundice, thrombocytopenia, and advanced skeletal maturation
- Usually resolves by 4–6 months.

Breastfeeding

- Maternal antithyroid drugs are also secreted in breast milk in small amounts, and therefore may rarely cause neonatal hypothyroidism
- If maternal daily dose ≥15 mg carbimazole or ≥150 mg propylthiouracil, split the dose and monitor baby's thyroid function postnatally. If lower maternal dose than this—no risk.

Diagnosis

- Monitor fetus, +/– cordocentesis for TFTs
- Cord blood for thyroid receptor antibodies (TSI + TII), TSH, and fT4 (free thyroxine)
- Check TSH and T4, 4–7 days after birth with clinical review.

Management

- If thyrotoxic, treat with antithyroid medication (usually propylthiouracil or carbimazole)
- Consider propranolol, iodine, steroids, sedatives, and exchange transfusion.

Calcium disorders

Hormones

- Calcitonin is secreted from the thyroid and acts to lower Ca^{2+}
- Vitamin D (calciferol) is produced from sunlight or diet. The liver converts it to 25(OH)D. It is then converted to active $1,25(OH)_2D$ (calcitriol) via 1α-hydroxylase enzyme activity in the kidneys. Calcitriol increases intestinal Ca^{2+} absorption
- PTH is secreted from parathyroid and acts to raise Ca^{2+}
- PTH →↑ Ca^{2+} reabsorption and phosphate excretion from kidneys, and Ca^{2+} and phosphate reabsorption from bone.

Fetal and neonatal bone metabolism

- Ca^{2+} moves across the placenta to enable bone mineralization in the fetus
- The majority of mineralization occurs in the third trimester and continues after birth
- At birth the placental supply stops and there is a normal physiological ↓ in plasma Ca^{2+} levels, associated with ↑ PTH
- Calcitonin levels remain high throughout pregnancy and after delivery
- Neonatal vitamin D reserves are maternal in origin. Vitamin D crosses and is activated by the placenta.

Hypocalcaemia

Definition

- Total Ca^{2+} <2.2 mmol/l
- Ionized Ca^{2+} <1.2 mmol/l.

Clinical presentation

- Congenital rickets, cardiomyopathy, stridor
- Irritability, seizures, apnoea
- ECG: prolonged QT and arrhythmia.

Causes

- Exaggerated physiological response
- Iatrogenic: steroids, diuretics, phosphate infusions, alkalosis
- Advanced metabolic bone disease (see ➋ Metabolic bone disease, pp. 384–5)
- Transient hypoparathyroidism of prematurity
- Magnesium deficiency
- Activating mutations of calcium-sensing receptors
- Other genetic causes: DiGeorge syndrome; HDR syndrome (hypoparathyroidism, deafness, renal abnormalities); glial cell missing, X-linked recessive hypoparathyroidism; PTH resistance; pseudohypoparathyroidism; Sanjad-Sakati syndrome (Middle East origin, congenital hypoparathyroidism)
- Metabolic disorders: mitochondrial disease
- Renal failure
- Vitamin D deficiency
- Perinatal asphyxia
- Maternal causes: pre-eclampsia, hypercalcaemia, vitamin D deficiency, hyperparathyroidism, diabetes.

Diagnosis
- Serum calcium, phosphate, magnesium, and electrolytes
- Urine calcium:creatinine ratio
- PTH
- ALP (alkaline phosphatase)
- 25-OH Vitamin D
- Blood gas.

Further investigations
- ECG.

Management
- If severe or symptomatic prescribe IV calcium 0.5 ml/kg 10% calcium gluconate solution (0.11 mmol/kg) over 10 minutes, or 24 hours if asymptomatic (**NB** Calcium infusions can cause chemical extravasation burns)
- If enterally fed, prescribe oral calcium supplements
- If receiving total parenteral nutrition (TPN) increase constituents of TPN
- △ Active vitamin D preparation, calcitriol or alfacalcidol (200–2000 IU/day)
- Treat any hypomagnesaemia.

Universal vitamin D supplementation
Vitamin D supplementation is recommended for preterm infants and children 6 months to 5 years of age.

DaliVit® contains 400 units (10 µg) of colecalciferol or ergocalciferol in 0.6 ml. Maintenance dose for neonate to 1 year: 200–400 units (0.3–0.6 ml) daily.

Hypercalcaemia

Definition
- Total Ca^{2+} >2.75 mmol/l
- Inonized Ca^{2+} >1.4 mmol/l.

Clinical presentation
- At birth: vomiting, constipation, polyuria, polydipsia, hypertension, irritability, seizures
- Older child: nephrocalcinosis, faltering growth, bone deformities.

Causes
- Iatrogenic causes: excessive calcium intake
- Hypophosphataemia
- Inactivating mutations of the calcium-sensing receptor: familial benign hypercalcaemia, neonatal severe hyperparathyroidism (fatal <6 months if untreated)
- Other genetic causes: Jansen's metaphyseal chondroplasia, hypophosphatasia, osteopetrosis, Williams syndrome, trisomy 21
- Macrophage activation (2° activation of vitamin D): subcutaneous fat necrosis (e.g. after therapeutic hypothermia), malignancy
- Metabolic disorders: lactase deficiency, disaccharidase deficiency, infantile hypophosphatasia

- Other endocrine causes: hypothyroidism, thyrotoxicosis, adrenal insufficiency
- Idiopathic hypercalcaemia of infancy.

Diagnosis
- Serum calcium, phosphate, magnesium, and electrolytes
- Urine calcium:creatinine ratio
- PTH
- ALP
- 25-OH vitamin D
- Blood gas.

Further investigations
- ECG
- Skeletal survey
- Renal ultrasound scan.

Management
- Avoid excessive calcium and vitamin D intake
- Ensure good hydration and consider IV fluids
- Consider loop diuretics, bisphosphonates, steroids (useful for subcutaneous fat necrosis), and calcitonin
- Cinacalcet may be useful for calcium-sensing receptor inactivating mutations
- Parathyroidectomy for neonatal severe hyperparathyroidism.

Further information

Ogilvie-Stuart A, Midgley P. *Practical neonatal endocrinology*. Cambridge University Press, UK, 2006.

Iatrogenic problems

Introduction

An iatrogenic problem is an illness that results from any diagnostic or thera-peutic intervention that is not attributable to an underlying disease process.

Iatrogenic problems are inevitable consequences of intensive care for the sick newborn. Decrease in the neonatal mortality rate has led to increasing numbers of neonatal intensive care unit (NICU) graduates, in particular sur-vivors of preterm birth. Many infants will sustain injury, usually non-serious but sometimes permanent, that has in its aetiology, an iatrogenic compo-nent (e.g. minor scarring from IV line sites).

The three major sources of iatrogenic injury are procedures, therapies, and medications.

Problems associated with procedures

- Pneumothorax (intubation, jugular central line; see ⮁ Femoral and internal jugular central venous line insertion, p. 516)
- Gastric rupture
- Airway trauma (intubation; see ⮁ Endotracheal intubation, pp. 494–5)
- Nasal septum damage (nasal intubation, nasal prong CPAP; see ⮁ Nasal intubation, p. 496)
- Anaemia (over-sampling, haemorrhage; see ⮁ aetiology, Anaemia, p. 398)
- Arterial thrombosis and distal ischaemia (central line, peripheral arterial line, cardiac catheterization; see ⮁ Thrombosis and thrombophilia, pp. 420–1)
- Cardiac tamponade (central line; see ⮁ Percutaneous central ('long') line insertion, pp. 514–15)
- Sepsis (lines, LP, urinary catheter; see ⮁ Lumbar puncture, pp. 520–1; ⮁ Transurethral catheterization, p. 528).

Catheter-associated infections are a significant cause of morbidity, particu-larly in preterms. Effective infection control, hand washing, and central-line care bundles can reduce the incidence of infection.

Problems associated with treatment

- Pneumothorax (PPV, CPAP)
- Chronic lung disease (PPV, see ⮁ Continuous positive airways pressure and nasal intermittent positive pressure ventilation, pp. 152–3)
- Subglottic stenosis (PPV/intubation, see ⮁ Endotracheal intubation, pp. 494–5)
- Retinopathy of prematurity (hyperoxia in preterms, see ⮁ Oxygen, p. 151)
- Necrotizing enterocolitis (formula feeding, see ⮁ Enteral feeds: general principles, p. 94)
- IVH (hypotension, hypoxia, hypercarbia, see ⮁ Brain injury in premature babies: germinal matrix haemorrhage–intraventricular haemorrhage, pp. 294–7)
- Pulmonary haemorrhage (fluid overload).

Problems associated with medication

- Medication error (incorrect drug or dose)
- Cholestatic jaundice (PN)
- Electrolyte and nutrient disturbances (IV fluids, PN)
- Fluid imbalance (IV fluids, TPN)
- Transfusion reaction (blood products)
- Intestinal ulceration/perforation (dexamethasone, ibuprofen, indometacin)
- Nephrocalcinosis (diuretics).

Medication errors can be reduced by encouraging safe prescribing habits (e.g. writing the word micrograms in full on drug charts), safe administration procedures (e.g. standardized infusions), and daily input from a neonatal/paediatric pharmacist. New technology can be beneficial, such as electronic prescribing systems and smart infusion pumps.

The general principles of management are timely intervention, good documentation, incident reporting, and open communication with parents.

There is a legal duty in the UK to inform and apologize to patients (parents) if there have been mistakes in their care that have led to significant harm (duty of candour).

Arterial thrombosis

Introduction

A thrombus may form at the tip of an arterial catheter where it has traumatized the endothelial lining. Thrombi likely form at the time of catheter insertion and may propagate, extending distally and proximally within the artery, as well as firing emboli into distal branches. The incidence of thrombi associated with catheters is uncertain.

Clinical features

- No symptoms/signs in many cases
- Poor peripheral perfusion, decreased temperature, mottling, discolouration, and loss of pulses in the affected limb
- Eventually leading to necrosis
- Reduced urine output, haematuria, and hypertension if the renal arteries are occluded
- Paraplegia and cardiac failure may occur with very large thrombi within the aorta
- Isolated intestinal perforation following embolization into the mesenteric circulation.

Management

Peripheral ischaemia may be due to transient arterial spasm or a large catheter in a small artery that compromises blood flow.

- If ischaemia develops immediately after catheter insertion, the most likely cause is arterial spasm. In this case, careful observation is all that is required until symptoms improve, usually within 30 minutes. Topical GTN patch to the affected area can be used
- If symptoms do not improve or worsen, the catheter may be impairing blood flow. If there is evidence of hypovolaemia, then correcting this can rapidly improve symptoms. Otherwise, the catheter should be removed, usually leading to quick resolution of symptoms without sequelae
- If ischaemia persists or occurs beyond the period of insertion, then a thrombus becomes more likely. Assess the extent of thrombus with US scan.

Treatment

- **Small thrombus with mild ischaemia**: supportive care, GTN patch, and monitor carefully
- **Moderate thrombus with moderate ischaemia**: perform cranial ultrasound scan and consider starting heparin infusion
- **Large thrombus with severe ischaemia or not responding to heparin**: consider *thrombolysis* (tissue plasminogen activator (tPA) or streptokinase) and continue heparin. Reassess every 4 hours including fibrinogen level. Maintain platelet count >50 and fibrinogen level >1 using blood products. Avoid traumatic procedures and consider sedation or muscle relaxant.

Close monitoring for haemorrhage from any site, including intracranial. Stop infusion immediately and correct any coagulopathy if there is haemorrhage. Contraindicated in infants <32 weeks gestation.

Heparin

Prevents thrombus propagation, while endogenous thrombolysis and relaxation of vasospasm takes place:

- Use lower doses for preterm infants
- Loading dose: 75 IU/kg over 10 minutes
- Initial maintenance dose: 15–28 IU/kg/h
- Measure activated partial thromboplastin time (APTT) after 4 hours, monitor efficacy, and adjust dose (Table 17.1)
- If there is significant haemorrhage, use protamine sulfate to reverse effects of heparin (see Table 17.2)
- Stop infusion when flow returns.

Tissue plasminogen activator

- Maintenance: 0.5 mg/kg/h
- *Low dose tPA* via local infusion can be given through a catheter when there is a high risk of bleeding (e.g. preterms or following cardiac surgery). A dose of 0.05 mg/kg/h can be administered for several days
- If symptoms have improved, stop tPA and commence heparin for 6 hours
- If there is significant haemorrhage, infuse cryoprecipitate and tranexamic acid (15 mg/kg IV over 10 minutes) to reverse the tPA
- Surgical thrombectomy is rarely required when there is no response to thrombolysis in a radiologically defined thrombus with severe ischaemia
- In extreme cases, necrosis develops and amputation is required
- If there are multiple thrombi at different sites, consider a thrombophilia screen
- Hypertension is managed in the usual manner (see ➔ Hypertension, pp. 226–7).

Table 17.1 Heparin dosing

APTT (s)	Bolus (IU/kg)	Hold (min)	Rate change (%)	Repeat APTT (h)
<50	50	0	+10	4
50–59	0	0	+10	4
60–85	0	0	0	24
86–95	0	0	−10	4
96–120	0	30	−10	4
>120	0	60	−15	4

APTT: activated partial thromboplastin time.

Table 17.2 Protamine dose

Time since last heparin dose (min)	Protamine dose (mg/100 IU heparin received)
<30	1
30–60	0.5–0.75
60–120	0.375–0.5
>120	0.25–0.375

Rate 5 mg/min, max dose 50 mg.

Extravasation injuries

Introduction

Around 4% of infants, mostly preterms, suffer extravasation leading to skin necrosis. Peripheral venous lines often rupture through the vessel wall or 'tissue' and central lines less often. Infusate may extravasate into subcutaneous and deep tissue, or pleural and pericardial spaces. Usually, a small amount of non-irritant fluid extravasates and causes few problems. However, large volumes or hypertonic solutions may cause severe damage to the soft tissue and skin leading to extensive skin loss followed by scarring and contracture. Central lines may extravasate causing pleural or pericardial effusions with serious consequences.

Staging system for extravasation injuries

Stage 1: painful IV site, no erythema and swelling, flushes with difficulty.
Stage 2: painful IV site, slight swelling, redness, no blanching, brisk CRT, and good pulse volume distally.
Stage 3: painful IV site, marked swelling, blanching, cool to touch, brisk CRT, and good pulse volume distally.
Stage 4: painful IV site, very marked swelling, blanching, cool to touch, CRT >4 s, decreased or absent pulse, skin breakdown or necrosis.

Management

- Identify the infusate
- Aspirate cannula and remove immediately
- Perform irrigation as soon as possible, if the extravasation is large, and causing ischaemia (i.e. stage 3 or 4) or the infusate is particularly irritant (e.g. PN, calcium or potassium containing infusion)
- Ensure adequate analgesia (e.g. lidocaine or morphine)
- Puncture the skin at multiple sites over the extravasation area using aseptic technique. If the area is particularly tense, a pair of opposing incisions can be made
- Introduce saline using a blunt needle or cannula in 2–5 ml aliquots up to 50 ml to flush out infusate, and massage out oedema
- Consider infiltration with hyaluronidase (500 IU)
- Dress and elevate the affected area and observe for signs of compartment syndrome
- Give antibiotics if there is evidence of infection
- Topical GTN has been used with limited evidence of efficacy
- Involve a plastic surgeon for moderate or severe injuries. Debridement or skin grafting is required in the most severe cases
- Photograph injury for clinical notes and inform parents.

Infants inadvertently receiving incorrect breast milk

The commonest root cause for infants receiving expressed breast milk from the wrong mother is sharing the same or similar surnames.

The main risk is exposure to blood-borne viruses, mainly hepatitis B and C (HBV and HCV), and HIV.

Prevention

- Bottles of breast milk should be labelled immediately after collection with the baby's name, hospital number, and date of collection
- Dispensing breast milk should be subject to a rigorous checking system similar to administering medications
- Computerized milk management systems are available.

Management

- Causes significant upset for family and staff and should be treated seriously and sensitively
- Aspirate milk from the infant's stomach if the milk was given recently
- Inform both the infant's mother and the donor mother as soon as practical after the incident. Maintain confidentiality by not sharing the identity of the donor mother with the infant's mother
- Gain consent and take blood to test for HBV, HCV, and HIV from the donor mother and recipient baby
- It is unusual, but if the donor mother refuses to be tested, a decision on treatment and follow-up is based upon antenatal serology and the recipient baby should be retested 3 months later
- Document the incident and discussions with parents
- Complete an adverse incident form.

Needle-stick injuries

The main risk is exposure to blood-borne viruses, mainly HBV, HCV, and HIV.

Prevention

- Wear gloves for all clinical procedures
- A useful tip is the person using the sharp is responsible for its disposal
- Dispose of all sharps in a designated sharps bin at the time and point of use
- Do not re-sheathe needles. Safety cannulas are available
- Sharps should be placed in a tray (including capillary tubes) when carried.

Management

- Rinse the injury thoroughly under warm running water
- Wash the site and encourage bleeding
- Report the incident to a senior team member to organize support
- Notify Occupational Health (or the Emergency Department, out of hours)
- Arrange for another team member (i.e. not the injured person) to take blood to test HBV, HCV, and HIV status from the infant after gaining consent from the parents
- If it is not possible to gain consent, then a stored sample can be used with the agreement of two consultants
- Above blood tests should also be taken from the injured person by Occupational Health (or a colleague, out of hours)
- Complete an adverse incident form
- Occupational Health will advise on the need for chemoprophylaxis and follow-up.

Further information

Ramachandrappa A, Jain L. Iatrogenic disorders in modern neonatology: a focus on safety and quality of care. *Clin Perinatol* 2008; **35**: 1–34.

Saxonhouse MA. Management of neonatal thrombosis. *Clin Perinatol* 2012; **39**: 191–208.

Stavroudis T, Miller MR, Lehmann CU. Medication errors in neonates. *Clin Perinatol*. 2008; **35**: 141–161.

Will A. Neonatal haemostasis and the management of neonatal thrombosis. *Br J Haematol* 2015; **169**: 324–332.

Neonatal transport

Introduction

In many countries, the delivery of neonatal care has become centralized with the formation of a number of perinatal clinical networks. Although good network planning can usually ensure that babies are born in the 'right' place, the requirement for emergency transfer for some is inevitable. Transporting vulnerable, sick, and sometimes extremely small newborn babies is not without risk.

Inter-hospital transport services

In the UK, organizing neonatal care into networks has resulted in better outcomes, with fewer out-of-area transfers and a greater number of extremely preterm babies being delivered in tertiary centres with neonatal intensive care unit (NICU) facilities. Regional transport teams are usually responsible for a defined geographical area, with dedicated staff and equipment, and offering a retrieval service from a centralized location (two-way transfer). A dedicated hotline may offer a standardized referral process, advice, and cot location.

When there is no transport team available, or for time-critical transfers when using a transport service would cause undue delay, staff from the referring or receiving hospital must carry out the transfer using their own equipment (one-way transfer). This may not only compromise staffing at the base hospital, but is more likely to increase the risk of adverse events during transport.

Indications for transfer

- Escalation of intensive care (e.g. Special Care Baby Unit to NICU for intensive respiratory support)
- Specialist assessment (e.g. cardiology or surgery)
- Local cot capacity is exceeded
- Local medical (usually nursing) staff insufficient
- Return or 'back' transfer from tertiary to local unit
- Intra-hospital transfer for an investigation (e.g. MRI scan) or treatment (e.g. surgery).

NB Antenatal transfer of pregnant mothers (*in utero transfer*) is likely to result in improved clinical outcomes than postnatal (*ex utero*) transfer, particularly for extremely preterm babies.

Elements of safe neonatal transport

- Preparation
- Stabilization
- Transfer
- Handover.

ACCEPT is a useful acronym to ensure safe and effective transfer.

Assessment

Initial assessment to identify the infant's needs. What support is needed and what is the most appropriate destination?

Control & Communication

Taking control of the situation requires someone to take responsibility for leading and managing the transfer. Effective communication between the referring and receiving units, transport teams, and family is vital to success.

Evaluation

Evaluate the infant's current condition and management. Optimize clinical condition as far as possible before transfer.

Preparation & Packaging

Prepare equipment, gases, fluids, and medication that may be needed during transfer. Ensure equipment is secure and the infant is comfortable.

Transfer

Appropriate monitoring and avoid unnecessary interventions.

Preparation

Anticipation

- Regular communication between transport team, referring hospital, and receiving hospital is essential
- Referring team and transport team should update the receiving hospital with significant changes in the condition of the infant in a timely fashion.

Communication

Good communication is essential from the first telephone call to the final handover.

Taking a referral request

- Ascertain the reason for the call (referral or advice)
- Obtain history and current condition of infant, and results of relevant investigations. A template is useful (Fig. 18.1 shows a sample neonatal transfer referral form)
- Give appropriate advice about further management
- Assess the need for specialty input (e.g. cardiology or surgery)
- Check bed availability before accepting an infant and suggest alternative units if no bed is available
- Inform the ambulance crew
- Maintain continuous contact and request to be informed if the baby's condition changes
- Document all telephone calls with the referring hospital, including any advice given and transfers accepted.

Personnel

- Specific personnel—depends on the infant's clinical condition and local procedures
- In general, it is safer to prepare for an infant that is more unwell than described in the transfer request
- Retrievals and transfer of unwell babies requires a minimum of a senior doctor (SpR/ST4+) or advanced neonatal nurse practioner (ANNP), and a nurse
- 'Return' transfers of infants to special care baby units, that have been stable for some time with little or no oxygen requirement, and no cardiovascular compromise may be transferred with a nurse and paramedic
- Extremely sick infants may require two experienced doctors (consultant and senior trainee) and a nurse
- An experienced driver/paramedic who is familiar with the vehicle and fixtures is an invaluable part of the team
- All staff must be familiar with the transport equipment. **NB** often different from that on the neonatal unit
- Know who to contact if there are difficulties at any stage. Most teams have a dedicated mobile telephone to take on transfers with an attending consultant on-call specifically for transfers.

NTS Referral Form

Date of Referral:	Time of Referral:	Ref No: 3014 _ _ _
Contacted via EBS: Yes No	EBS Operator:	Conference Call: Yes No

Please tick one of the options below:				
Emergency		Elective Referral	File sheet in diary	Enquiry	Once dealt with file in Red Tray

Referring Hospital:		Ward:	
Contact Name:		Consultant:	
Telephone Number:		Ex or Bleep:	

Baby Details			
Name:	D.O.B:	Birth Weight:	
Gestation:	Time of Birth:	Current Weight:	
NHS No:	Day:	Sex:	

Date of Transfer:		Team used: BT01 BT02
Team location at time of call: At base On another call Pre-booked Other :		

Clinical Details
Details of referral:
Antenatal History & Delivery (brief history)

Respiratory State: Ventilated CPAP N.Cannula Oxygen SV					The following info is needed for the MINT score:		
Vent mode:	Pressures:	ETT Size:		ETT Length:		Apgars: /1min /5min /10min	
I Time:	Rate:	Latest Gases: (A)rterial (V)enous (C)ap				Congenital Abnormalities:	
FiO_2:	Sats:	Time					
BM:	Mean BP:	Site	A V C	A V C	A V C	Lines:	
Fluids:		PH				1.	3.
		PCO_2				2.	4.
Feeding:		PO_2				Temperature:	
Sedation & Paralysis:		HCO_3				Antibiotics:	
		BE				Inotropes:	
Relevant Blood Results:						Infection Issue: Yes No	

You MUST answer this question!

IS THIS TRANSFER TIME CRITICAL?

(See overleaf for definitions)

YES   NO

PTO:

Advice given to referring unit:	Advice followed: Yes / *No	* If No provide reason

Chargeable Journey: Yes / No (charging sheet sent to LAS) Total Time:		Form completed by:
Accepting Hospital:	Ward:	Transfer Cancelled: Yes No (Reason)
	Contact Name:	
Consultant:	Telephone Number:	Consultant on-call for NTS:
Personnel on board: Doctor/ANNP:	Nurse:	Paramedic:
Consultant:		Observer:

Fig. 18.1 Neonatal transfer service (NTS) referral form.

Choice of vehicle
- Mode of transfer depends upon the infant's clinical condition, urgency of transfer, and geography of the journey
- Use of a helicopter or fixed wing aircraft should be considered when journey time to the referring hospital exceeds 2 hours by road
- Air transfer requires specialist staff, a great deal of organization, and is expensive. The physiological effects of altitude must be considered, which include hypoxia, barometric effects, noise, vibration, and hypothermia
- Air transfer is a highly specialized retrieval service and beyond the scope of this handbook.

Equipment
- Take equipment to deal with every eventuality and never rely on equipment being available at the referring hospital
- All equipment needs to checked and operational before departing
- Make an estimate of the oxygen requirement for the transfer:

O_2 required (l) = Flow (l/min) $\times$ FiO_2 $\times$ journey time (minutes) $\times$ 2

Including allowance for possible delays:

'F' cylinder = 1360 l and 'E' cylinder = 680 l

If possible, prepare drug infusions before departure to save time at the referring hospital.
- All staff should be trained in the use of all transport equipment
- See ➔ Transport equipment checklist, pp. 480–1, for a list of recommended items.

Stabilization

- Aim to optimize the baby's clinical condition before transfer
- Measures to stabilize for transfer should be instituted as early as possible
- The referring hospital should be advised to start this process when making the referral
- On arrival, take a handover from the referring team
- Make your own thorough assessment of the infant and continue the stabilization process.

Airway

- Is the airway **patent?** Is the airway **secure** (for transport)?
- **Consider likely indications for elective intubation for transfer:** <30 weeks gestation, signs of respiratory distress, increasing O_2 requirement, apnoeas, increasing PCO_2, signs of shock, airway anomaly
- Have a lower threshold for intubation than in hospital. If there is any doubt whether the infant will be able to maintain their airway during transfer then it is best to electively intubate and ventilate before departing.

Breathing

- Is ventilation adequate?
- Consider administering **surfactant** before departure (if appropriate)
- Carefully assess any **pneumothoraces** and give thought to drainage, as they may increase in size and become clinically significant during transfer. Replace underwater drains with one-way flutter valves as these are more portable
- Review **chest** X-ray (including checking endotracheal tube (ETT) and central line positions).

Switch to the transport ventilator

- Most transport ventilators cannot provide high frequency oscillatory ventilation (HFOV) or patient-triggered ventilation (PTV), so the infant needs to be switched to continuous mandatory ventilation and stabilized before transfer
- Use the settings on the unit ventilator as a guide, especially if the infant has been stable on these settings
- Connect to the transport ventilator and check there is good chest movement and O_2 sats are stable
- Check **blood gas** and correct any problems before departure
- Ensure **good suction** of the airway before departure as using portable devices during movement is generally less effective
- When ready to depart **switch from wall O_2 supply to a cylinder.**

Does the infant require inhaled nitric oxide (iNO) during transfer?

- Stopping iNO therapy abruptly can result in rebound worsening of pulmonary hypertension. Therefore, infants receiving iNO or who have stopped iNO recently should have iNO available for transfer
- iNO delivery during transfer requires a specialized set up and an **experienced clinician** (see nitric oxide delivery, in ❍ Stabilization, p. 475).

Circulation

- Is there **adequate vascular access**? Are all lines **secure** (for transfer)?
  - one peripheral IV line is advisable for infants requiring special care and at least two lines if more unstable, as a safe approach is to assume one line will fail during transfer and therefore it is prudent to place a 'spare' line and consider central access
- How will **blood pressure be monitored**?
  - place an arterial line if there is any concern about cardiovascular status
- Is **perfusion adequate**?
  - ensure an adequate and stable BP before departure. Consider starting inotropes if hypotensive. (see ⟳ Collapse and shock, pp. 186–7)
- In infants with circulatory problems or who are sedated or ventilated, place a urinary catheter to accurately measure urine output
- **Check Hb** and transfuse before departure if anaemic (see ⟳ Anaemia, pp. 398–400)
- **Check coagulation** and administer blood products before departure if coagulopathic (see ⟳ Neonatal clotting abnormalities, pp. 412–15)
- If <24 hours of age, take a **maternal blood sample** for cross-matching at the receiving hospital
- Consider dinoprostone infusion if duct-dependent heart disease suspected

Disability

- Assess pupil size and reactivity, and other neurological signs
- All intubated infants should have sedation, and many should be muscle relaxed to make ventilation easier and reduce the chance of accidental extubation
- Look for seizures and manage accordingly (see ⟳ Neonatal seizures, pp. 290–3)
- Is the infant adequately cushioned/protected within the incubator?

Thermoregulation

- Switch the ambulance heating on before loading the incubator
- Initial incubator temperature guidance:
  - *>2500 g*: 33°C
  - *1500–2500 g*: 35°C
  - *1000–1500 g*: 36°C
  - *<1000 g*: 39°C
- Use heating packs and bubble-wrap (avoid gloves filled with hot water).

Asphyxiated newborns can be cooled during transport if there is careful monitoring of core temperature (see ⟳ Therapeutic hypothermia, pp. 288–9). Passive cooling may be provided by reducing incubator temperature, opening portholes, and adjusting covering. Active cooling needs specialized securable equipment.

Metabolic

- **Stop enteral feeds** for transfer and commence maintenance fluids if necessary
- Ensure **blood glucose** is adequate (approx. 3–12 mmol/l) and stable
- **Check U&Es** and correct any serious disturbances
- Place nasogastric/orogastric tube.

Head-to-toe
Perform a brief exam to confirm pertinent findings and ensure nothing has been overlooked.

Investigations
- Review relevant X-rays and laboratory results
- Obtain copies of case notes, charts, and X-rays to take to receiving unit.

Family support
Meet with the family and bear in mind the following:
- Give **information about the baby's illness** and management. Explain the reason for transfer. Assess their understanding of the situation
- **Avoid painting an unrealistically optimistic picture** and do not be afraid to say that you do not know the answer to certain questions about outcome
- **Do not make negative comments** about the care given by the referring team
- **Obtain agreement** for transfer if possible
- Give **information about the destination** (contact telephone numbers, directions to NICU, parking, accommodation, etc.)
- Parents cannot always accompany the infant in the ambulance for a number of reasons (limited space, insurance of passengers).

Communication
- Ensure you have relevant **telephone numbers** before departing from referral hospital (referring and receiving units, and parents)
- Once the baby has been assessed, **inform the ambulance crew** how long the stabilization period is expected to take so that they are able to refuel and rest
- Before departure, inform the **receiving unit** of the infant's condition and requirements (e.g. ventilation, infusions), and estimated time of arrival.

Documentation
Document the stabilization period, including any procedures undertaken and discussions with parents.

Stabilize or 'scoop and run'?
In certain circumstances, it may be more important to transfer early and reach the specialist centre sooner ('**scoop and run**'), rather than delay transfer in an attempt to further stabilize the infant.

This occurs in two specific situations:
- When nothing can be done to further improve the infant's condition for transfer
- When the outcome from specialist treatment at the receiving hospital is **time-critical** and would be jeopardized by waiting for stabilization (e.g. surgery, or procedure such as balloon atrial septostomy, or ECMO).

This decision must be made after discussion with the receiving unit, sub-specialists, and family, and considering the potential risks and benefits.

Nitric oxide delivery
- A portable iNO circuit can be set up as follows: a small gas cylinder fitted with a flow regulator (set at 0.5 bar) feeds a flow-meter (0–500 l/min) that connects with the inspiratory limb of the ventilator circuit. In addition, an NO monitor needs to be incorporated into the ventilator circuit close to the patient
- Calculate the flow required using the formula:

  [NO required (ppm) × flow in ventilator circuit]/NO in cylinder (ppm)

- Purge the delivery system before connecting to patient
- Remember to connect NO circuit to the bagging circuit during resuscitation
- Use an environmental NO sensor to monitor for leaks, although exhaust fumes may give a false alarm.

Transfer

Moving to the ambulance

- Secure the trolley and all other equipment within the ambulance (ask ambulance staff if you are unsure about how to do this)
- Ensure the infant is as comfortable as possible (e.g. using straps and a 'nest')
- Change equipment over to ambulance **power and gas supplies**
- Ensure all passengers are using **seatbelts**
- Consider **anti-emetics** prior to departure if you suffer from motion sickness.

Monitoring

- HR and electrocardiogram (ECG): movement will cause interference and artefact in the ECG trace. This can be minimized by placing electrodes on bony prominences and ensuring good contact between electrodes and skin
- RR: do not rely solely on the monitor to assess ventilation, but regularly check for chest movement
- Pulse oximetry: causes of poor signal include movement, poor peripheral perfusion, bright ambient lighting, and electromagnetic interference. If there is suspicion of a shunt, monitor both pre- (right hand) and post-ductal (left arm or lower limbs) saturations
- BP: non-invasive BP for well infants and invasive BP for sicker infants. Non-invasive BP devices are affected by vibration and motion, and will tend to overestimate at low pressures and underestimate at high pressures. However, they will still give valuable trend information. Remember to use an appropriate sized cuff. If the invasive BP reading changes suddenly, check the level of the transducer
- Skin and core temperature
- Transcutaneous PO_2 and PCO_2: attach sensors and check correlation with blood gas measurements after moving into the transport incubator just before departure. Readings that become increasingly incongruous with the infant's condition may be due to sensors detaching from the skin during transfer.

Care during the journey

- *Constant vigilance* is required because infants can deteriorate rapidly and without warning. This may be due to either the infant's clinical condition or equipment failure (e.g. dislodged endotracheal tube or IV cannula)
- *Perform regular assessments* of the infant's condition in a systematic manner—ABC (airway, breathing, circulation), especially when moving to and from the ambulance
- Avoid unnecessary interventions, but if required the ambulance should be stopped in the interests of safety
- If in doubt, call for advice from more senior medical staff using a mobile phone.

Airway and breathing
- Continuous monitoring of pulse oximetry and regular checks of chest movement
- Check the blood gas with a portable analyser if the infant's condition deteriorates significantly
- You may need to use higher FiO_2 and higher pressures for the duration of the transfer as movement often compromises ventilation
- Address a sudden fall in oxygen saturation in the usual way, but pay particular attention to disconnected or dislodged equipment (see ⟳ Conventional ventilation, pp. 154–5).

Circulation
- Ensure there is easy access to an IV line to administer drugs or fluid on the move
- Consider continuous blood pressure monitoring
- Movement during transport can compromise cardiac output. Consider fluid boluses if the infant becomes hypotensive and start/increase inotropic support if there is no response (see ⟳ Collapse and shock, pp. 186–7).

Disability
- Monitor for seizures and manage accordingly (see ⟳ Neonatal seizures, pp. 290–3)
- Assess pupil size and reactivity if there is any significant change in the infant's condition.

Thermoregulation
- Monitor skin and core temperature
- Maintain temperature using a hat and gel mattresses, as well as increasing incubator and vehicle environmental temperature
- Avoid opening portholes unless absolutely necessary.

Suctioning
If continuous low-level suction is needed (e.g. infants with oesophageal atresia with a Replogle tube) there are two options:
- Intermittent suction with a portable (high-flow) device every 5–10 minutes *or*
- Use a Y-connector to introduce a hole in the circuit that reduces the suction (low-flow).

Documentation
Make a written record of physiological parameters and any problems and interventions.

Vehicle speed
- Acceleration and deceleration during transfer have a detrimental effect on cardiac output, ventilation, and intracranial pressure
- Inform the ambulance crew of the urgency of the transfer and the need (or lack of need) for 'blue lights'
- In most cases, there is little benefit to travelling at high speed with 'blue lights', but the risk of adverse incidents, such as dislodged tubes, injury to staff, patients, and the public is greatly increased

- Using 'blue lights' should be considered when:
  - road traffic is significantly delaying transfer
  - the infant is being transferred for a time-critical intervention (e.g. neurosurgery)
  - the infant is unstable during transport and decreasing transit time might significantly improve outcome, but balance versus risks.

Handover

Handover needs the full attention of both the transfer and receiving teams.
- Both teams need copies of discharge summary, charts, investigation results, and transport team care records
- Ensure the family is updated.

Difficult decisions

Redirection to palliative care

The nature of neonatal transport means some infants are in a terminal condition by the time of retrieval. In these unfortunate cases, a decision should be made whether to withhold or withdraw/not escalate intensive care and redirect to palliative care at the referring hospital (where the parents may be closer to home and have built a rapport with staff) or to transfer to a specialist centre (an unfamiliar setting, but where the parents may feel 'everything has been done'). Every case is different and careful discussion is needed with the parents and staff at both the referring and receiving units.

Death during transport

If an infant is receiving prolonged cardiopulmonary resuscitation during transfer, the same principles for discontinuation apply as for an in-hospital cardiac arrest.

If death occurs during transfer, proceed to where the parents are most likely to be (usually on the way to the receiving unit). These deaths require referral to the coroner.

Transport equipment checklist

Airway and ventilation equipment

- Transport incubator fixed to trolley
- Transport ventilator, ventilator tubing, and bagging circuit
- Self-inflating bag, valve, facemasks
- Intubation equipment (ETT, introducer, laryngoscope, blades)
- Stethoscope
- Oxygen cylinders
- Portable suction device and suction catheters, including Yankauer
- Nitric oxide kit (ventilator circuit and monitors)
- Nitric oxide cylinder.

Drugs and fluids

- Resuscitation drugs (adrenaline, atropine, sodium bicarbonate), inotropes (dobutamine, dopamine, noradrenaline), sedatives (morphine), muscle relaxants (suxamethonium, pancuronium), anticonvulsants (phenobarbital, paraldehyde), surfactant, calcium gluconate, furosemide, phytomenadione, glucagon, mannitol
- Fluids (maintenance fluids, 0.9% saline, 10% glucose, 4.5% human albumin solution)
- Portable infusion pumps—at least three are needed and more if transporting a sick infant. They should be light-weight, accurate, able to administer boluses, and have a long-life battery.

Vascular access and sampling equipment

- Cannulas
- Syringes
- Umbilical catheter sets
- Lancets.

Monitoring equipment

- Portable monitors (ECG, oximetry, temperature) with visible, as well as audible alarms
- BP transducers
- Portable blood gas analyser (e.g. I-Stat and cartridges)
- Portable glucometer.

Miscellaneous

- Expressed breast milk (EBM)/special formula milk and cool bag
- Warming devices (hat, blankets, gel packs).

Staff

- Patient notes, X-rays, and recording charts
- Transfer letter
- Mobile telephone
- Warm jackets and high-visibility jackets for staff
- Directions to referring hospital
- Snacks
- Anti-emetics
- Parents' contact information
- Torch.

Defibrillators

Rarely needed in newborns. Paramedic ambulances will carry a defibrillator, usually an automatic external defibrillator (AED). Special care is needed when using a defibrillator during transport to keep clear of electrical contacts.

Further information

Barry P, Leslie A. (eds) *Paediatric and neonatal critical care transport*. BMJ Books, London, 2009.

Medical Devices Agency. *Transport of neonates in ambulances*. Department of Health, Guidance of the TINA-Project, London, 1995.

National Institute for Health and Care Excellence (2010) NICE Quality standard 4 (QS4). *Neonatal transfer services*. In: *Neonatal specialist care*. ℘ www.nice.org.uk/guidance/qs4/chapter/Quality-statement-4-Neonatal-transfer-services

Neonatal Transfer Service London Resources. ℘ www.london-nts.nhs.uk/professionals/

NHS England. *Service Specification Neonatal Intensive Care Transport*. 2012. ℘ www.england.nhs.uk/commissioning/wp-content/uploads/sites/12/2015/01/e08-serv-spec-neonatal-critical-transp.pdf

Karlsen KA, Trautman M, Price-Douglas W, Smith S. National Survey of Neonatal Transport Teams in the United States. *Pediatrics*. 2011; **128**: 685–691.

Task Force on Interhospital Transport. *Guidelines for air and ground transport of neonatal and pediatric patients*, 2nd ed. American Academy of Pediatrics, New York, USA, 1993.

Family support, consent, and end of life care

Introduction

Admission of any baby to the neonatal unit is likely to be stressful for the family.

Difficulties for parents when a baby requires neonatal unit admission

- Mother may be unwell and/or physically exhausted from the pregnancy and following delivery
- Grief due to not having a healthy baby
- Feeling powerless to help their baby
- Feelings of guilt that their actions/inactions have caused the illness/ problem leading to admission
- Difficulty forming a normal relationship with their baby due to the restrictions of medical care
- Unfamiliar environment
- Sometimes receiving complex and worrying information regarding their baby's condition
- Travel to and from hospital, especially if other children at home
- Financial difficulties due to not being able to work, travel, and childcare costs.

Key messages

- Listen to and register the concerns of parents
- Empower parents by involving them in care-giving and decision-making
- Facilitate mutual social and emotional attachments between parents and baby
- Foster trust with families through openness and transparency
- Adopt a non-judgemental and impartial attitude
- Provide clear, consistent, and accurate information in a timely manner
- Avoid giving conflicting medical opinions
- Avoid commenting on management decisions of others
- Ensure complete documentation of every discussion with parents
- Aim to resolve disagreements through open discussion, only using the legal process as a last resort.

Communicating with families

The first meeting

- Sit with parents in a quiet room and leave your pager outside/turn mobile phone off if possible. Have a member of nursing staff with you and other family to support parents
- This may be the start of a relationship lasting months or years, and requires a polite and respectful introduction (e.g. 'Hello, my name is…'). Explain your role in the team; ask how the parents would like to be addressed; etc.
- Keep information simple and in manageable amounts. Consider using diagrams and multimedia. Signpost them to useful resources (e.g. Bliss Family Handbook, patient support websites)
- Beware of giving false hope (use 'we need to see how he does over the next few hours' or 'I can't give you a definite answer at this stage', rather than 'everything is fine') but remain appropriately positive (sometimes all parents have is hope)
- Use an interpreter if appropriate and avoid communicating through relatives if possible
- Do not appear hurried
- Avoid medical jargon.

Further discussions

- Foster a partnership between family and medical teams
- Give information in a timely manner
- Important discussions should include a consultant and nurse known to the parents, and as few others (observers) as possible
- Explore family dynamics and belief systems
- Liaise with social workers to understand the family situation if necessary
- Be vigilant for signs of postnatal depression in a vulnerable mother who is being prevented from forming a normal bond with her baby. Psychiatric/psychological support may be helpful
- Do not give confidential information to relatives other than parents unless there is consent to do so.

When a baby is acutely unwell

This can be a time of great uncertainty and there may not be definite answers to give parents. Aim to be informative and sensitive, for example, 'We are supporting his breathing with a ventilator and we are giving him medicines to support his heart. He is very unwell at the moment, but he is in the right place, and we will continue to do everything we can to help him.'

When a baby is chronically unwell

Good communication is vital with families of long-stay babies. Weekly meetings with the lead consultant are a good way of updating parents and addressing their concerns.

When a parent is a healthcare professional

Aim to treat parents in the same manner as you would treat any other parents. It may be useful to state that this is your intention at the first meeting in order to allow them to take the role of parents. Do not assume that they understand everything that is happening—their expertise may lie in a different specialty.

Consent to treatment

Informed consent should be gained, ideally by the person performing the procedure and, at the very least, by someone competent to perform the procedure.

It is best practice to obtain consent for every procedure and examination whenever possible.

If the parents are present at the bedside, always ask for consent before a procedure.

If the parents are not present, *implied consent* is often assumed for *life-saving interventions* (e.g. endotracheal intubation, needle thoracocentesis) and *minor procedures* with minimal risks (e.g. blood sampling and vitamin K administration).

When the parents are absent, consent for *invasive procedures* can be problematic. In general, *time-critical* interventions are often undertaken without formal consent from parents (e.g. lumbar puncture for suspected meningitis). If there is no time pressure then the procedure should be delayed until formal consent is obtained.

Parents may give consent verbally over the telephone, but it is always desirable to have written consent. Ensure verbal consent is clearly documented and involve two staff members for invasive procedures.

Parental responsibility confers the right to give consent on behalf of the infant. The birth mother has parental responsibility. The father has parental responsibility if he is married to the mother or has acquired it through legal process. Only one parent has to give consent to proceed legally but it is preferable to have the agreement of both parents.

In rare cases (in UK law), the High Court has powers to make certain orders regarding children where parental responsibility has been removed or is absent. Social services and the hospital legal department should provide advice in these circumstances.

Cultural and religious beliefs

Occasionally, parents' belief systems may be at odds with the best interests of the baby as perceived by the medical team. These situations are often not clear-cut and should be dealt with sensitively. A typical example is a child of a Jehovah's Witness: explore the parent's beliefs, as some parents may allow use of selected blood products, such as fresh frozen plasma and even blood if there is risk of death. However, the medical team has a duty of care to administer blood products if there is risk of death or permanent injury, even if parents do not consent.

End of life decisions

Modern neonatal intensive care allows us to sustain life even in situations where there may be no benefit for the baby. Decisions to continue, limit escalation, or withdraw/withhold intensive care should reflect the best interests of the baby but also take the views of the family into consideration.

Benefits of any management strategy must outweigh the potential risks not only measured by survival and other clinical indices, but also by quality of life.

The Royal College of Paediatrics and Child Health (RCPCH) framework outlines situations where withdrawal of life-sustaining treatment and redirection towards palliative care may be appropriate:

- When life is limited in **quantity**: if treatment is unable or unlikely to prolong life significantly it may not be in the child's best interests to provide it (i.e. brain stem death, imminent death, or inevitable death)
- When life is limited in **quality**: this includes situations where treatment may be able to prolong life significantly but will not alleviate the burdens associated with illness or treatment itself:
  - burdens of treatments—where the treatments themselves produce sufficient pain and suffering so as to outweigh any potential or actual benefits
  - burdens of the child's underlying condition—here the severity and impact of the child's underlying condition is in itself sufficient to produce such pain and distress as to overcome any potential or actual benefits in sustaining life
  - lack of ability to benefit—the severity of the child's condition is such that it is difficult or impossible for them to derive benefit from continued life.

Key questions when considering redirection of care:
- Are there any potentially treatable problems that have not been excluded?
- Is there sufficient evidence to make a firm prognosis?
- Do the parents fully understand the prognosis?
- Do the parents have adequate support?
- Is there a potential conflict of opinion between the medical team and the parents?

Reaching consensus

Parents should be actively involved in decision-making. Withdrawal of intensive care should be a consensus reached by the medical team and the family whenever possible.

Treatment should usually be continued until any conflict is resolved. Initiate resuscitation in acute situations until senior help arrives or more information becomes available (except in special cases, such as extreme prematurity (i.e. <23 weeks gestation) or severe congenital anomalies, such as anencephaly). Antenatal counselling can be important in helping to reach an agreement with parents before delivery.

The key to reaching consensus is parents understanding and realizing that further treatment would be futile. Often understanding evolves over time through several discussions with the medical team. It is important to give parents enough time to discuss important changes in management whenever possible. Emphasizing that the medical team has reached consensus and is taking the lead on difficult decision-making may help some parents understand when it is appropriate to consider redirection of care.

Limiting intensive care or avoiding escalation of the level of care is sometimes an appropriate interim step. For example, agreeing that extensive resuscitation, such as chest compression and IV adrenaline, are not appropriate but active treatment of other problems, such as resolving endotracheal tube blockages or providing airway suction may be.

Clearly document discussions with parents and decisions to withhold, withdraw, or limit intensive care.

There are times when parents may wish to continue intensive care against the advice of the medical team. This most often occurs when parents have firm cultural beliefs regarding end of life decisions or where communication has been ineffective. However, there is no ethical basis for continuing life support at the parents' request if it is clear that there is no benefit to the baby. Furthermore, the medical team is under a legal obligation to act in the best interests of the baby. In this situation, it is important to explore the reasons behind the parents' views, and suggest that they discuss the situation with family or friends, or seek religious/spiritual advice.

It may be necessary to offer parents a second opinion from within the team or a different hospital. The hospital clinical ethics committee or mediation service may also be useful.

It is extremely unusual to need to resort to a legal process in order to resolve conflict between medical teams and parents in neonatal care. The process begins by consulting the hospital legal team and may progress after presenting the case to a High Court.

The British Association of Perinatal Medicine (BAPM) has suggested the following categories of candidate conditions for perinatal palliative care:

- Category 1: An antenatal or postnatal diagnosis of a condition which is not compatible with long term survival (e.g. bilateral renal agenesis or anencephaly)
- Category 2: An antenatal or postnatal diagnosis of a condition which carries a high risk of significant morbidity or death (e.g. severe bilateral hydronephrosis and impaired renal function)
- Category 3: Babies born at the margins of viability, where intensive care has been deemed inappropriate
- Category 4: Postnatal clinical conditions with a high risk of severe impairment of quality of life and when the baby is receiving life support or may at some point require life support (e.g. severe hypoxic ischaemic encephalopathy)
- Category 5: Postnatal conditions which result in the baby experiencing 'unbearable suffering' in the course of their illness or treatment (e.g. severe necrotizing enterocolitis, where palliative care is in the baby's best interests).

Support of babies and families during withdrawal of intensive care and provision of palliative care

Carefully consider each family's needs as this will be different for everyone and be variable across different cultures. Where there is a choice, parents should be given information regarding alternatives and be supported by a multi-disciplinary team to make their own decisions (e.g. location, who is present, timing, etc.).

An experienced member of the nursing staff can guide the family through the process and act as the primary contact with the medical team.

If the duration is expected to last days then consider transfer to a hospice or home under the care of a specialized palliative care team.

- Most units have a 'bereavement pack' with advice on local procedures to follow, documentation check lists, and other useful information
- Move baby and family to a separate/side room if possible. If not possible, use screens and provide as much privacy as possible
- Encourage parents to hold baby and be involved in care as appropriate and respecting family's wishes
- Devote sufficient time to support parents with genuine sensitivity and empathy, and treat them with respect and dignity
- Inform the parents that the baby may die very soon (i.e. minutes) after being taken off the ventilator, but that this may take hours or days and involve colour changes, laboured breathing, gasping, and other signs of life for a variable period of time
- Remove as much intensive care equipment as possible (i.e. vascular lines and catheters)
- Take tissue samples for diagnostic purposes if necessary and consent has been obtained for this
- Consider discontinuing monitoring, medications, and investigations
- Allow time and space for the gathering of family member or friends
- Offer the chance to bathe and make hand/foot-prints, photographs, take a lock of hair, and provide other mementos according to family's wishes
- Arrange baptism or other religious service if requested
- Keep the baby comfortable using positioning, skin care, mouth care, feeding, analgesia including paracetamol, buccal midazolam, morphine increased as needed, anticonvulsants as needed, glycopyrronium bromide or hyoscine to decrease secretions as needed. Be clear with parents about the purpose of medication
- Withdrawal of intensive care and redirection to palliative care can continue despite recent use of muscle relaxants, but not if they have been administered immediately before a planned withdrawal of intensive care
- It is unlawful to administer a medication with the primary intent to cause or shorten time to death
- Intermittently examine and auscultate for heart sounds and certify death in the usual manner
- An experienced doctor should complete the death certificate and explain the causes to parents as appropriate

- The body should be moved to a cold room or mortuary <4–6 hours after death
- Ask about religious or cultural considerations that should be respected. For example, Muslim parents may wish burial to take place within 24 hours; Sikh parents may not wish toys or clothing with animals near the baby at the time of death. Hospitals usually have an on-call member of the spiritual care department to give advice
- Provide parents information on how and where to certify death. If a baby is born with signs of life before 24 weeks the parents must register both the birth and death
- There should be local procedures for informing relevant healthcare professionals, including GP, health visitor, midwife, Child Death Overview Panel (CDOP)
- Deaths may be reported to the coroner for a number of reasons, usually because the cause of death is not known or, sometimes, because there is a suspicion of trauma or medical negligence
- Neonatal organ donation has been facilitated on rare occasions but this is complicated by difficulties around diagnosing brain stem death in the newborn.

Post mortem (PM) examination

A hospital PM examination should be offered to all parents after the death of a newborn baby. The PM may provide significant information regarding the cause of death in ~60–80% of cases and may have implications for future pregnancies. Reassure parents that a PM does not involve mutilation or unnecessary retention of organs. PMs in neonates are usually carried out by a perinatal pathologist and tissue samples and other material may be retained according to parental consent. The parents will be asked what they would like to happen to this material, including tissue blocks and slides. The charity Sands and the Human Tissue Authority have developed a standardized consent form and support booklets for this purpose. The options for parents are complete PM, a limited PM, or an external PM. A complete PM consists of an external examination with photos and X-rays, an internal examination of the organs usually through a longitudinal incision from the top of the sternum to just above the pubic bone, and another incision around the back of the scalp. Small samples of tissue are taken from the organs for microscopic examination the and sometimes fixed in formalin to enable examination. In a limited PM only certain areas of the body are examined (e.g. chest and neck, abdomen or head). Limited and external PM may not pick up some abnormalities. The role of PM MRI is currently being evaluated. A PM ordered by the coroner does not need parental consent.

Bereavement follow-up care

Each neonatal unit should have a follow-up programme for bereaved families. Parents may also access resources through their GP including counselling and psychological support and other support groups (e.g. via Sands). Meetings with an obstetrician and geneticist may also be useful. It is important to remember that staff may require additional support. Formal staff debriefing following the death of a baby may be useful and counselling services should be available for staff if required.

Further information

Association for Children's Palliative Care. *A Neonatal Pathway for Babies with Palliative Care Needs*. ACT, 2009. ★ www.togetherforshortlives.org.uk/assets/0000/7095/Neonatal_Pathway_for_ Babies_5.pdf

Beauchamp T, Childress J. *Principles of biomedical ethics*, 6th ed. Oxford University Press, Oxford, UK, 2008.

BAPM. *Consent in neonatal clinical care: Good practice framework*. British Association of Perinatal Medicine, London, 2004.

Henley A, Schott J. Stillbirth and Neonatal Death Society. Guide for consent takers. *Seeking consent/ authorisation for the post mortem examination of a baby*. Sands, London, 2012.

Larcher V, Craig F, Bhogal K, Wilkinson D, Brierley J. Making decisions to limit treatment in life-limiting and life-threatening conditions in children: a framework for practice. *Arch Dis Child* 2015; **100** (S2): s1–s23.

Mancini A, Uthaya S, Beardsley C, Modi N. Royal College of Paediatrics and Child Health. *Practical guidance for the management of palliative care on neonatal units*. RCPCH, London, 2014.

Schott J, Henley A, Kohner N. Stillbirth and Neonatal Death Society. *Pregnancy Loss and the Death of a Baby: Guidelines for professionals*. Sands, London, 2007.

Organizations

Stillbirth and Neonatal Death Society. ★ www.uk-sands.org

Child Bereavement UK. ★ www.childbereavement.org.uk

Practical procedures

Endotracheal intubation

Indications
- Obtain definitive and secure airway to provide respiratory support
- Administration of surfactant.

Equipment
- Laryngoscope + straight blades (size 00 for extreme preterms, 0 for moderate preterms, 1 for term infants)
- Continuous heart rate and O_2 saturation monitoring
- Endotracheal tubes (ETT) including a size above and below (see Table 20.1) with introducer (optional)
- Ventilation equipment and gas supply—appropriate size facemask + self-inflating bag or breathing system (e.g. Neopuff/Ayre's T-piece)
- Fixation device (many types used), or ties and flange
- Suction system with Yankauer sucker/10 FG (black) suction catheter
- IV access and appropriate drugs for intubation (in elective cases)
- End-tidal CO_2 probe and monitor or colorimetric device
- Ventilator ready to use (tubing, connectors, settings).

Procedure
Requires careful supervision until competent. Prepare ETT and insert introducer if required (not protruding from end) and bend around connector. Hold laryngoscope in left hand, open blade, and check light source.
- **Step 1: position** the baby supine with head in midline and slightly extended (can use a rolled-up nappy under neck)
- **Step 2: suction** the oropharynx to clear secretions
- **Step 3: pre-oxygenate** baby for 1–3 min and ensure vital signs stable
- **Step 4: elective intubations:** administer drugs for intubation, e.g. **fentanyl** (5 µg/kg), **atropine** (20 µg/kg), then **suxamethonium** (2 mg/kg). **NB** Muscle relaxants should only be used by someone competent to manage airways
- **Step 5: insert blade** in the midline
- **Step 6: lift the epiglottis** using a vertical movement of the laryngoscope to reveal the vocal cords (see Fig. 20.1), gastric tube may provide a guide
- **Step 7: hold ETT** in right hand, introduce into right corner of mouth and **pass the tip of the ETT through the cords** under direct vision until the thick black mark lies just past the cords (1–2 cm). An assistant continuously monitors O_2 sats and heart rate, and advises when to resume mask ventilation (at 30 s, or if bradycardic or sats and HR falling precipitously) and return to step 1

Table 20.1 Recommended endotracheal tube (ETT) size and insertion length

Gestational age (weeks)	Weight (g)	ETT size, internal diameter (mm)	Oral insertion length
23–24	<600	2–2.5	5.5
25–27	700–1000	2.5	6–6.5
30–34	1000–2000	3.0	7–7.5
34–38	2000–3500	3–3.5	7.5–8
>38	>3500	3.5–4.0	8.5–9.0

Tracheal intubation

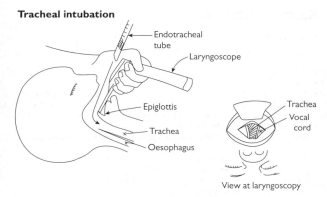

Fig. 20.1 Anatomy of the airway.

- **Step 8:** remove introducer, attach the bagging system to the ETT and start ventilating
- **Step 9:** check for **correct placement** by observing for **good chest movement**, improving O_2 sats, auscultating for bilateral and equal breath sounds in chest, absence of breath sounds over stomach, and rise in end tidal CO_2. If there is no improvement in sats and heart rate then remove the tube and start bagging without delay, and return to step 1
- **Step 10:** firmly hold the ETT at the lips. **Fix the ETT** with a preformed fixation device or suturing flange to ETT, and tying flange to a hat
- **Step 11: trim ETT** to reduce dead space
- **Step 12: connect to ventilator** and **observe** chest movement
- **Step 13:** check ETT position using **CXR** (tip between clavicles and carina, overlying T2–3)
- **Step 14: document** in case notes: view of cords, number of attempts and problems during procedure, size of ETT and length from tip to lips.

Helpful hints

- If in doubt that tube is in the correct place, take it out
- **ETT length:** approx. weight + 6 cm at lips, less reliable under 1 kg (see Table 20.1)
- Overextending the neck can obscure the view of the cords
- Cricoid pressure (gentle downward pressure on the cricoid cartilage) may improve view of the cords
- Do not use excessive force to pass the ETT through closed or tight cords
- If air entry is greater on the right, slowly withdraw ETT until air entry is equal.

Complications

- Local trauma to mouth, oropharynx, or nasopharynx
- Pneumothorax
- Airway oedema and subglottic stenosis.

Nasal intubation

Procedure
- Appropriate for term infants needing longer duration of respiratory support
- Follow the same principles as for oral intubation
- Lubricate an ETT
- Pass ETT through a nostril (take care that the nose does not remain blanched), aim vertically and use rotary motion. If this is difficult, try passing a nasogastric tube (NGT) then pass ETT over it
- Visualize the cords as for oral intubation
- Grip the end of ETT with Magill forceps and, under direct vision, pass it through the cords
- If an oral ETT is present, ask an assistant to remove this just before passing the nasal tube through the cords
- Fix using Y-shaped/trouser leg sticky tape around ETT on to a hydrocolloid dressing over the lips and cheeks.

Needle thoracocentesis

Indications
- Emergency drainage of a suspected tension pneumothorax
- Drainage of a pneumothorax in a baby too unstable for chest drain insertion
- Exclude a pneumothorax when unable to ventilate a baby *in extremis*.

Equipment
- Alcohol swab
- 21 G (green) or 23 G (blue) butterfly
- Universal container
- Sterile water or 10 ml syringe with 3-way tap.

Procedure
- **Clean skin** with alcohol swab at entry site (2nd intercostal space in the mid-clavicular line)
- **Immerse** the end of the butterfly tubing in a universal container containing water
- **Insert** the needle at 90° to the chest and advance slowly until air bubbles through the water. Aiming slightly lateral may reduce the risk of leaving an open track on removal. (Alternatively, attach a 3-way tap to the end of the butterfly and gently aspirate air then close tap to patient and expel air from syringe.)
- When bubbling has stopped, **remove the needle** and cover site with a **non-occlusive dressing**
- Insert a chest drain (see ➲ Intercostal (chest) drain insertion, pp. 498–9) as soon as possible.

Pericardial effusion drainage

Indications

- Cardiac tamponade confirmed by echocardiography
- Unexplained cardiac arrest in a baby with a central venous line or post-cardiac surgery.

Equipment

- Alcohol swab
- Cannula 22 G (blue)/20 G (pink); or needle 21 G (green)/23 G (blue)
- 10 ml syringe.

Procedure

- Discuss with neonatologist and cardiologist
- Perform under **US guidance** if possible and with continuous ECG monitoring
- **Clean the skin** at the xiphisternum with an antibacterial swab and allow to dry
- **Insert the needle** with syringe attached at 30° angle to the skin just below and left of the xiphisternum. See Fig. 20.2
- **Slowly advance** the needle, whilst aspirating, aiming for the left shoulder
- Stop when there is 'flashback' and **aspirate** up to 10 ml
- **Withdraw the needle** and monitor closely.

Complications

- Cardiac chamber puncture
- Cardiac arrhythmias
- Pneumothorax and pneumopericardium.

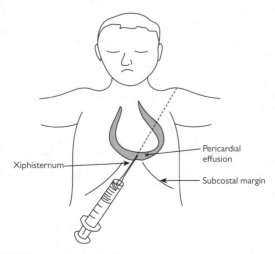

Fig. 20.2 Drainage of pericardial effusion.

Intercostal (chest) drain insertion

Indications
Drainage of pneumothorax or pleural effusion.

Equipment
- Sterile gown and drapes
- Antibacterial cleaning solution and saline
- Local anaesthetic (lidocaine 1%), 5 ml syringe, and 25 G (orange) and 23 G (blue) needles for term babies
- Chest drain insertion pack
- Intercostal drain (8–12 F), straight or pig-tail drains
- Guidance for selecting drain size is the bigger the better: <2.5 kg = 8F, 2.5–3.0 kg = 10 F, 3.0–3.5 kg = 12 F, >3.5 kg = 14 F
- Skin closure strips (e.g. Steri-Strips™)
- Adhesive dressing
- Scalpel
- Suture
- Underwater collection bottle sometimes on suction.

Procedure
Aseptic technique using adequate sedation and analgesia. Avoid using the trochar included with most drains.
- **Position** the infant with the arm fully abducted and chest elevated on the side of insertion by 45° to horizontal for pneumothoraces or supine for pleural effusions
- **Clean skin** with antibacterial cleaning solution
- Infiltrate insertion site (usually 4th intercostal space mid-axillary line but depends on imaging) with **local anaesthetic** (lidocaine 1%) and wait 2 minutes to take effect
- Make a small (1–2 cm) **skin incision** parallel to and at the upper border of the rib below (avoiding the neurovascular bundle and breast bud)
- **Bluntly dissect** through muscle layers down to the pleura by gently pushing with artery forceps, and repeatedly opening them parallel and perpendicular to the ribs
- **Open the pleura** with a small nick of the scalpel
- **Introduce the drain** with a 3-way tap into the pleural space using forceps and quickly advance 2–3 cm to avoid air being entrained
- For pneumothoraces, aim anteriorly and apically; for effusions, aim posteriorly, and basally
- Pig-tail drains are inserted using the Seldinger technique without dissection. They can be less traumatic and more secure, but block more easily
- **Connect the drain** to the underwater collection bottle and observe for bubbling/swinging with respiration
- **Close the skin incision** tightly around the drain using sutures
- **Suture the drain to the skin** by repeatedly encircling and knotting around drain
- Apply **adhesive dressing** around drain site to make an airtight seal
- Perform **CXR** to check drain position and assess for improvement of the pneumothorax/effusion.

Complications
- Malposition
- Haemorrhage
- Infection
- Lung parenchymal injury
- Pericardial injury
- Thoracic duct injury
- Phrenic nerve injury
- Scarring.

Intercostal drain removal

Procedure

Remove drains when bubbling and swinging has stopped for at least 12–24 hours. If unsure whether a drain is still needed, clamp the drain and observe over the next 6 hours for re-accumulation clinically and/or perform CXR.

- Remove dressing and cut fixing sutures
- Withdraw the drain and rapidly pinch the wound closed with fingers (wearing sterile gloves). Time with expiration if possible
- Use skin closure strips and adhesive dressing to close the incision and make an airtight seal (sutures are occasionally needed)
- Observe for signs of re-accumulation and perform CXR if concerned.

Blood sampling: heel pricks

The choice of route depends upon the volume of blood required:
- Small volumes (<2 ml) heel pricks. Heel pricks are useful to conserve veins in long-term patients
- Intermediate volumes (>2 ml) venepuncture
- Large volumes (>5 ml and difficult access) venepuncture and sometimes arterial stab.

Remember to label specimens correctly, hand-label specimens for group and save/cross-match. Common samples include:
- **EDTA**: FBC, group and save/cross-match, DNA analysis
- **Lithium heparin (or bottle with** clot activator and serum gel separator **(check local requirements)**: U&Es, liver function, bone profile, chromosomes
- **Citrate**: coagulation studies
- **Oxalate**: glucose.

Equipment
- Automated lancet
- Paraffin oil
- Cotton wool.

Procedure

Ensure the foot is warm and well perfused (massage foot or place next to glove filled with warm water for few minutes).
- Clean the heel with an antibacterial swab and allow to dry
- Smear a small amount of paraffin over the puncture site
- Use an automated lancet to pierce the skin at a point along the lateral or medial margins of the plantar hind foot (avoid the calcaneal area due to risk of osteomyelitis; see Fig. 20.3)
- Gently milk the foot from toes to heel to encourage bleeding and collect blood as it forms droplets directly into bottles
- Pressure with cotton wool to stop the bleeding.

Helpful hints
- Alcohol swabs and paraffin oil may affect blood glucose measurements
- Excessive force may falsely elevate potassium and lactate levels as well as cause bruising and discomfort
- Capillary blood gases are less reliable taken from cold or poorly perfused feet.

Complications
- Bruising
- Infection (superficial and osteomyelitis).

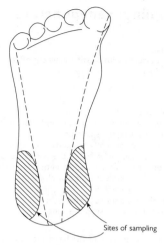

Sites of sampling

Fig. 20.3 Sites for heel prick.

Blood sampling: venepuncture

Equipment
- Antibacterial swab
- Winged needle, butterfly with plastic tubing cut off, or needle, 21 G (green) or 23 G (blue)
- Cotton wool.

Procedure
- Identify a suitable vein
- **Clean the skin** with an antibacterial swab and allow to dry
- Stabilize the vein by pulling the skin taut
- Hold the limb and squeeze gently, proximally, or apply a tourniquet
- **Insert the needle** at an angle of 30° to the skin, bevel upwards, and advance slowly until a vessel is pierced and there is flashback of blood
- Hold the needle still and **collect drops of blood** directly into bottles, while maintaining the tourniquet
- **Remove the needle** and dispose in sharps bin
- Pressure with cotton wool to **stop bleeding**.

Helpful hints
- Common sites include **dorsum of the hand and foot**. The **antecubital fossa** and **long saphenous vein** at the ankle should be spared for central access
- If blood stops flowing, the needle may have migrated out of the vein, move the needle very slowly forward and backwards until flow resumes
- Consider whether inserting a cannula and collecting blood would be more appropriate.

Blood sampling: arterial stab

Equipment
- Alcohol swab
- Butterfly with plastic tubing cut off or needle, 25 G (orange)
- Cotton wool.

Procedure
Common sites are the **radial, ulnar, posterior tibial**, and **dorsalis pedis arteries**. Occasionally brachial and femoral arteries are used.

Do not access more than one artery in each limb and document all attempts, even if unsuccessful.
- Identify the artery by **palpation** or by using a **fibre-optic ('cold') light**
- **Clean the skin** with an antibacterial swab and allow to dry
- **Check adequate collateral circulation** using firm pressure to occlude the artery and assessing distal perfusion
- Hold the limb in the **anatomical position** (marked flexion/extension can impair blood flow), keep the leg abducted and flexed when accessing the femoral artery
- **Insert the needle** at an angle of 30° to the skin and advance slowly until the artery is hit
- Hold the needle still and **collect drops of blood** directly into bottles
- **Remove the needle** and dispose in sharps bin
- Firm and prolonged pressure with cotton wool to **stop bleeding**.

Helpful hints
- Use only if large volumes of blood needed and other routes are difficult
- There are a limited number of sites and can only be used a limited number of times so consider whether an arterial line is appropriate.

Complications
- Haemorrhage
- Infection
- Thrombosis
- Distal ischaemia.

Peripheral venous cannulation

Indications

Administration of fluids and drugs.

Equipment

- Antibacterial swab
- 24 G (yellow) cannula
- Extension set flushed with saline
- 5 ml syringe with saline
- Clear dressing/Steri-Strips™
- Splint
- Cotton wool.

Procedure

- Identify a suitable vein (common sites include **dorsum of hands and feet, antecubital fossa, long saphenous vein** at ankle and temples of **scalp**) a fibre-optic ('cold') light is helpful in preterms, shave the scalp with a safety razor
- **Clean the skin** with an antibacterial swab and allow to dry
- Stabilize the vein by pulling the skin taut
- Hold the limb and squeeze gently, proximally, or apply a tourniquet
- **Insert the cannula** at an angle of 30° to the skin, bevel upwards, and advance slowly until a vessel is pierced, and there is flashback of blood into the hub
- **Advance the plastic** Teflon® cannula into the vein and **remove the stylet**
- **Collect blood** directly into bottles or aspirate using needle and syringe
- **Fix the cannula** to the skin with tapes/Steri-Strips™, whilst occluding the vessel with pressure proximally
- Attach the extension set and **flush with saline**
- Cover with a **non-encircling clear dressing**
- Use a **splint** to immobilize the limb and bandage if the baby is active.

Helpful hints

- Practice makes perfect but many units adopt a **three strikes and out** policy—i.e. stop after three attempts and ask for help
- Peripheral veins should be used initially and spare larger veins for central access (e.g. long saphenous and antecubital fossa veins).

Complications

- Bruising
- Infection
- Extravasation of infusate.

Peripheral arterial cannulation

Indications

Invasive blood pressure monitoring and frequent blood sampling.

Equipment

- Antibacterial swab
- 24 G (yellow) cannula
- 5 ml syringe with saline
- 3-way tap and extension set (primed with saline)
- Skin closure strips
- Clear dressing
- Splint
- Heparinized saline infusion
- Blood pressure transducer set (primed with saline).

Procedure

First choice: radial, ulnar, posterior tibial, and dorsalis pedis arteries.

Second choice: axillary and femoral arteries.

Do not access more than one artery in each limb and document all attempts, even if unsuccessful.

- **Allen's test:** confirms there is collateral blood supply to the hand when the ulnar artery is to be cannulated. Pressure on the radial and ulnar arteries causes blanching of the hand that pinks up when each artery is released alternately
- **Palpate** the artery and visualize its course. A **fibre-optic ('cold') light** is helpful in preterms
- **Clean the skin** with an antibacterial swab and allow to dry
- **Insert** the cannula at an angle of 30–45°
- **Slowly advance** the cannula until flashback of blood is seen in the hub
- **Advance** the Teflon® cannula into the artery and remove the stylet
- Apply firm pressure to the artery proximally while attaching an **extension set and 3-way tap** to avoid excessive blood loss
- **Secure the cannula** to the skin with Steri-Strips™, apply a clear dressing, and **splint** the limb in a comfortable position
- Flush with saline and attach **transducer** and prescribe **heparin infusion** (1 U/ml at 0.5–1 ml/h)
- Observe for **signs of distal ischaemia.**

Helpful hints

- The artery may be **transfixed** by entering the artery and passing through the posterior wall. Slowly withdraw the cannula until flashback of blood is seen and advance the plastic cannula
- **Arterial spasm** may occur immediately following cannulation causing a transient reduction in blood flow, presenting as 'damp' trace of arterial wave form or duskiness of extremities, wait for flow to normalize and apply GTN patch to improve distal perfusion. If perfusion does not improve then remove the cannula.

Complications

- Haemorrhage
- Infection
- Thrombosis and distal ischaemia.

Umbilical arterial catheterization

Easiest on first day of life and possible up to 5–7 days after delivery.

Indications

Secure and in-dwelling vascular access for frequent blood sampling, invasive blood pressure monitoring, or to perform exchange transfusion.

Equipment

- Sterile drapes and gown
- Umbilical catheter set (scalpel holder, artery forceps, non- and toothed forceps, dilator, needle holder, pot, swabs)
- Antibacterial solution (e.g. chlorhexidine)
- Cord ligature
- 10 ml syringe
- 3-way tap
- Umbilical catheter
- Suture
- Blood pressure transducer.

Procedure

Aseptic technique. An assistant is essential during cleaning to hold the cord and to help maintain asepsis during central access procedures.

- Open the catheter set onto a trolley and add other equipment while maintaining a sterile field
- Wash hands, put on sterile gown and gloves
- Attach 3-way tap to the catheter and prime with saline
- **Clean the umbilical stump and surrounding skin** with antibacterial cleaning solution
- Arrange drapes around the umbilicus creating a sterile field, allowing access to vascular lines and airway should it become necessary
- Loosely **tie the cord ligature** around the base of the stump with artery forceps ready to clamp the stump if blood loss becomes difficult to control
- **Cut the cord horizontally**, cleanly and 1–2 cm from the base of the stump with a scalpel
- Grip the Wharton's jelly with toothed forceps and **identify the umbilical vessels** (arteries: two, small/2 mm, protruding and muscular; vein: single, larger, thin walled)
- Gently **pass the dilator** or fine forceps into the artery, and use a circular motion to dilate the vessel opening
- Gently **introduce the catheter** holding it with non-toothed forceps
- Insert the catheter to the desired length and **aspirate** blood to check correct position
- **Fix the catheter** with a suture through the stump (avoiding the vessels) and tied around the catheter
- Alternatively, use tape in an H shape from the abdominal wall to the catheter and tie suture to tape
- **Label** with 'arterial' label or red button on 3-way tap
- Attach **an extension set and transducer** then flush

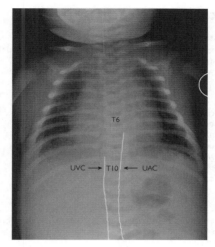

Fig. 20.4 X-ray showing positions of umbilical catheter tips.

- Prescribe **heparin infusion** (1 U/ml at 0.5–1 ml/h)
- Check tip position on an **X-ray**, ideally 'high' (T6–10) or 'low' (below L3) to avoid coeliac axis, renal, and mesenteric arteries. See Fig 20.4.
- Catheters can be pulled back using a similar aseptic technique, but never advanced due to the risk of infection
- **Document** procedure in case notes (size and length of catheter, blood loss, lower limb perfusion, complications)
- Observe for **signs of impaired blood flow to the buttocks and lower limbs.**

Helpful hints
- **Size of catheter** depends upon size of baby (<1500 g = 3.5 Fr; 1500–2500 g = 4 Fr; >2500 g = 5 Fr)
- **Length to be inserted** = 3 × weight (kg) + 9 cm + stump length (cm)
- Monitor the infant's condition, whilst covered by drapes
- Sometimes there is resistance at the base of the stump because the artery initially runs caudally, pull the stump towards the baby's head and aim the catheter caudally
- Using excessive force may create a false passage within the cord.

Complications
- Haemorrhage
- Peritoneal perforation
- Ischaemia and thrombosis
- Infection.

Umbilical venous catheterization

Indications
- Secure vascular access for frequent blood sampling, drug and fluid administration, or to perform exchange transfusion
- Emergency administration of drugs and fluid during resuscitation.

Equipment
- Sterile drapes and gown
- Umbilical catheter set (scalpel holder, artery forceps, toothed forceps, dilator, needle holder, swabs)
- Antibacterial cleaning solution
- Cord ligature
- 5 ml syringe
- 3-way tap
- Umbilical catheter
- Suture.

Procedure
- Umbilical arterial catheterization (UAC) insertion is often more difficult and may be attempted first
- Aseptic technique
- Same approach as insertion of UAC. See Fig 20.5.

Helpful hints

> **Length to be inserted** = 2 × weight (kg) + 5 cm + stump length (cm)

- Monitor the infant's condition whilst covered by drapes
- Using excessive force may create a false passage within the cord
- If there is resistance at 2 cm, the UVC may be in the portal sinus. Withdraw slightly and reinsert
- Tip of line should lie in the inferior vena cava, but not in the right atrium or liver
- If inserted during resuscitation it should be done as cleanly as practically possible and replaced under sterile conditions once on the NNU.

Complications
- Haemorrhage
- Peritoneal perforation
- Arrhythmias (if tip in the heart)
- Infection.

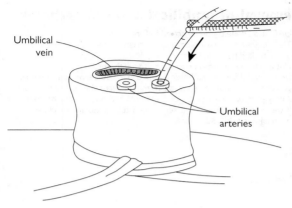

Fig. 20.5 Umbilical catheterization.

Removal of umbilical arterial catheter

- UAC should ideally be removed before 10 days
- Tie a loose cord ligature around the base of the stump in case of uncontrolled haemorrhage
- Cut any fixing sutures and mobilize the catheter
- Slowly withdraw the catheter and pause for 30 seconds at the final centimetre to allow arterial spasm that reduces the risk of haemorrhage
- Apply pressure with gauze for 5 minutes and observe for haemorrhage
- If there are concerns about sepsis then cut the tip and send for microbiology (MC&S).

Percutaneous central ('long') line insertion

Indications
Long-term administration of drugs, fluid, or parenteral nutrition.

Equipment
- Measuring tape
- Sterile gown and drapes
- Central venous line pack (<1000 g = 1 Fr; >1000 g = 2 Fr)
- Dressing pack (forceps, swabs, pot)
- Antibacterial cleaning solution (e.g. chlorhexidine)
- 10 ml syringe and saline and 21 G (green) needle
- Skin closure strips
- Clear dressing.

Procedure
Aseptic technique requiring an assistant. Common sites are: **antecubital fossa, axillary, saphenous,** and **scalp** veins.
- **Estimate** desired insertion length: measure from site of entry along the course of the vein to the top of the sternum (superior vena cava) or xiphisternum (inferior vena cava) as appropriate
- Wash hands, put on sterile gown and gloves
- Prime the central line with saline
- **Clean the skin** with antibacterial solution before applying sterile drapes
- **Insert the needle/cannula** provided in the pack into a vein until blood flows or insert a cannula large enough to hold the central line
- **Advance** the **central line** using non-toothed forceps to the desired length (the limb may have to be manipulated to allow the line to pass the angle at the shoulder/groin)
- Depending on the type, the **needle can be withdrawn over the line and the hub screwed together, or the needle/cannula pulled or snapped apart,** taking care not to withdraw the line, and press on insertion site to control haemorrhage
- **Secure the line to the skin** using skin closure strips, coil the remainder of the line taking care not to kink it, place sterile hydrocolloid dressing patch or gauze under the hub to prevent skin damage, and apply a clear dressing
- Check line tip position using X-ray (small lines that are radiolucent may require contrast). Line tip should lie within a large vein, ideally the vena cava and outside the heart.

Helpful hints
- Make a sterile tourniquet from a rolled piece of gauze
- Small bore lines require high pressure pumps
- Malposition is common. If any doubt in position of line tip, ask for senior review
- If the line becomes blocked, try to flush with 10 ml syringe or instil urokinase (1 ml of 5000 U) and lock for 15 minutes; high pressure may damage the line.

Complications
- Haemorrhage
- Pericardial tamponade
- Arrhythmias
- Thrombosis
- Infection
- Extravasation
- Air embolism.

Femoral and internal jugular central venous line insertion

Indications

Short-term administration of drugs, fluid, or parenteral nutrition (e.g peri-operatively).

Equipment

- As in ➋ Percutaneous central ('long') line insertion, pp. 514–15.
- Central line insertion sterile pack
- Central line catheter pack (7.5 F 10–15 cm triple lumen or other suitable line).

Procedure

Aseptic technique requiring assistant.

- Wash hands, put on sterile gown and gloves
- Attach 3-way taps to each lumen of the line and prime with saline
- **Clean the skin** with antibacterial solution before applying sterile drapes
- Insert using the Seldinger technique.

Femoral vein

- **Femoral vein landmarks:** aim just medial to the pulsation of the femoral artery (midway between anterior superior iliac spine and symphysis pubis) at the inguinal ligament in the groin. **Insert the needle and syringe** at 30–45° angle and aiming for the umbilicus whilst aspirating.

Internal jugular vein

- Position the baby supine with a 20° tilt, head down, and the head turned away from the side of insertion
- **Insert needle and syringe** at the junction of the sternal and clavicular heads of sternocleidomastoid muscle, anterior, and lateral to the carotid artery at a 30° angle, aiming for the nipple
- When there is blood flashback, **remove the syringe**
- Ensure blood flows freely and **pass the guide wire through the needle** (it should pass easily) and advance a few cm. If the guide wire gets caught, withdraw slightly, rotate, and re-advance
- **Remove the needle over the guide wire** while controlling blood loss at the puncture site with a swab (take care not to withdraw the wire inadvertently)
- Larger bore lines require a **dilator** to be passed over the guide wire and into the vein to widen the lumen using a corkscrew movement
- **Insert the line over the guide wire** (keep an eye on the distal end of the guide wire at all times and ensure it's not advanced excessively)
- **Remove the guide wire**
- **Fix the line** to the skin with sutures and a clear dressing
- Check line tip position with an **X-ray**.

Intraosseous access

Indications
Difficult vascular access during resuscitation in a collapsed infant for blood sampling, fluid, and drug administration.

Equipment
- Antibacterial swab
- 18 G intraosseous needle
- 10 ml syringe
- Extension set flushed with saline
- Gauze
- Tapes.

Procedure
- **Clean the skin** with antibacterial swab and allow to dry
- **Insert the needle** at 90° into the flat part of the upper, anteromedial tibia (1 cm below the tibial tuberosity)
- Screw the needle until there is an unmistakable crunch when passing through the cortex and remove the trochar or use a specifically designed drill
- **Aspirate** bloody marrow, check blood glucose and send remainder for analysis
- **Fix with tape** and stabilize with gauze
- **Attach extension set** and administer drugs/fluids.

Helpful hints
- Alternative site is the anterolateral surface of femur, 2 cm above the lateral condyle
- Administer fluids by pushing a syringe because of resistance to passive flow in the marrow
- Watch for swelling on the lateral and posterior leg, a sign that the line is no longer within the bone marrow
- Rarely performed in preterm infants; spinal needles can be used instead of intraosseous needles.

Complications
- Fractures
- Infection
- Malposition
- Growth plate injury.

Exchange transfusion

Indications
- Severe hyperbilirubinaemia
- Disseminated intravascular coagulation
- Severe anaemia
- Severe metabolic disease.

Equipment
- Central arterial and/or venous access and peripheral venous access
- O negative blood, fresh (<5 days old), CMV negative, leuco-depleted, irradiated if the baby had *in utero* transfusions, with PVC 50–55% (i.e. not packed cells)
- Blood-giving sets (and warming coil)
- 3-way taps
- Blood discard container
- Recording sheet
- Discuss with parents due to risk of serious complications.

Procedure
- NBM before and until there is no further risk of another exchange (due to the risk of NEC)
- Vascular access to withdraw and transfuse blood, ideally UVC and UAC
- Usually perform double volume exchange for haemolytic disease, circulating blood volume = 80 ml/kg (term), 100 ml/kg (preterm), i.e. 160 ml/kg in term infants
- **Withdraw blood in 5–20 ml aliquots** over 5 min/aliquot
- Aliquots: <28 weeks = 5 ml; 28–32 weeks = 10 ml; 32–36 weeks = 15 ml; >36 weeks = 20 ml
- **Infuse blood** over total exchange time
- Assistant to record carefully on a sheet each aliquot that is removed and given
- **Check bloods** (gas, glucose, bilirubin, Ca, U&Es, FBC) at start, midway, and end-points
- Closely monitor vital signs throughout procedure.

Ideally, withdraw through arterial line and replace continuously via UVC. If UVC is the only access then withdraw and replace alternately. Use a closed circuit technique to prevent air embolus.

Complications
- Mortality 1–4%
- Thromboembolism
- Infection
- Hypovolaemia or circulatory overload
- Acid–base and electrolyte disturbances (metabolic acidosis, hypoglycaemia, hyperkalaemia, hypocalcaemia)
- Coagulation disturbance (thrombocytopenia)
- Transfusion reactions
- Hypothermia
- Necrotizing enterocolitis
- Air embolism
- Cardiac arrhythmias.

Dilutional exchange transfusion

Indications
Polycythaemia.

Equipment
- As for exchange transfusion
- Replace with 0.9% saline instead of blood

Volume to replace = total blood volume × (observed PCV
− desired PCV)/observed PCV

PCV = packed cell volume, desired PCV usually 0.55.

Procedure
- Withdraw blood as for exchange transfusion and replace with saline
- Closely monitor throughout procedure, and check blood at start, midway, and end.

Lumbar puncture

Indications
- Investigation of CNS infection or abnormal neurology
- Decrease intracranial pressure in communicating hydrocephalus.

Contraindications
- Severe cardiorespiratory disease
- Coagulopathy
- Thrombocytopenia (Plt <50)
- Local infection at lumbar puncture (LP) site.

Equipment
- Antibacterial cleaning solution
- Sterile dressing pack
- 22 G 1.5-inch spinal needle
- Three universal containers and one fluoride oxalate bottle to measure glucose
- Sterile manometry pack
- Dressing or adhesive spray, e.g. OpSite®.

Procedure
- **Position** the baby in the left lateral position and palpate the anatomical landmarks (the L4 intervertebral space lies in the midline at the level of the iliac crests), keep the back perpendicular to the bed. See Figs. 20.6 and 20.7
- **Aseptic technique**
- **Clean the back** with antibacterial solution
- Monitor the baby's condition throughout the procedure and abandon if baby becomes unstable
- **Assistant gently flexes the spine** by holding shoulders and legs to open the intervertebral spaces
- **Insert the needle** in the L3/L4 intervertebral space or one space below, aim for the umbilicus, keeping the needle parallel to the floor
- **Advance slowly** to a depth of 0.5–1 cm, there may be a sharp decrease in resistance or 'give' as the ligamentum flavum is pierced in term infants but not in small or preterm babies
- **Remove the stylet and collect drops of cerebrospinal fluid (CSF)**, 5–8 drops in each universal container, labelled with the order collected and send for microbiology (MC&S) and/or virology and protein; 3 drops in fluoride bottle (for glucose/lactate). Send an extra container to measure amino acids or other special tests
- If LP is performed as a neurological investigation or to decrease intracranial pressure then opening pressure should be measured (before CSF is taken off) by attaching a **manometer** to the needle hub
- **Replace stylet, withdraw needle**, and apply pressure with gauze before applying a dressing or using an adhesive spray.

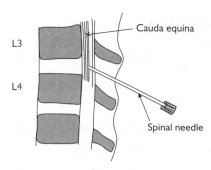

Fig. 20.6 Lumbar puncture anatomy.

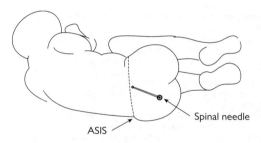

Fig. 20.7 Lumbar puncture anatomy.

Helpful hints
- An experienced assistant to hold the baby improves the chances of success
- If CSF is not forthcoming when the stylet is removed, slowly withdraw whilst gently rotating the needle
- If blood flows from the needle when the stylet is removed, collect a few drops to see if it clears
- If unsuccessful, attempt in the intervertebral space below.

Complications
- Infection
- Haemorrhage
- Headache.

Ventricular tap

Indications
- Removal of CSF in a baby with rapidly increasing head circumference when LP is ineffective.

Equipment
As for LP + safety razor.

Procedure
- **Perform under ultrasound guidance** to determine angle and depth of insertion
- Tap the side of the larger ventricle or, if equal, the right (non-dominant) side
- **Shave the hair** around the point of insertion (lateral angle of the anterior fontanelle)
- Aseptic technique
- **Position** the baby supine and an assistant holds the head still in the midline
- Monitor the infant's condition throughout the procedure
- **Clean the skin** with antibacterial solution
- **Insert the needle and advance** at the angle, and to the distance estimated from scanning, aiming for the inner canthus of the opposite eye, there may be a 'give' when entering the ventricle
- **Remove the stylet and measure pressure** with manometer and collect samples as for LP
- **Drain 10–15 ml/kg CSF** at a rate of 1–2 ml/min in cases of hydrocephalus and re-measure pressure
- **Replace stylet, withdraw needle,** and apply pressure with gauze before applying a dressing or using an adhesive spray
- Send samples for microbiology (MC&S), and measure protein and glucose.

Helpful hints
- Use the same needle track if repeating the procedure.

Complications
- Infection
- Haemorrhage
- Trauma to brain parenchyma leaving a needle track.

Cerebrospinal fluid reservoir access

Indications

As for ventricular tap.

Procedure

- Aseptic technique
- Clean overlying skin with antibacterial solution
- Grip the reservoir to stabilize between thumb and index finger. Insert a 21 F (green) butterfly attached to 10 ml syringe at 90° to the skin until the resistance is felt at the floor of the reservoir
- Slowly aspirate **10–15 ml/kg** CSF at a rate of 1–2 ml/min
- Remove the butterfly and apply pressure with gauze before applying a dressing or using an adhesive spray
- Send samples for microbiology (MC&S) and measure protein and glucose.

Nasogastric and orogastric tube insertion

Indications
Enteral feeding and bowel decompression.

Equipment
- Feeding tube (<1000 g = 4 Fr; >1000 g = 6 Fr; for decompression = 8–10 Fr)
- Lubricant gel
- Hydrocolloid dressing and tape
- pH paper and syringe.

Procedure
- **Estimate length for insertion** (NGT—from nares to ear to midway between xiphisternum and umbilicus; OGT—from mouth to midway between xiphisternum and umbilicus)
- **Position** baby supine, head in midline, and **insert lubricated tube** into nose/mouth. Look down on baby and hold head firmly
- Aim downwards, towards the bed, to traverse the nasal passages
- **Advance quickly**, to the desired length
- **Tape** tube to cheek (NGT) or chin (OGT) over hydrocolloid dressing.

Checking tube position
- **Aspirate from tube and test** with pH paper (gastric secretions are acidic)
- If there are no secretions, wait 30–60 minutes, for sufficient gastric secretions to be produced
- If NGT needs to be used sooner, perform X-ray to confirm tip is in the stomach.

Complications
- Gastrointestinal erosions or perforations
- Malposition in airway leading to aspiration.

Nasojejunal tube insertion

Indications

Enteral feeding when gastric feeding is not tolerated.

Equipment

As for OGT/NGT.

Procedure

- Estimate length to stomach: from nares to umbilicus
- **Estimate total length for insertion**: from nares to ankle
- **Position** baby on right side and insert lubricated tube into mouth
- **Advance tube** quickly to the desired distance or as near as possible
- **Inject 2 ml of saline** through the tube when it reaches the stomach to aid peristalsis
- **Secure tube** (see 🔗 Nasogastric and orogastric tube insertion, p. 524)
- **Insert OGT** (see 🔗 Nasogastric and orogastric tube insertion, p. 524)
- **Check position** of NJT and OGT with X-ray, the tip should lie beyond the pylorus and cross the midline.

Helpful hints

- If unsure about position, commence feeds and aspirate OGT. If milk aspirates from the OGT then the 'NJT' is in the stomach
- Tubes initially at the pylorus may be left to migrate into the small bowel with peristalsis over the next few days.

Complications

Gastrointestinal erosions or perforations.

Abdominal paracentesis

Indications
- Obtain sample of ascitic fluid for microbiology and biochemistry (diagnostic)
- Reduce intra-abdominal pressure by removing ascitic fluid (therapeutic) to improve ventilation.

Equipment
- Undertaken under US guidance except in an emergency
- Antibacterial solution and saline
- Sterile dressing pack
- Cannula 24 G (yellow), or needle 23 G (blue)/21 G (green)
- 10 or 20 ml syringe.

Procedure
- Aseptic technique
- **Position** the baby supine and attempt to **percuss fluid level**
- **Clean the lower abdomen and flank** with antibacterial solution
- **Insert the needle with syringe** attached under US guidance in the left iliac fossa and **advance slowly whilst aspirating** until there is flashback of fluid
- **Aspirate** 10–20 ml/kg of fluid
- **Withdraw needle** slowly and cover puncture site with dressing
- Record volume and colour of aspirate and send samples to microbiology and biochemistry.

Complications
- Bowel puncture
- Infection
- Haemorrhage
- Fluid balance and electrolyte disturbance.

Peritoneal dialysis catheter insertion

Indications

- Renal failure with severe hyperkalaemia, acidosis, or fluid overload needing short-term dialysis. Catheters for anything longer than brief dialysis should be inserted surgically
- Involve a **nephrologist**, and specially trained staff are needed to perform dialysis.

Equipment

- Antibacterial cleaning solution
- Local anaesthetic (e.g. lidocaine 1%) + 5 ml syringe + 23 G (blue) needle
- Sterile dressing pack
- Peritoneal dialysis catheter and insertion pack
- Peritoneal dialysis fluid
- Peritoneal dialysis catheter drainage set
- Suture
- Clear dressing.

Procedure

- Aseptic technique
- **Clean skin** with antibacterial solution
- Infiltrate insertion site with **local anaesthetic**
- **Insert the peritoneal dialysis catheter using the Seldinger technique**
- **Insert introducer needle** attached to syringe through abdominal wall, whilst aspirating in the left iliac fossa, midway between umbilicus and anterior superior iliac spine until there is a fluid flashback
- Remove the syringe **and** thread guide wire through needle; withdraw needle leaving guide wire; pass dilator over guide wire then withdraw before passing peritoneal dialysis catheter over guide wire; and finally remove guide wire
- **Suture peritoneal dialysis catheter to the skin**, cover with dressing, and **attach to the peritoneal dialysis drainage set**.

Complications

- Bowel puncture
- Infection
- Haemorrhage
- Fluid balance and electrolyte disturbance.

Transurethral catheterization

Indications
- Monitoring urine output/fluid balance
- Urinary retention
- Obtain uncontaminated urine to send to microbiology.

Equipment
- Sterile dressing pack
- Urinary catheter (3–5 Fr) recommended by nephrologists/urologists; or feeding tube (4–6 Fr) or umbilical catheters (3 Fr) in small infants
- Sterile lubricant gel
- Tape.

Procedure
- Aseptic technique
- If sample required for microbiology have a universal container ready for a clean catch sample, as spontaneous urination during the procedure is not uncommon
- **Position** the baby supine with an assistant holding the legs with hips abducted
- **Clean the external genitalia** and perineum with antibacterial solution (do not retract the foreskin in males)
- **Insert the lubricated catheter/feeding tube** through the urethral meatus (difficult to directly visualize in males) and **advance slowly** until urine flows from the catheter
- **Attach catheter to collecting system**
- **Fix catheter to anterior abdominal wall** and one leg with tape (penis pointing upwards in boys).

Complications
- Urethral trauma, haematuria, and urethral stricture
- Infection.

Suprapubic aspiration of urine

Indications
Obtain uncontaminated urine to send to microbiology.

Equipment
- Antibacterial cleaning solution (e.g. chlorhexidine)
- Sterile dressing pack
- 23 G (blue) needle
- 10 ml syringe
- Universal container.

Procedure
- Confirm bladder contains urine by **palpation** or **US scan**
- Have a universal container ready for a clean catch sample, as spontaneous urination during the procedure is not uncommon
- Aseptic technique
- **Position** the baby supine with an assistant holding the legs with hips abducted
- **Clean the skin** of lower abdomen with antibacterial solution
- **Insert needle with attached syringe** at 90° to the abdominal wall, 1 cm above the symphysis pubis in the midline. See Fig. 20.8
- **Advance needle slowly** to depth of 1–2 cm, while **aspirating continuously** until urine is aspirated
- **Remove needle** and apply pressure to puncture site
- Test at cot-side with urinalysis dipstick and send remainder to microbiology (MC&S).

Complications
- Bladder trauma and haematuria
- Bowel puncture.

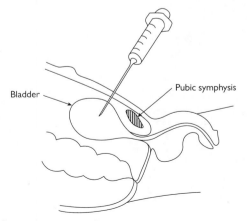

Fig. 20.8 Suprapubic aspiration of urine.

Further information

British Association of Perinatal Medicine. *Consent in neonatal clinical care: Good practice framework*. BAPM, London, 2004.

British Association of Perinatal Medicine. *Use of central venous catheters in neonates, a framework for practice*. BAPM, London, 2015.

Kempley, S. Neonatal endotracheal intubation: the 7-8-9 rule. *Arch Dis Child Educ Pract Ed* 2009; **94**: 29.

Rennie, J.M. (ed.). Practical procedures. In: Rennie J. (ed.) *Rennie & Roberton's Textbook of Neonatology*, 5th ed. pp. 1259–1292. Churchill Livingstone, London, 2012.

Normal values, therapeutic drug levels, and useful formulae

Introduction

It is important to acknowledge that normal values and therapeutic drug levels used in local guidelines may differ between centres. Therefore, those suggested in this chapter are given as ranges. Please refer to local guidelines as appropriate.

Normal neonatal blood biochemistry values

See Table 21.1.

Table 21.1 Normal neonatal blood biochemistry values

Alanine aminotransferase (ALT)	<60 U/l	
Albumin	32–48 g/l	May be lower in preterm or small for gestational age babies
Aldosterone	166–2900 pmol/l	Less useful than urine assay; correct potassium prior to taking sample
Alkaline phosphatase (ALP)	180–400 U/l	Normally lower if >3 weeks of age
Alpha-fetoprotein	Neonates: 50,000–150,000 µg/l >1 month: 100–10,000 µg/l	
Alpha-1-antitrypsin	0.9–2.1 g/l	Consider checking phenotype if levels low
Ammonia	<50 µmol/l	
Aspartate aminotransferase	<110 U/l	
Bilirubin (conjugated)	<10 µmol/l	See ➔ Conjugated hyperbilirubinaemia, p. 391
Bilirubin (unconjugated)	<17 µmol/l (>4 weeks)	See ➔ Non-physiological jaundice in Neonatal jaundice, p. 386 See ➔ Treatment of jaundice, pp. 388–9
Calcium	<48 h: 1.8–2.3 mmol/l >48 h: 2.2–2.7 mmol/l Ionized: 1.1–1.3 mmol/l	
Chloride	95–108 mmol/l	
Cholesterol	<4.53 mmol/l	
Copper	3–11 µmol/l	
Cortisol	<700 nmol/l	Delay measuring until >24 h old Random level >560 nmol/l suggests hypopituitarism unlikely. If low or borderline, discuss further investigations with local paediatric endocrinology unit

Table 21.1 (Contd.)

C-reactive protein (CRP)	<10 mg/l	
Creatinine kinase (CPK)	<390 U/l	Likely to be higher if <72 h age or after seizures
Creatinine	<44 µmol/l	
Creatinine clearance	7 ml/min/1.73 m² (at 26 weeks gestation) 26 ml/min/1.73 m² (at term)	See ➲ Useful formulae, p. 542 Values are those expected at given gestational ages
Follicle-stimulating hormone (FSH)	Male <15 U/l Female <38 U/l	
Galactose-1-phosphate uridyl transferase (Gal 1-PUT)	300–470 U/kg Hb	
Gamma glutamyl transferase (GGT)	<385 U/l	
Glucose	2.6–6.6 mmol/l	See ➲ Hypoglycaemia: overview, pp. 372–3; ➲ Hypoglycaemia: management, pp. 374–5; and ➲ Hyperglycaemia, p. 376
17-α-hydroxyprogesterone	<10 nmol/l	May be as high as 30 nmol/l in sick preterm babies
Immunoglobulins IgG IgA IgM	2.73–16.6 g/l 0–1.0 g/l 0–2.16 g/l	
Insulin	<145 pmol/l	See ➲ Hyperglycaemia, p. 376
Lactate	<2.5 mmol/l	
Luteinizing hormone (LH)	Male <23 U/l Female <20 U/l	
Magnesium	0.75–1.15 mmol/l	
Manganese	9.1–27.3 mmol/l	
Methaemoglobin	<5 g/l or <3% total Hb	See ➲ Persistent pulmonary hypertension of the newborn, pp. 122–3
Osmolality	275–295 mmol/l	May be lower if <5 days of life
Parathyroid hormone (PTH)	10–65 ng/l	
Phosphate	1.62–3.10 mmol/l	

(Continued)

Table 21.1 (*Contd.*)

Potassium	3.5–4.5 mmol/l	
Progesterone	<6 nmol/l	
Pyruvate	80–150 µmol/l	
Renin	<14.0 ng/l/s	
Selenium	0.4–0.75 µmol/l	
Sodium	135–145 mmol/l	
Testosterone	Male <6.6 nmol/l Female <1.0 nmol/l	
Thyroid stimulating hormone (TSH)	0.5–5.0 mU/l	Baby should be >4 days old when first checked
Thyroxine (T4)	100–250 nmol/l	Baby should be >4 days old when first checked. Levels may be significantly lower in preterm babies during the first few weeks
Total protein	45–75 g/l	
Triglycerides	<1.8 mm/l	
Troponin T	0.001–0.06 ng/ml	
Urea	2.9–5.0 mmol/l	
Vitamin A	0.7–2.10 µmol/l	
Vitamin D (25-OH vit D)	20–80 nmol/l	
Vitamin E	12–46 µmol/l	
Zinc	10–22.2 µmol/l	

Normal neonatal urine biochemistry values

See Table 21.2.

Table 21.2 Normal neonatal urine biochemistry values

Calcium	0.2–1.6 mmol/l	Preterm
	<0.6 mmol/l	Term
Creatinine clearance	7–22 ml/min/1.73m^2	<1 week postnatal age
	10–28 ml/min/1.73m^2	1–2 weeks postnatal age
	11–34 ml/min/1.73m^2	2–4 weeks postnatal age
Fractional excretion of sodium	Measure if oliguric	Low (<3%) suggests pre-renal cause (<6% in preterm)
		High (>3–6%) suggests a renal cause
Sodium	Varies depending on corrected gestational age (higher in preterm babies <32 weeks gestation), sodium intake and losses	Measure routinely in babies with a stoma. If <20 mmol/l in babies with significant stoma losses, consider increasing sodium supplements
Potassium	2–28 mmol/l	Preterm
	<5 mmol/l	Term
Sodium:potassium ratio		If <3:1 in babies with significant stoma losses, consider increasing sodium supplements

Normal neonatal blood haematology values

See Table 21.3.

Table 21.3 Normal neonatal blood haematology values

Haemoglobin (Hb)	28 weeks gestation	110–170 g/l
	34 weeks gestation	120–180 g/l
	Term	140–210 g/l
Haematocrit (Hct)	28 weeks gestation	0.30–0.40
	34 weeks gestation	0.35–0.50
	Term	0.40–0.65
Reticulocyte count	At birth	$200–300 \times 10^9$/l
	<4–6 weeks	$<5 \times 10^9$/l
	>4–6 weeks	$5–250 \times 10^9$/l
Total white blood cell (WBC) count	<48 h	$20.0–40.0 \times 10^9$/l
	>48 h	$5.0–15.0 \times 10^9$/l
Neutrophil count	<48 h	$6.0–26.0 \times 10^9$/l
	>48 h	$1.8–10.0 \times 10^9$/l
Lymphocyte count	<1 week	$2.0–6.0 \times 10^9$/l
	>1 week	$2.0–15.0 \times 10^9$/l
Platelet count		$150–400 \times 10^9$/l
PT (ratio or INR)	Preterm	12.5–13.0 secs (1.0–1.2)
	Term	12.0–13.0 secs (1.0–1.1)
APTT (ratio)	Preterm	50.0–54.0 secs (1.0–1.8)
	Term	42.5–43.0 secs (1.0–1.2)
Fibrinogen		1.6–4.0 g/l
D-dimer		<200 ng/ml
Glucose-6-phosphate dehydrogenase (G6PD)		4.5–13.6 units/g Hb

Normal neonatal cerebrospinal fluid values

See Table 21.4.

Table 21.4 Normal neonatal CSF values

White blood cell (WBC) count	Preterm	$\leq 27 \times 10^6/l$
	Term (>37 weeks)	$\leq 20 \times 10^6/l$
Protein	Preterm	≤ 1 g/l
	Term (>37 weeks)	≤ 0.6 g/l
Glucose	2.1–3.6 mmol/l	If blood glucose taken at same time normal

Therapeutic drug levels

See Table 21.5.

Table 21.5 Therapeutic drug levels

Amiodarone	1–2.5 mg/l
Digoxin	0.8–2.2 µg/l
Flecainide	200–400 µg/l
Flucytosine	40–60 mg/l
Gentamicin:	
trough	<1 mg/l
peak	6–10 mg/l)
Phenobarbital	9–25 mg/l
Phenytoin	6–15 mg/l
Vancomycin:	
trough	5–10 mg/l
infusion	>15 mg/l at 12 h; 15–25 mg/l at 24 h and every 3 days thereafter

Useful formulae

ET tube length at lips (cm)
Orotracheal tube: weight of baby (kg) + 6

Umbilical catheter lengths (cm)
- **UAC length**: $3 \times$ birth weight (kg) + 9 (for high position T6–T10)
- **UVC length**: $(0.5 \times$ UAC length$) + 1$

Respiratory formulae
NB Use mmHg for PO_2 and PCO_2 unless stated otherwise.
- Mean airway pressure (MAP)

$$MAP = PEEP + \{(PIP - PEEP) \times [Ti/(Ti+Te)]\}$$

- Oxygenation index (OI) =

$$\left[\text{Mean airway pressure} \times FiO_2 \text{ (as \%)}\right]/[PO_2 \text{ (in kPa)} \times 7.6$$

$$(\text{>25 indicates severe respiratory failure; consider ECMO >40})$$

- Ventilation index (VI) =

$$PCO_2 \times RR \times PIP/1000$$

$$\left(\begin{array}{l}\text{N.B. } PCO_2 \text{ in mmHg } (1 \text{ kPa} \approx 7.5 \text{ mmHg}), \text{ PIP in } cmH_2O; \\ \text{values >100 = severe respiratory failure}\end{array}\right)$$

- Alveolar – arterial oxygen difference (A-aDO_2) =
  $(716 \times FiO_2) - (PCO_2/0.8) - PO_2$

NB PCO_2 and PO_2 in mmHg; values >600 mmHg = severe respiratory failure.

Biochemistry
- Anion gap = $(Na^+ + K^+) - (HCO_3^- + Cl^-)$
  (normal <12–17)
- Osmolality (serum) = 2Na + glucose + urea
  (normal: 270–295 mmol/l)
- Creatinine clearance = (urine creatinine × urine flow rate) ÷ plasma creatinine (see Table 21.2)
- Fractional excretion of sodium (FENa) = (urine Na/serum Na) × (serum creatinine/urine creatinine) × 100 (see Table 21.2)
- Glucose delivery (mg/kg/min) = [IV rate (ml/h) × dextrose concentration (%)] ÷ [weight (kg) × 6].

Index

S